JOB HAZARD ANALYSIS

JOB HAZARD ANALYSIS

A GUIDE FOR VOLUNTARY COMPLIANCE AND BEYOND

SECOND EDITION

JAMES ROUGHTON

NATHAN CRUTCHFIELD

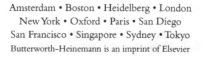

Amsterdam • Boston • Heidelberg • London
New York • Oxford • Paris • San Diego
San Francisco • Singapore • Sydney • Tokyo
Butterworth-Heinemann is an imprint of Elsevier

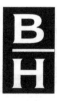

Butterworth-Heinemann is an imprint of Elsevier
The Boulevard, Langford Lane, Kidlington, Oxford OX5 1GB, UK
225 Wyman Street, Waltham, MA 02451, USA

Notices
Knowledge and best practice in this field are constantly changing. As new research and experience broaden our understanding, changes in research methods, professional practices, or medical
treatment may become necessary.

Practitioners and researchers must always rely on their own experience and knowledge in evaluating and using any information, methods, compounds, or experiments described herein. In using
such information or methods they should be mindful of their own safety and the safety of others,
including parties for whom they have a professional responsibility.

To the fullest extent of the law, neither the Publisher nor the authors, contributors, or editors,
assume any liability for any injury and/or damage to persons or property as a matter of products
liability, negligence or otherwise, or from any use or operation of any methods, products, instructions, or ideas contained in the material herein.

British Library Cataloguing-in-Publication Data
A catalogue record for this book is available from the British Library

Library of Congress Cataloging-in-Publication Data
A catalog record for this book is available from the Library of Congress

ISBN: 978-0-12-803441-5

For information on all Butterworth-Heinemann publications
visit our website at http://store.elsevier.com/

Typeset by Thomson Digital
Printed and bound in US

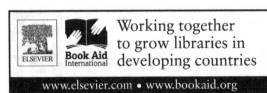

Working together
to grow libraries in
developing countries

www.elsevier.com • www.bookaid.org

DEDICATION

I dedicate this book to my loving wife, who has been my friend and partner for 45 years. She has always been patient with me in my endeavors to enhance the safety profession and has always given me the freedom to pursue my dreams.

I also owe a lot to the safety professionals whom I have met throughout the many years of my career who have helped me in many aspects of learning my profession. Their professionalism, continued friendship, insights and encouragement, and feedback have been very valuable to me.

I am also grateful to all of the social media gurus who have inspired me in my interest on learning how to use social media to be more productive.

James Roughton

My efforts for this book are dedicated to lifelong learners with whom I have been associated throughout my professional life – Dr Michael Waite, William Montante, and James Roughton; the Georgia Safety, Health, and Environmental Conference Board; fellow consultants from my brokerage life; and the consultants, risk and safety managers who are on the "front lines" in the continual effort to improve organizations and workplace.

I am grateful to have learned and benefited from them all.

Nathan Crutchfield

CONTENTS

ABOUT THE AUTHORS

James is an experienced Safety Professional with an in-depth knowledge in the use of Social Media to help improve the productivity. He is an accomplished speaker, author, and writer, develops and manages his own web sites that provide a resource network for small businesses at http://www.safetycultureplusacademy.com.

Three of his most notable books include, Safety Culture: An Innovative, Leadership Approach, Developing an Effective Safety Culture: A Leadership Approach, and Job Hazard Analysis and A Guide for Voluntary Compliance and Beyond. He is an active board member and web master for the Georgia Conference – www.georgiaconference.org.

He is the past President of the Georgia of the ASSE; Past Chair – Gwinnett Safety Professionals, Past Adjunct Professor Safety Technology Lanier Tech, Georgia Tech, and currently an adjunct Professor in Columbia Southern University. He has received awards for his efforts and was named the Georgia Chapter ASSE Safety Professional of the Year 1998–1999, Project Safe Georgia Award, 2008, and received the Georgia Safety, Health, and Environmental Conference's Earl Everett distinguished Service Award, 2014.

**James Roughton, MS, CSP, CRSP, R-CHMM,
CIT, CET, Certified Six Sigma Black Belt**

Nathan is an independent consultant whose professional history encompasses a full range of risk control program design, development, implementation, and evaluation. He has provided expertise to a broad array of clients that include public entities, associations, and general industry.

He was awarded the National Safety Council's "Distinguished Service to Safety Award" in 2001 and served on the National Safety Council Board of Directors in 1993–1995 was a Vice President, with a major risk management and insurance brokerage for over 20 years. He has been a speaker at various risk and safety conferences throughout his career. He has served on the Executive Board of the Georgia Safety, Health, and Environmental Conference. He received the Georgia Safety, Health, and Environmental Conference's Earl Everett distinguished Service Award, 2014.

Nathan Crutchfield, CSP, CPCU, ARM, ARP

FOREWORD

In this second addition of "Job Hazard Analysis, A Guide for Voluntary Compliance and Beyond", we continue to follow a hands-on, comprehensive approach to build and enhance a job hazard analysis (JHA) process. From our experiences since the first edition, we are even more convinced that JHA provides the critical link between risk assessment and an effective safety system.

In our discussions about new concepts, we wanted to keep an emphasis on creating and sustaining an effective safety culture, as discussed in our book, "Safety Culture, An Innovative Leadership Approach." We believe the new perspectives bring together a wider array of new concepts and techniques. We see safety as a result of many dynamics of the ever-changing organizational environment. It is an ecosystem where changes and operational conditions can occur quickly.

Since the first edition, more emphasis has been placed on the use of risk management concepts. We have long held that when the JHA process incorporates risk-assessment criteria within its hazard analysis, it becomes the foundation for effective implementation of a safety system's elements.

We have included insights and materials derived from human performance improvement concepts to add new dimensions to the analysis of a job. The basic structure we developed continues to follow the one outlined in our first edition, use of the risk matrix and cause and effect diagrams for job component assessment, and use of the tools found in a Six Sigma process.

In addition to the hazard, risk recognition, and JHA development concepts, a brief overview of Six Sigma tools is provided for use as part of a continuous improvement effort for a safety system. Many different uses of specific tools such as diagrams, charts, analysis techniques, and methods provide step-by-step help to establish a process that can continually improve.

We have found that while we are from different professional backgrounds, that is, manufacturing and risk management, we have similar experiences in a wide range of diverse industries. This difference in perspective has allowed us to create diverse points of view based on our personal histories. Both of us have lived the experience, from both the inside and outside of organizations. We have seen both, the good and the bad in the process and program design, administration, and leadership of safety systems. We believe that this edition will continue to provide the tools, methods, and concepts that meet the challenge of sustaining an effective safety system within an organization.

The authors hope that this book is used by the leadership, safety professionals, safety educators, and students of safety management for developing the focal point for a successful safety system, the JHA.

James Roughton, MS, CSP, R-CRSP,
R-CHMM, CET, CIT, Six Sigma Black Belt

Nathan Crutchfield, MBA, CSP, CPCU, ARM, ARP

PREFACE

The truth is that we may not be doing our jobs in the safest possible way or even conducting our personal business in a safe manner all of the time. We tend to put ourselves at risk each day and so often do not know it because we have done something at-risk so many times it just becomes the right way of doing things.

It is the intent of our book to help you discover way to prevent loss-producing events from occurring.

CHAPTER 1, WHY FOCUS ON THE JOB HAZARD ANALYSIS PROCESS

Based on our opinion and lessons learned through experience, we have found that the job hazard analysis (JHA) is "The Centerpiece and Critical Link" to ensure a solid foundation for the safety system. A safety system can be defined as "... the formal, top-down business approach to managing risk, which includes a systemic approach to manage safety, including the necessary organizational structures, accountabilities, policies, and procedures."

The overarching safety system goal is to ensure an effective safety culture exist within an organization. A true safety culture can only exist when the leadership team fully embraces and understands how jobs, their steps and tasks are defined, administered, and completed as a whole unit. "A safety culture goes beyond simply managing a basic series of required programs for regulatory compliance. The design of job(s), step(s), and task(s) must take into consideration the variations in cultures and account for the inherent hazards and associated risk that must be managed and controlled."

CHAPTER 2, UNDERSTANDING HUMAN PERFORMANCE IN THE JOB HAZARD ANALYSIS PROCESS

The development of a JHA must include elements that go beyond just listing a job's steps. While not part of the actual JHA, organizational, and human performance elements and issues directly influence the effective implementation of the process. Even with an in-depth understanding of how to develop a JHA, getting the leadership team and employees to buy into the effort involves more than a mechanical, rote filling out of a document.

CHAPTER 3, INTRODUCING JHA INTO THE ORGANIZATION

The JHA is still viewed as an additional activity not a fundamental part of an overall safety system. As with the issue found in quality control where the effort was to fix defects and not the cause of defects, loss-producing events still focus on the immediate cause and not the reduction of risk found within the system.

Various levels of activities must be considered in order to improve the existing the safety system. After decades of research and insights within the safety profession, the misconception still remains that the majority of injuries are due to unsafe acts or human error. Why? Improving safety efforts are still in many cases restricted to trying to change employee behavior through incentive programs, games, or low value activities such as exhortations (lecturing), posters, and the like.

CHAPTER 4, LEADERSHIP TEAM AND EMPLOYEE PARTICIPATION

Organizations have a "built-in" resource that can be utilized in the JHA process. This resource is its employees who have the direct experience about the job, its required steps and related tasks. When engaged and motivated, employees can be excellent problem-solvers as they are closest to the "what, when, why, and how" of required actions that must be accomplished.

CHAPTER 5, PREPARING FOR THE HAZARD AND RISK ASSESSMENT

An important objective of a JHA process is to assist the leadership team and employees in understanding and improving their knowledge of hazards and associated risks. A hazard and risk assessment is accomplished by conducting structured surveys that are designed to review the organization's operations. An analysis is completed of the assessment survey findings to establish the nature and potential impact of activities, potentially unsafe practices, and any history of at-risk or loss-producing events that may have occurred.

CHAPTER 6, HAZARD ANALYSIS AND REVIEW OF ASSOCIATED RISK

Untold thousands of interactions are occurring every day in the average organization. The JHA process can aid in these interactions, for example, job requirements, specific activities, the required steps, and tasks of a job, etc.

JHA provides the blueprint for designing and customizing surveys and inspections to be used within the safety system. It enhances the ability of an organization to anticipate and understand how job elements (steps and task(s)) combine and interact with each other.

CHAPTER 7, ENHANCING THE SAFETY MANAGEMENT SYSTEM IN MANAGING RISK

Organizations are dynamic and are always in a state of flux and can change due to many types of internal and external influences. These influences are always present and do not always act consistently.

The premise is that the JHA when considered the centerpiece for a safety system provides the critical linkage between all aspects of a Safety Management System. The view of the JHA as the linkage is used to provide essential information for the leadership team and employees about the scope and severity of hazards and risk exposure. With this information, the leadership team can then better weigh the impact of changes in job related tasks and select more informed decisions as loss-producing consequences are made visible.

CHAPTER 8, DEFINING ASSOCIATED RISK

The concept of risk must be clearly defined and included as a major element in the JHA process. Using only loss-related data that is solely based on injuries, incident rates, and/or damage does not provide a full understanding of the potential for loss-producing events. This data only provides a snapshot of what has occurred. To understand how risk affects an organization, a risk assessment must be conducted. A risk assessment determines where hazards and associated risk may exist but may or may not have resulted in a loss-producing event.

CHAPTER 9, PLANNING FOR THE JOB HAZARD ANALYSIS

One goal for the job hazard analysis (JHA) process is to become self-sustaining and effective. That goal first begins by establishing a JHA committee that can provide experience, expertise, and assistance in developing the process. A properly structured committee working on the JHA process increases the effectiveness of the safety system.

For the JHA to become an integral part of the organization's planning and daily management activities, a focused committee approach provides leadership and can guide the necessary activities if given the tools and authority to make change.

Before starting the JHA development, determine and carefully consider who is going to be on the development committee. Experienced employees actually doing the job should be involved for a comprehensive job steps and tasks development. The insights and perspectives of all employees should be considered as solid insights from unlikely sources may come out of the process.

The JHA process involves developing an inventory of jobs and a search for nonroutine jobs that may be hidden from view. The use of the JHA committee and employees can improve the depth and scope of the JHA portfolio. The JHA process can restore the feel of the workplace as it identifies how things are getting done and how hazards and associated risk are controlled.

CHAPTER 10, BREAKING THE JOB DOWN INTO INDIVIDUAL COMPONENTS

The job hazard analysis (JHA) process begins by selecting designated jobs, ranked in order by priority, and ends with standard operating procedures (SOP.) Used this way, the JHA process provides a baseline for the development and refinement of SOPs, safety protocols, work instructions, and guidelines.

Consider the job as a whole system when breaking it down into individual components of action steps and the tasks required within each step. The suggested method to structure the JHA is through the use of the Ishikawa or "Fishbone" diagram. This creates a cause and effect graphic diagram of the job, its steps and tasks along with the tools, equipment, materials, environment, administrative documents, and employees exposed to the job.

CHAPTER 11, PUTTING THE PUZZLE PIECES TOGETHER

A successful job hazard analysis (JHA) will involve collecting job data, developing the job steps and tasks, creating cause and effect diagram(s), the hazard assessment, and using a risk matrix to identify probability, and severity. The JHA should be cross referenced against documents in human resources, quality control, process management, security, maintenance, and other departments that may have safety related criteria to prevent confusion or conflicts. Programs under the safety system should be clearly linked to the JHA for ease of reference.

CHAPTER 12, ASSESSING TRAINING NEEDS

Training is a professional discipline that requires knowledge about multiple learning theories, presentation skills, survey and assessment, current research on human performance, and various learning strategies. It is not just a PowerPoint© presentation and should be implemented with a strategy that understands the nature of organization and the workforce.

Organizations have the responsibility to ensure that their employees are trained to achieve its objectives and that each employee understands the hazards of their work environment and how to protect themselves from specific hazards. An in-depth knowledge of the job hazard analysis (JHA) process should be developed and used by the leadership team and employees. Without this basic training, it will be difficult to establish an effective and efficient JHA process, which adds value to the organization with overall operational improvement.

CHAPTER 13, BASIS ELEMENTS OF A SAFETY SYSTEM

A safety system supports the development of the job hazard analysis (JHA) process by providing a structure for its use. The safety system is a critical "filter" that allows the communication of essential information and knowledge between the various parts of the organization. An organization consists of many processes that should be coordinated if the organization's intended goal are to be effectively met.

CHAPTER 14, BECOMING A CURATOR FOR THE SAFETY SYSTEM

As the focal point for safety-related information, the safety professional is the organization's memory regarding the documentation of hazards, associated risk, safety system performance, regulatory compliance, job hazard analysis (JHA), etc. This means that the one in charge of the organizations resources, you need to ensure that they are accurate with timely safety-related information. In addition, you must be able to track and locate information as quickly as possible to get it into the hands of the appropriate decision makers for further action.

From day one, a library and filing methodology and structure is adopted that will organize all resources. These resources will include hard copies and e-copies of materials, websites information, reports, loss data, risks assessments, electronics books, and much more. The objective is to have a system that can access and retrieve the specific information for a timely and quick response to risk and hazardous situations or request for assistance.

CHAPTER 15, EFFECTIVELY MANAGING A JHA PROCESS USING SIX SIGMA

Organizations follow a structured methodology to get things done. The methodology may be informal or industry best practice or may be based on some combination of concepts. The end product or service drives the process and dictates what equipment, technology, skill levels, raw materials, etc. are necessary. The requirements of a safety system are directly parallel to those required to maintain the quality of products and services.

While the JHA can be used for specific targeted use (incident investigations, PPE selection, training development, etc.), it must viewed as a beneficial tool for the ongoing overall process.

A number of concepts can be useful when developing a JHA. Six Sigma is essentially an array of problem solving and assessment tools.

APPENDIX 1: JOB HAZARD ANALYSIS OSHA 3071

The job hazard analysis (JHA) is a valuable tool for providing enhanced training for all employees in the appropriate steps, and task of their jobs.

However, as we started to learn how to develop a JHA many years ago, the only guidance that we found was the public domain document, "Job Hazard Analysis OSHA 3071," which was a great resources at that time. Based on our experience, we decided to include this document as an appendix so that end users could experience the beginning of the JHA process.

As we progressed developing JHAs, we discovered that there were not many new and innovative ways available in regards to defining how the job, it's steps, and tasks were structured. This is the reason that we wrote this book, to go beyond any voluntary compliance, to fill the gaps in the JHA process, as we consider that the JHA is "The Centerpiece and Critical Link" of a solid foundation for the safety system.

ACKNOWLEDGMENTS

For their assistance in researching, discussing the concepts, developing and writing this book, we would like to acknowledge the essential people and organizations that made the endeavor possible.

Dr Mike Waite and William Montante, CSP, for their friendship, insights, and discussions on the nature and scope of safety systems. They have lead the way in thought leadership for improvement of safety and risk concepts.

Presenter Media for the use of their graphics used to emphasize concepts and thoughts through the book. We cannot thank them enough for the quality of their products and service.

We made every effort to ensure that all references are cited and appropriately identified.

Sources of quotations, material, and references are listed in the bibliography at the end of each chapter.

ACRONYMS

ABC	Above and beyond compliance
ABSS	Activity-based safety system
ADA	Americans with Disabilities Act
ANSI	American National Standard Institute
ASSE	American Society of Safety Engineers
BBS	Behavioral-based safety
BMP	Best management practices
CFR	Code of Federal Regulations
CPR	Cardiopulmonary resuscitation
CTD	Cumulative trauma disorders
EMR	Experience modification rate
EMTs	Emergency medical technicians
FAA	Federal Aviation Administration
HPI	Human performance improvement
ILCI	International Loss Control Institute, Inc.
JHA	Job hazard analysis
JSA	Job safety analysis
LPN	Licensed practical nurses
LVN	Licensed vocational nurses
LWDIR	Lost workday incident rate
MSD	Musculoskeletal disorders
MSDS	Material safety data sheet
NIOSH	National Institute of Occupational Safety and Health
OIR	OSHA incident rate
OSHA	Occupational Safety and Health Administration
PEP	Performance evaluation program
PPE	Personal protective equipment
SOPs	Standard operating practices
SWAMP	Safety without a management process
VPP	OSHA's Voluntary Protection Program
WCCR	Workers compensation cost per hour worked

INTRODUCTION

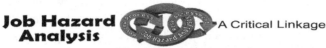

Job Hazard Analysis — A Critical Linkage

The Centerpiece

Why Focus on the Job Hazard Analysis?

- Detects Existing and/or Potential Hazards and Consequences of Exposure
- Assesses and Develops Specific Training Needs and Requirements
- Aids In Recognizing Changes in Procedures, Tools, Machine/Equipment, etc.
- Defines The Potential for Specific At-Risk Events
- Identifies Preventive Measures Necessary to Modify or Control Associated Risk

What are The Benefits of a Job Hazard Analsys?

- Helps To Detect And Reduce Potential Loss-Producing Events
- Provides Instruction On How To Safely Perform The Tasks Within Each Step and Task
- Employees, Teams, And Supervisors Know Better How The Total Job Is Done
- Job Methods Improve, Efficiency Increases, Quality Is Enhanced, Costs Are Reduced
- Employees Are Kept Closely Involved In Safety Efforts

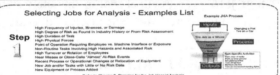

Selecting Jobs for Analysis - Examples List

Step 1

- High Frequency of Injuries, Illnesses, or Damage
- High Degree of Risk as Found In Industry History or From Risk Assessment
- High Duration of Task
- High Physical Forces
- Point of Operation Requiring Employee vs. Machine Interface or Exposure
- Non-Routine Tasks Involving High Hazards and Associated Risk
- High Turnover or Rotation of Employees
- Near Misses or Close-Calls "Almost" At-Risk Events
- Recent Process or Operational Changes or Relocation of Equipment
- New Job and/or Tasks with Little or No Risk Data
- New Equipment or Process Added

Refer to Chapter 9, Planning for the Job Hazard Analysis

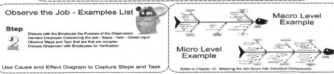

Observe the Job - Examples List

Step 2

- Discuss with the Employee the Purpose of the Observation
- Inerview Employee Concerning the Job - Steps - Task - Obtain Input
- Observe Steps and Task that are that are complex
- Discuss Observatin with Employees for Verification

Use Cause and Effect Diagram to Capture Steps and Task

Macro Level Example

Micro Level Example

Refer to Chapter 10, Breaking the Job Down Into Individual Components

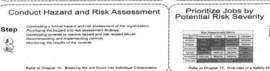

Conduct Hazard and Risk Assessment

Step 3

- Conducting a formal hazard and risk assessment of the organization.
- Prioritizing the hazard and risk assessment findings.
- Developing controls to resolve hazard and risk-related issues
- Recommending and implementing controls.
- Monitoring the results of the controls

Refer to Chapter 10, Breaking the Job Down Into Individual Components

Prioritize Jobs by Potential Risk Severity

Refer to Chapter 13, Overview of a Safety Management Systems

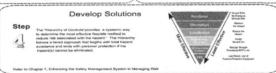

Develop Solutions

Step 4

The "Hierarchy of Controls" provides a systemic way to determine the most effective feasible method to reduce risk associated with the hazard." The Hierarchy follows a tiered approach that begins with total hazard avoidance and ends with personal protection if the hazard(s) cannot be eliminated.

Refer to Chapter 7, Enhancing the Safety Management System in Managing Risk

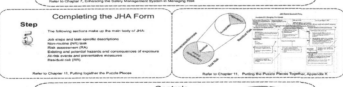

Completing the JHA Form

Step 5

The following sections make up the main body of JHA:

- Job steps and task-specific descriptions
- Non-routine (NR) task
- Risk assessment (RA)
- Existing and potential hazards and consequences of exposure
- At-risk events and preventative measures
- Residual risk (RR)

Refer to Chapter 11, Putting together the Puzzle Pieces

Refer to Chapter 11, Putting the Puzzle Pieces Together, Appendix K

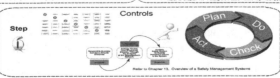

Controls

Step 6

Refer to Chapter 13, Overview of a Safety Management Systems

This Infographic is based on Research by James Roughton and Nathan Crutchfield. The user must have permission to use.

"Life is filled with opportunities for practicing the inexorable, unhurried rhythm of mastery, which focuses on process rather than product, yet which, paradoxically, often ends up creating more and better products in a shorter time than does the hurried, excessively goal-oriented rhythm that has become the standard in our society." – "Mastery" by George Leonard, published by the Penguin Group, 1992

This is what this book is about, using a structured, methodical approach to job hazard analysis (JHA) in lieu of just focusing on individual programs.

THE VALUE OF THE JHA

The intent of this second edition of "Job Hazard Analysis, A Guide for Voluntary Compliance and Beyond" is to continue the development of a process that can be integrated into the safety system and bring increased value to an organization. JHA as an essential tool in the safety system can establish more effective job procedures when effectively and routinely used.

WHAT IS A JOB HAZARD ANALYSIS?

JHA is used to assess the existing and potential hazards of a job, understanding the consequences of risk, and act as an aid in helping identify, eliminate, or control hazards. JHA is a tool used to focus and break down a specific job, define its required steps and tasks and identify its inherent hazards and risks. JHA focuses on the relationship between:
- the employee.
- the job as a whole unit.
- the steps that make up the job.
- the tasks that are defined in each step.
- the tools, materials, and equipment being used.
- existing and potential hazards.
- the consequences of exposures to those hazards.
- potential at-risk events associated with each task.
- existing policies and procedures.
- the nature of the physical environment that the job is complete within.

By assessing all of the components of a job, a comprehensive overview is developed that allows one to focus on the essential areas where changes may be needed. By using a comprehensive JHA process, the foundation for a more effective safety culture is established. Our approach uses both quality and risk management concepts and incorporates human performance concepts into its model. This JHA process links the safety system with risk assessment.

CHAPTER ONE

Why Focus on the Job Hazard Analysis Process

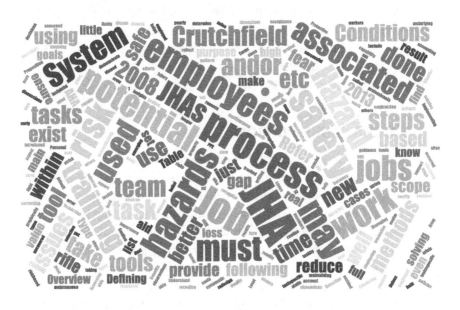

"We Report it – You Decide"

—*Fox News Broadcast*

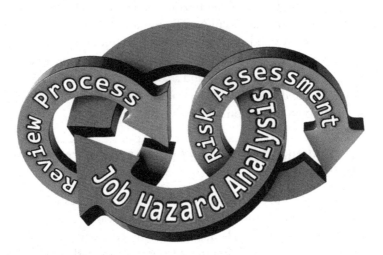

Job Hazard Analysis. http://dx.doi.org/10.1016/B978-0-12-803441-5.00001-5

"We do not want production and a safety program, or production and safety, or production with safety. But, rather, we want safe production."

—Dan Petersen

Chapter Objectives

At the end of this chapter, you should be able to:

- Discuss the importance and benefits of the JHA to the safety culture.
- Compare and contrast the benefits and drawbacks of a JHA process.
- Discuss how to build a case for having a JHA process.
- Discuss how JHA brings focus and respect for the job.
- Discuss the challenges to the JHA process.

1.1 JHAs' MAIN PURPOSE

JHA's main purpose is to aid the safety system to:

- Ensure that all members of an organization can recognize and understand real or potential operational hazards, their associated risk, appropriate actions, and controls, necessary to reduce the potential for injury or loss.
- Provide guidance to employees at all levels of the organization so they can demonstrate the importance of correcting potential hazards that they may be routinely exposed to, as well as how to protect themselves and others (Roughton & Crutchfield, 2013).

Based on discussions with safety professionals, when writing "Safety Culture: An Innovative Leadership Approach", safety efforts must be viewed as an "emerging property" that results from the interactions of all elements of an organization. In this view, the JHA becomes a crucial process element necessary to support the safety culture (Roughton & Crutchfield, 2013).

By being proactive and implementing, a JHA process throughout the organization, the leadership team, and employees can develop a better understanding of task-specific hazards and associated risk. Based on this belief, hazards and associated risk can only be tracked, identified, and controlled by using an ongoing proactive comprehensive JHA process.

1.2 DEFINING THE VALUE PROPOSITION CASE FOR JHA PROCESS

JHA process provides a multipurpose toolkit that can be used for more than just improvement of the safety system. It can provide insights on every aspect of how jobs are designed and how efficiently and effectively hazards and associated risks within the various steps and tasks are controlled.

This knowledge can also be used to improve job quality by increasing the greater potential for reducing human errors.

A properly designed JHA can be used as a comprehensive training aid to ensure that all employees know the primary requirements of each assignment and how to make safe choices when performing the required steps and tasks. When JHA is used on a consistent and routine basis, it provides a structured method for developing and maintaining an effective safety system. In turn, a more consistent safety system provides more effective hazard control for work methods. JHA can be used in conjunction with many elements of the safety system such as inspection programs, incident investigations, job observations, as well as for general problem-solving activities.

1.3 WHY IS THE JHA IMPORTANT?

JHA is used to close the gaps that can develop between what is actually being done, as jobs are completed and requirements to implement a successful safety system. When conducting a JHA, an in-depth understanding of tasks-specific physical and mental skill requirements is developed, as the step-by-step and task-by-task analysis is done.

Obvious hazards are identified through JHA process and less obvious hidden hazards become visible as the systematic analysis of each job step and related task are confirmed and reviewed. By combining the identification of potential loss-producing events with a risk analysis, better preventive measures and controls are defined. A uniform JHA approach provides a consistent method for developing effective employee selection and training programs that better ensure that a safe and effective work methods are employed. Refer to Table 1.1 for a list of why JHAs are important.

Table 1.1 Why are JHAs important?

The following list describes various reasons why are JHAs important. JHAs can assist in:
• detecting existing and/or potential hazards and consequences of exposure.
• assessing and developing specific training needs and requirements.
• providing the leadership team with an understanding what each employee should know about how to effectively perform his/hertheir job.
• recognizing changes in procedures, tools, machine/equipment, etc. that may have occurred.
• defining the potential for specific at-risk events and potential loss-producing events.
• identifying preventive measures necessary to modify or control associated risk.
• providing the opportunity to evaluate any residual risk.

(Conducting a Job Hazard Analysis (JHA), n.d.).

Caution! Personal protective equipment (PPE) and training are not and should not be the default solution for every hazard or safety related issue. Use of JHA provides a more insightful approach that opens up more opportunities or alternatives for a safe work environment improvement. Refer Chapter 7 for a discussion on techniques and methods to use in selecting hazard and associated risk control methods.

"The JHA process provides a better method to identify opportunities for improvement in the safety system and can help provide the foundation for a hazard and risk-based analysis. As this structured process is followed, issues may be uncovered that may require the leadership team to make decisions if a specific task should be avoided or modified" (Roughton & Crutchfield, 2008).

Refer to Figures 1.1 and 1.2.

1.4 BENEFITS OF DEVELOPING A JHA PROCESS

By comprehensively and routinely using JHA as a tool, performance-based measurements can be established to determine if jobs are correctly using the proper controls, procedures, and protocols. Performance-based measurements without an understanding of how jobs are completed and accomplished may not be providing a full picture of where problems or issues exist. As a result, the potential to identify loss-producing events can remain hidden from both the employees and the leadership team.

If implemented correctly, JHA has the potential for improving the following:
- Properly selecting materials, equipment, and tools necessary to complete a job, and reduce the hazards and associated risk within the steps and task where those items are being used.

By using a structured approach that graphically maps out all of the components of a job's step(s) and task(s), interactions can be assessed for improvements that can be more readily implemented. In many cases, a full job "retooling" or redesign may not be necessary as it may be found that minor changes can be made that reduce a potential loss-producing event within the job.

The review of materials, tools, and equipment may find disconnects between purchasing, accounting, job requirements, and required employee

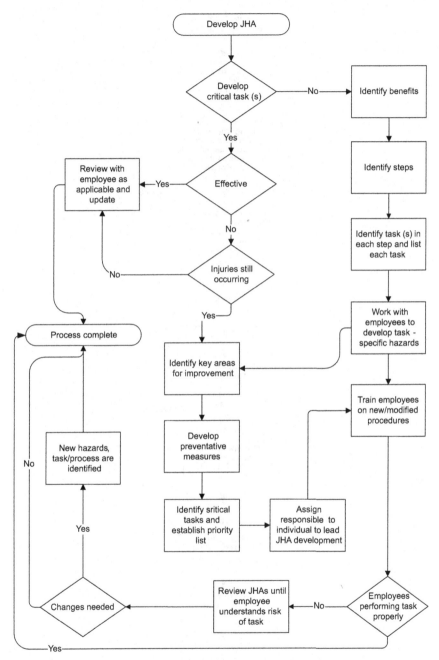

Figure 1.1 *High Level Overview of the JHA Development Process. Based on and adapted using Roughton and Crutchfield (2008).*

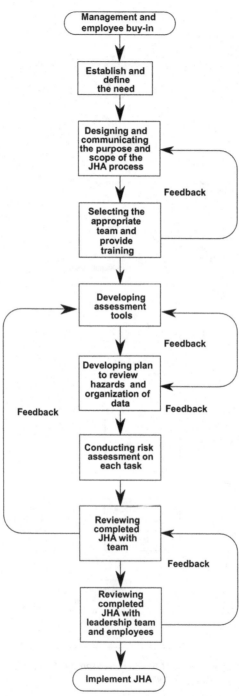

Figure 1.2 *Overview of the JHA Implementation Process. Based on and adapted using Roughton and Crutchfield (2008).*

capability, and needs. What is believed to be a good idea in the implementation of new tools, materials, or equipment may be found to be increasing safety issues and problems.

- Identifying specific policies, procedures, protocols, rules, and training requirements that can be matched against what is actually required, thereby closing the gap between mandated administrative criteria and what is actually taking place to get the assigned jobs completed.

Jobs evolve and change over time. Guidelines that once were effective may no longer reflect the reality of what is being done. The JHA process provides a periodic review of the job steps and tasks to ensure that controls are effective and in place.

- Identifying the necessary skills, both mental and physical requirements that take into consideration human performance improvement challenges.

Unless all the components of a job are assessed, the potential for human error can increase. The JHA process can take into account the limits of what employees can and cannot do. This knowledge can be linked with hiring, training, and supervision procedures, and needs. To tell employees to "work safe" or hold them accountable for poorly designed jobs leads to the abyss of never being able to improve the effectiveness of even a rudimentary safety system.

- Improving the workplace environment.

The job must be accomplished in a work environment that has been assessed in all its dimensions. For example, areas for consideration include inadequate lighting, noise, vapors, dust, housekeeping, and maintenance requirements, etc. If the conditions surrounding a job are not assessed, obstacles are put into place that can prevent the efficient and effective completion of the job.

- Developing specific goals and objectives.

If employees have goals set for them and their job has obstacles built into how the job must be accomplished, an underlying mental negativity can develop. The JHA process should bring into light, where those issues and obstacles exist.

It must be kept in mind that the work environment is not static and conditions change as new technology, procedures, etc. are introduced. Without a JHA process that routinely reviews the components and elements of the safety system, one may find that there may be misalignment of the required interactions that hide or mask hazards and associated risk.

"Supervisors can use the findings of a JHA to eliminate and/or prevent hazards, thereby helping in reducing injuries; providing a safer and more effective work method for a given task; reduced workers' compensation costs, and helps to increase productivity. The analysis can be a valuable tool for training new employees in the tasks required to perform their jobs safely" (Roughton & Crutchfield, 2008).

"The JHA provides a consistent reminder for all new, relocated, and/or seasoned employees. It can be applied to specific job steps or tasks that have been modified. It can be used as an awareness tool for those who need updated training and/or site-specific review of non-routine task" (How to Identify Job Hazards, n.d.; Roughton & Crutchfield, 2008).

1.5 BUILDING THE CASE FOR A JHA PROCESS

Most organizations have the tendency to operate in a reactive mode and only making changes when serious conditions dictate or experience has shown that change is necessary. Change is made in many cases only after a severe loss-producing event creates a crisis and unmasks conditions that now become unacceptable. A primary objective of the JHA process is to increase the potential for identifying hazards or increased risk before a job has begun and/or a loss-producing event happens. The JHA process aids in building an increased resilience against acceptance of hazards if used early in any job design stage and as part of an ongoing activity.

The Corps of Engineers uses a form of the JHA process called Activity hazard analysis (AHA) on all construction sites. "Before beginning each work activity involving a type of work presenting hazards not experienced in previous project operations or where a new work crew or sub-contractor is to perform the work, the Contractor(s) performing that work activity shall prepare an AHA" (Army System Safety Management Guide, 2008).

A comprehensive implementation strategy is needed that continuously emphasizes the value of the JHA process and how it can improve the overall organization by avoiding or reducing the impact of unnecessary injuries and damage. One technique is to use the JHA and its concepts as a problem-solving tool. As stated earlier, when the JHA is used consistently and routinely, it can be gradually incorporated into job design, purchasing criteria, training assessments, incident investigations, etc., becoming an integral part of the general safety process.

1.6 GAINING GREATER RESPECT FOR THE JOB

The JHA provides an understanding of what employees are actually doing and what they must contend with while coordinating the activities necessary to complete an assignment. This can bring a greater respect and understanding of what must be done to organize and complete a job's steps and tasks effectively.

> "Does an employee's perception of an existing and/or potential hazards and consequences of exposure differ from that of the employer? The employee sees a hazard and wants it fixed immediately. The employer may respond to this issue quickly and address the hazard but is often slowed down by internal structures, budget restraints, proper corrective actions, priorities, etc. Answers to critical questions must be clearly defined:
> Is the safety issue real?
> How large is the risk?
> What are the options?
> What is the best way to correct the identified risk?
> Who is going to correct the hazard?
> How long will it take to develop and implement preventative measures?
> How much will it cost?
> Is there need for additional training?
> One must remember that risk is based on probability even with a blatant hazard; no loss-producing events may have been developed" (Roughton & Crutchfield, 2008).

The JHA gives insight on how much decision-making leeway and task flexibility can be given to employees to complete a job. Jobs with high hazards and severe potential for loss have little or no flexibility in how they can be accomplished. A strict set of guidelines, procedures, protocols, and rules must be followed in this type of case.

On the other extreme, jobs exist that allow almost total employee flexibility with the determining what steps and procedures should be followed. These would be those jobs that are identified with limited low hazards and associated risk and with little unintended consequences.

1.7 CHALLENGES TO JHA PROCESS

JHA is not just a tool limited to determining the criteria required to complete a job. It is a part of an overall network useful to the leadership team and employees in communicating how things are being done and determining whether the desired methods and/or techniques are being used within the desired work process criteria.

JHAs can serve as a conduit that increases the speed of communications for safety issues and concerns to the leadership team. A disconnect or gap can exist between what the leadership team believes is happening and what is really going on and actually being done without this conduit. This gap of "What is" versus "What is thought to be" is the result of:

- "Scope-drift" – gradual unrecognized changes. "Scope drift is a rifle sighting term describing the condition where your telescope is not aligned with the rifle barrel. When aiming at a target through an unaligned rifle scope, you will miss your target every time" (Roughton & Crutchfield, 2013).
- Employees are allowed to take short cuts. Conditions are in place that allows employees to take short cuts without understanding the consequences of the exposure.
- Changes are created in the work environment because of various and possibly gradual modifications to tools, equipment, materials, facilities, etc.
- Lack of having a quality workplace and not having an environment that is well designed, well maintained, and properly managed.

1.8 JHAs REQUIRE EFFORT AND TIME TO IMPLEMENT

A primary consideration in the implementation of the JHA process is that it requires time to complete. Given that time is generally limited due to various organizational constraints, a thorough understanding of potential organizational constraints must be considered when devising a JHA process and planning its implementation. Job requirements, how production hours are utilized, available skills, and capabilities of employees must be considered. As hazards and associated risk are an intangible concept to many people that do not study them as a profession, the need for JHAs may not be immediately visible.

Second, the fear that "something" may be found that requires correction and resources not available must be addressed at the beginning of an implementation. The current workplace environment and financial health of the organization can drive this fear. Once hazard related issue(s) are out in the open and properly prioritized as to scope of risk to employees, alternative solutions can be assessed and budgets can be developed based on knowledge of job.

"To move the JHA from just occasional use, its strength as part of any continuous improvement process must be made clear to leadership and employees as to its potential for improving the work environment" (Conducting a Job Hazard Analysis (JHA), n.d.; Roughton, 1995).

SUMMARY

The JHA process provides a multipurpose toolkit that can be used for more than just improvement of the safety process. It can provide insights on every aspect of how jobs are designed and how efficiently and effectively hazards and associated risks within the various steps and tasks are implemented. This knowledge can also be used to improve job quality by increasing the greater potential for reducing human errors.

By comprehensively and routinely using the JHA as a tool to identify hazards and associated risks, performance-based measurements can be established to determine if jobs are being performed correctly using the proper controls, procedures, and protocols. Performance-based measurements without an understanding of how jobs are completed and accomplished may not be providing a full picture of where problems or issues exist. As a result, the potential for severe loss can remain hidden from both the employees and the leadership team.

A primary objective of the JHA process is to increase the potential of identifying hazards or increased risk before a job has begun and/or a loss-producing event occurs. The JHA process aids in building an increased resilience against acceptance of hazards if used early in any job design stage and as part of an ongoing activity.

A comprehensive implementation strategy is needed that continuously emphasizes the value of the JHA process and how it can improve the overall organization by avoiding or reducing the impact of unnecessary injuries and potential damage. One technique is to use the JHA and its concepts as a problem-solving tool.

The JHA provides an understanding of what employees are actually doing and what they must contend with while coordinating the activities necessary to complete an assignment. This can bring a greater respect and understanding of what must be done to organize and complete a job's steps and tasks effectively can be achieved by using JHA concepts.

The JHA provides insight on how much decision-making leeway and task flexibility can be given to employees to complete a job. Jobs with high hazards and severe potential for loss have little or no flexibility in how they can be accomplished. A strict set of guidelines, procedures, protocols, and rules must be followed in this type of case.

The JHA is not just a tool limited to determining the criteria required to complete a job. It is a part of an overall network useful to the leadership team and employees in communicating how things are being done and determining whether the desired methods and/or techniques are being used and within the desired work process criteria.

JHAs can serve as a conduit that increases the speed of communications for safety issues and concerns to the leadership team. A disconnect or gap can exist between what the leadership team believe is happening and what is really going on and actually being done without this conduit.

A primary consideration in the implementation of the JHA process is that it requires time to complete. Given that time is generally limited due to various organizational constraints, a thorough understanding of potential organizational constraints must be considered when devising a JHA process and planning its implementation.

CHAPTER REVIEW QUESTIONS

1. Discuss the main purpose of a safety system and why it is important.
2. What does JHA process provide?
3. Why are JHA's important?
4. What does the JHA have the potential for improving?
5. Discuss why is important to get employees involved in the JHA process.
6. What is one primary objective of the JHA process?
7. Why is a comprehensive implementation strategy necessary for the JHA process?
8. How does JHA bring better focus and respect for the job?
9. Discuss how does JHA act as a form of communication?
10. What type of fear might exist when developing a JHA process?

BIBLIOGRAPHY

Conducting a job hazard analysis (JHA). (n.d.). Oregon Occupational Safety and Health Division (Oregon OSHA), Public Domain, Permission to Reprint, Modify, and/or Adapt as necessary. Retrieved from http://bit.ly/WXGJhK

How to identify job hazards. (n.d.). Saskatchewan Labour, Occupational Health & Safety, Partners in Safety. Retrieved from http://bit.ly/Z3mCS9

Roughton, J. (1995). Job hazard analysis: an essential safety tool. *J. J. Keller's OSHA Safety Training Newsletter*, 2–3.

Roughton, J., & Crutchfield, N. (2008). *Job hazard analysis: A guide for voluntary compliance and beyond. Chemical, petrochemical & process.* Elsevier/Butterworth-Heinemann. Retrieved from http://amzn.to/VrSAq5

Roughton, J., & Crutchfield, N. (2013). *Safety culture: An innovative leadership approach.* In B. Heinemann (Ed.). Butterworth Heinemann. Retrieved from http://amzn.to/1qoD4oN

Safety Management System. (2008). Federal Aviation Administration (FAA), *Manual – Version 2.1, Public Domain.* Retrieved from http://1.usa.gov/WSds8S

System Safety Management Guide. (2013, August). Department of the Army, Pamphlet 385–16, Public Domain. Retrieved from http://bit.ly/11f0gib

CHAPTER TWO

Understanding Human Performance in the Job Hazard Analysis Process

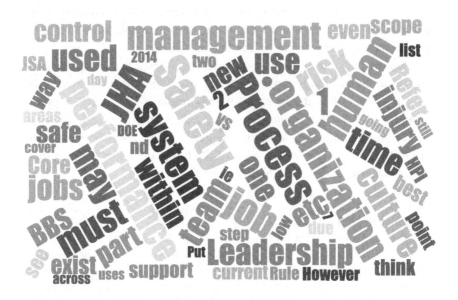

"I have never met a man so ignorant that I couldn't learn something from him."

—Galileo Galilei

Chapter Objectives

At the end of this chapter, you should be able to:

- Discuss how the JHA process fits into the overall organization.
- Discuss how the JHA communicates information through the organization.
- Explain how the culture of the organization impacts job completion.
- Discuss and explain the basic concepts of human performance improvement (HPI).
- Outline the importance of understanding the types of performance.
- Explain the importance of reducing human error potential.

Job Hazard Analysis. http://dx.doi.org/10.1016/B978-0-12-803441-5.00002-7

2.1 BASIC OVERVIEW

Jobs in an organization are part of an overall complex system of human interactions and ongoing change coupled with varying and potentially conflicting goals and objectives. The JHA process requires a strategy that provides for an administrative structure, employee time, and a budget for the implementation of recommended hazards and associated risk controls. As with any new process, a buy in from the leadership team and employees is necessary as the process must be able to show tangible added value in improving the organization as well as making jobs safer.

When introducing the JHA system, the main obstacle may be the leadership team questioning implementation, based on the perception that things are going well and why extra effort is needed. Many safety programs are traditionally based on injury frequency reduction due to regulatory record keeping requirements. If injury frequency is low then the perception is "risk" must be low or under control. If things are under control then resources will be allocated to "higher priorities."

Case Study # 1
Organizations must set priorities. Safety may be an espoused value but it must be translated into something tangible. A dialog was once overheard between a general manager and a safety director. Safety Director, "I need more of your support." General Manager, "You have my support. What do you want?" Be prepared to have an answer if found in a similar position!

Espoused Values
"Corporate values and morals important to an organization. Espoused values contribute to the development of normal standards of the organization for how it conducts business now and in the future" (Espoused Values, n.d.).

2.2 PROFESSIONAL RESPONSIBILITY

The safety professional must research and develop an understanding of how an organization operates, its motivations, and reason for being. They must have an appreciation of what must be done to reach the organizational goals and objectives. While what a safety professional does is crucial (at least to the safety professional), other professional disciplines (human resources, security, quality control, sales, operations, etc.) feel the same about their discipline and its needs. This mindset sets up potential competitive conflicts for time, financial budgets, use of employees, and other resources as each discipline attempts to maximize its influence on the organization. This interaction and its overall effect is what drives and defines an organizational culture.

> *"...culture is created and sustained by a network of communications in which meaning is generated. The culture's material embodiments include artifacts and written texts, through which meaning is passed on from generation to generation."*
>
> **(Capra & Luisi, 2014)**

2.3 THE JHA – A COMMUNICATION TOOL

JHA should be considered more than a tool used to define individual activities. It should be considered part of the overall hazard and associated risk communication. The JHA defines what is to be communicated about ongoing activities and must be viewed as an essential part of the safety system. Its format and use encapsulates the scope of operational hazards and their associated risks found directly within an activity. If used routinely and consistently, it provides the conduit for in-depth logical discussions about hazard avoidance, reduction, and control that are necessary.

The JHA provides an effective communication tool that can be used for a variety of purposes; for example, training, operational reviews, employee selection, and specific job design. To be most effective, it must be routinely used and flexible enough to adjust to the ongoing changes within the workplace.

JHAs provide an understanding of hazards at their point of beginning - the location where job actions are completed. JHAs communicate to the leadership team and employees the potential for injury and the controls that are required. The use of the JHA also improves the potential for removing obstacles hindering the effectiveness of activities that reduce the severity of loss-producing events.

2.4 IMPLEMENTATION STRATEGY

The organization may have an established planning process that allows the leadership team to organize, budget, and account for all activities that are considered of value. Projects that are not considered of value are not budgeted and not supported with resources. A critical step in developing a JHA process is to ensure that the information presented follows the same format for project management and budgeting that are used by the organization, i.e., you need to speak the same language.

The following is a list of areas for consideration that must be addressed before implementation of a JHA process:

- Budget: What resources are needed and what is the cost?
- Time requirements: How many JHAs are to be developed and what is the time frame for completion? This provides an indication of resources required.
- Team approach: Is a team approach to be used? Who will be needed to do the work?
- Leadership team: Does the leadership team understands the intent of the project and has signed off on a team charter?
- System measurement: Is the JHA development incorporated into the leadership team and employee goals and objectives? Is it part of an annual human resources merit review?
- Training: How much training is required for employees and the leadership team?
- Format and curation: What media and format are to be used and where will they be stored? Curation will be discussed in more detail in Chapter 14.
- Safety system: How will the JHA process fit within the existing safety system?
- Sustaining the process: After developing the JHA process, what will be required to keep it up to date and sustained? Who will be defined as the champion? Who will be assigned the responsibility?

2.5 DEFINING THE TERM "JOB"

The term "job" has changed over the years from being a specific limited activity to an overall definition as a "job title," which may cover a number of various activities and responsibilities. Consider the following definitions:

Definition 1: A job is "a piece of work, especially a specific task done as part of the routine of one's occupation" (Job, n.d.).

Definition 2: "Anything a person is expected or obliged to do; duty; responsibility" (Job, n.d.).

A traditional JHA uses Definition 1. The job is broken down into steps and hazards identified for each step. Control for each hazard is then implemented without the benefit of knowing about task and associated risk. The "job" itself is then considered safe if the person doing the work uses the controls determined by the analysis.

A job as defined by Definition 2 could have a number of JHAs completed for each assigned "Job" as defined by Definition 1. The potential exist for the accumulative effects of multiple "jobs" and their interactions to be overlooked. The traditional method does not take into account time and the accumulative effects of multiple "jobs" being done by that particular "job" title.

One way of describing the two types of job definitions is as a parent and child concept. This concept is used in computer programming for overall theme development where the parent is the primary theme that should not be changed (the way that a website is to be viewed). This ensures that the important features of the main theme are not overwritten when the various "child" themes are updated.

If the same concept is applied to the JHA development, the parent becomes the primary overall job analysis that takes into account all of the overlapping or similar job tasks. It provides a baseline for the overall assigned responsibilities and activities. The parent JHA contains the core elements that create the function and are universal to that job. The child JHAs provides hazard and risk assessment and defined controls for each required specific individual activity.

For example, a situation where five pieces of equipment operate exactly the same would develop one generic JHA, i.e., the parent that would cover the equipment hazard analysis. However, differences or potential variations in how specific tasks are performed can develop no matter if the equipment is similar in nature. The child JHA would provide for these potentially additional hazards and associated risk in the analysis of the steps and tasks required.

2.6 COMPARING JHA AND JSA

The terms "job hazard analysis (JHA)" and "job safety analysis (JSA)" are used somewhat interchangeably. A variety of other terminology such as job task analysis (JTA), activity task analysis (ATA), and others are used depending on the industry and organization.

Case Study #2

One of the authors was involved in a project with an ergonomist to find control methods for cumulative trauma disorders, i.e., muscle strains, stress, back injuries, etc.

During the project, many discussions were held concerning how to approach the current conditions. It became apparent that an issue with definitions had developed.

To resolve the differences in terminology, they developed a flow diagram outlining the differences between the JHA and JSA. The result of the brainstorming session was that the term "JSA" became the parent and was used to cover potential accumulative traumas that can occur over time. JHAs became the children and used for individual job actions specific to a point in time. The flowchart combined the differences between a JHA and JSA (Figure 2.1).

The concept of defining JHA versus JSA over time provided for a multidimensional approach to the analysis of a job.

By adding time as an element of the analysis, health and accumulative trauma potential can be better factored into the analysis. As a point of reference, the JHA process team must understand how time will be weighted as a factor in the analysis of the job.

2.7 HUMAN PERFORMANCE PRINCIPLES

One of the issues with the structure of the traditional JHA is that it implies that all hazards can be controlled looking only at the job steps (Job Hazard Analysis, 3071, 2002). Additional elements must be considered in reviewing a job or families of jobs for mental and physical requirements, the potential for human error (which too many times becomes the selected default problem), and the impact of technology.

The key to the process is to understand that people have their own perceptions, personal and professional experiences, and/or knowledge, preferences, skills, and ability.

According to Reason, as cited in the *HPI Handbook*, "It is crucial that personnel and particularly their managers become more aware of the human potential for errors, the task, workplace, and organizational factors that shape their likelihood and their consequences. Understanding how and why unsafe acts occur is the essential first step in effective error management" (US DOE, 2009a).

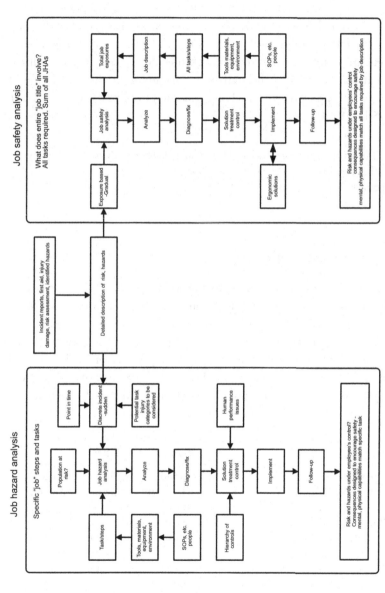

Figure 2.1 *Overview of the Concept of the Job Hazard Analysis Versus the Job Safety Analysis. Based on and Adapted from Research and discussions with other safety professional.*

The *HPI Handbook* identifies five principles that should guide the safety system and in turn the JHA process:
- "People are fallible, and even the best people make mistakes.
- Error-likely situations are predictable, manageable, and preventable.
- Individual behavior is influenced by organizational processes and values.
- People achieve high levels of performance because of the encouragement and reinforcement received from leaders, peers, and subordinates.
- Events can be avoided through an understanding of the reasons mistakes occur and application of the lessons learned from past events (or errors)" (US DOE, 2009a).

"…human performance can only be realized when individuals at all levels of the organization accept these principles and embrace concepts and practices that support them" (US DOE, 2009a).

2.8 ERROR PRECURSORS

Potential error precursors, (existing conditions that increase error rates) should be assessed as to their impact on safe job completion. For example, time pressure to complete a job can result in the employee expected to take short cuts or accept risk as part of the job. "Error precursors are unfavorable prior conditions…that increase the probability for error during a specific action" (US DOE, 2009a). Refer to Table 2.1 for a comparison on human error precursors concerning task demands and individual capabilities and

Table 2.1 Human error precursors – task demands and individual capabilities

Task demands	Individual capabilities
Time pressure (in a hurry)	Unfamiliarity with task/first time
High workload (large memory)	Lack of knowledge (faulty mental model)
Simultaneous, multiple actions	New techniques not used before
Repetitive actions/monotony	Imprecise communication habits
Irreversible actions	Lack of proficiency/inexperience
Interpretation requirements	Indistinct problem-solving skills
Unclear goals, roles, or responsibilities	Unsafe attitudes
Lack of or unclear standards	Illness or fatigue; general poor health or injury

Source: US DOE (2009a)

Table 2.2 Additional human error precursors – work environment and human nature

Work environment	Human nature
Distractions/interruptions	Stress
Changes/departure from routine	Habit patterns
Confusing displays or controls	Assumptions
Work-arounds/out of service instrumentation	Complacency/Overconfidence
Hidden system/equipment response	Mind-set (intentions)
Unexpected equipment conditions	Inaccurate risk perception
Lack of alternative indication	Mental shortcuts or biases
Personality conflict	Limited short-term memory

Source: US DOE (2009a)

Table 2.2 for additional human error precursors concerning work environment and human nature.

The HPI principles along with an understanding of human error precursors can be used to enhance the development of the JHA process. If a fundamental attribute of humans is that they can make mistakes and make wrong decisions then it becomes important to ensure that job requirements are properly analyzed and designed.

The necessary steps and tasks should be evaluated with the intent of reducing or eliminating as many error-provoking precursors as possible in combination with hazard controls. If "error-likely situations are predictable, manageable, and preventable," then the JHA becomes the foundational tool for the potential control these situations.

2.9 DEFINING ORGANIZATIONAL CULTURE

Organizations are subject to errors made at any level and by anyone in the course of everyday operations. The use and application of the JHA provides an aid in reducing the potential for error by assessing critical hazards and associated risk in as many aspects of an activity as possible.

One thing to remember is that an organization is a series of emerging properties that are the result of its many components blending together or at the very least colliding or interfering with the safety system (Roughton & Crutchfield, 2013).

A strong organizational culture takes into account the potential for improving human performance. The objective of a strong culture within the overarching organizational culture is to aid in reducing the potential for human error. The nature of the organization's culture and its acceptance of risk can be assessed by determining the status and emphasis on the safety system.

> "...a pattern of shared basic assumptions that the group learned as it evolved its problems of external adaptation and internal integration. Over time this pattern of shared assumptions has worked well enough to be considered valid and, therefore, to be taught to new members as the correct way you perceive, think, and feel in relation to those problems" (US DOE, 2009a).

An initial assessment should review how the organization currently develops and designs jobs required meeting its daily goals and objectives. The JHA process must be customized to ensure that it fits within the current methods and concepts used to solve problems.

When implementing a JHA process, the organizational elements at a minimum must be reviewed include:

- The current safety system. Does the organization use a national or international standard? Refer to Chapter 7 or other approaches used that incorporate the JHA into overall guidelines or standards? If the organization has developed its own safety system, what is its scope and does it currently have a JHA element?
- The level of employee and leadership team training. What is the scope and depth of job-specific training? Does the training incorporate a comprehensive safety aspect into the training content? If not, why?
- Who is responsible for job design and development? Is the process centralized or decentralized and how is it monitored and supervised?

2.10 SHIFT IN PERCEPTION

HPI principles provide a new dimension for the JHA process. The traditional safety process focuses primarily on injury reduction, an effort that has had considerable success over time. It stresses a behavioral approach aimed at observable acts or active errors that can be immediately seen (US DOE, 2009a). HPI focuses on the reduction of both potential active errors as well as latent errors (Figure 2.2).

2.11 LEVELS OF CULTURE DEFINED

An understanding of the organizational culture will aid in determining the priorities and values actually held by the organization and provide insights on the best methods to implement the JHA process.

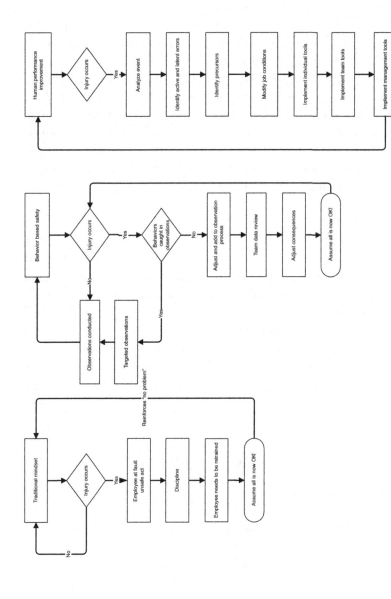

Figure 2.2 *Overview of Human Performance Model Versus Traditional Models, Employee vs Leadership Team Behavior. Based on Human Performance Improvement Handbook.*

According to Schein (Roughton & Crutchfield, 2013; US DOE, 2009a), three organization culture levels should be considered:

- Artifacts. "…the visible organizational structures and processes. These are the tangible things seen as you move within operations or facilities and review the environment of the organization." For example, things you see, visible structures and processes, Inspection findings (maintenance, housekeeping, orderliness, etc.
- Espoused Values. "…the content of the various strategies, goals, core philosophies that are used by the leadership team to guide the organization." For example, what is said and how said, strategies, goals, philosophies, posters, safety slogans, mission statements, policies/procedures, etc.?
- Underlying Assumptions."…are the unspoken rules followed by all employees of the organization." For example, how things are actually done, day-to-day beliefs, etc.

(US DOE, 2009a)

The correlations between the levels of culture will give an indication of how the organization operates. Do inspections identify "artifacts" that indicate that the espoused values are or are not true values to the organization? Do underlying assumptions show consistency between the espoused values and artifacts?

For example, if the espoused value says "We will be a safe and healthy workplace" but inspections and observations show many safety violations, poor maintenance, and/or no true safety efforts, then the underlying belief system is not in alignment with the espoused values (Roughton & Crutchfield, 2013).

2.12 ORGANIZATIONAL STRUCTURE

The organizational structure may change the strategy used to implement the JHA process. As part of the review of the organizational culture, how it organizes personnel, assigns responsibilities and authorities, and allocates resources must be assessed.

The safety professional or person tasked with managing the safety system can report into many different departments and levels of an organization. Understanding the organizational structure and how it has established responsibilities and duties gives insights on how it communicates.

Seabrook stated "Recent injury and illness trends within companies and their global supply chains indicate that overall incident rate improvement has slowed and rates of fatal and serious injuries have remained steady for a number of years. Clearly, a different approach is required if further improvements are to be made."

As cited in Risk Assessment Institute (n.d).

2.13 JOB COMPLEXITY - EVEN FOR "SIMPLE JOBS"

Too often it is heard that a specific job is "simple" and that it doesn't take a "rocket scientist" to do it. This type of statement demeans the employee assigned to do the task as well as establishes a mindset that it is a throwaway job that does not need review. As simple jobs can be usually completed without loss, a mindset of "no loss equals no risk" develops even though hazards and inherent risk can be hidden within a job's steps and tasks.

This mindset allows the development of situations where the leadership team is blindsided by a serious or severe loss-producing event stemming from what appeared to be a very simple job. The first rule for the development of a JHA process is to never assume that because a job looks simple that it does not incorporate inherent hazards buried within it that have some element of risk with the potential for injury or damage in some form. The JHA can demonstrate that even if a job looks simple, it can still be very complex and require a large number of steps and tasks to be completed.

Lesson Learned # 1

In presenting supervisory JHA workshops and in coordination with the safety manager, actual jobs were selected for analysis based on their frequency of injury, cost of injury claims, or general concern about the potential for a loss-producing event. In just about every workshop session, a "surprise" was uncovered that was known by employees but not known to the organization's leadership team or the safety manager.

JHAs developed by the supervisors found jobs required more steps and tasks than expected. In addition, tools, equipment, materials had in various cases gradually changed over time resulting in the need for different training, standard operating procedures, and methods for what was currently in place.

2.14 OVERLAPPING AND SIMILAR JOB ACTIVITIES

As a first step in the JHA process, a job inventory is completed with a preliminary review that rank orders jobs by their perceived or known potential hazards and associated risk.

This can provide insights on jobs completed in the same vicinity or work area and how they are coordinated and managed. Hazards and associated risk within one job may have an impact on adjacent or nearby activities, similar to the parent child concept discussed earlier. For example, would be the use of a flammable chemical may be controlled in one job but an activity or operation nearby contains a possible ignition source. Overlapping job activities are very common in construction or when routine maintenance is being completed while a production process is ongoing.

2.15 TYPES OF PERFORMANCE

Several types of performance must be considered when reviewing jobs for further analysis. The nature of the job performance requirements can impact the nature of the JHA process. Jobs can easily combine elements of each of three performance types, skill based, rule based, and knowledge based:

2.15.1 Skill-Based Performance

Skill-based performance requires "highly practiced largely physical actions in a familiar situation in which there is little conscious monitoring." "Errors are primarily from execution errors, involving action slips and lapses in attention or concentration" (US DOE, 2009a). The origination of the traditional JHA appears to be for this type of work. Types of jobs that are primarily skill-based require minimum thought or decision making. Once the steps and hazards are established, controls are put into place, and the job is monitored to ensure that all implemented controls remain in use. The JHA can be simple and straightforward.

2.15.2 Rule-Based Performance

Rule-based performance requires following preset solutions then taking prearranged specific actions. This performance uses an "If-Then" decision-making process. If "X" occurs, then "Y" is required (US DOE, 2009a). The JHA defines scenarios where standard operating procedures, rules, guidelines, and structure are essential. Errors can possibly occur when rules or protocols are misinterpreted or established procedures not followed or understood.

2.15.3 Knowledge-Based Performance

Knowledge-based performance "is a response to a totally unfamiliar situation (no skill or rule is recognizable to the individual)" (US DOE, 2009a). At this performance level, a JHA should be completed for each new experience with unique issues or problems to ensure controls are implemented. The overall job requirements become the parent and a portfolio of experiences developed for future use and periodically reviewed for similarities. This experience-based knowledge provides an understanding of types of hazards that could be created and how they might combine to increase the risk severity.

As no rules may be present to guide knowledge performance, emphasis is on problem solving, in-depth hazard identification, prejob planning and briefing, and peer-review for recommended controls (US DOE, 2009b). The JHA would be developed before the job begins to define various scenarios showing the steps of each approach and what various worst case situations might occur.

2.16 HUMAN ERROR POTENTIAL

In theory, if jobs are designed logically and employees trained on how to do the job then it is assumed that safety will naturally follow. In this scenario, safety is a destination to be achieved. This approach assumes that a job can be developed without the potential of latent (built-in) human errors from the overall design of the production system. It assumes a design team was able to predict all the many variations of what might be needed to complete a job. The further assumption is that this team has a solid grasp of hazard identification and risk assessment. Latent error (build-in) potential is highly probable and is why safety management systems such as ANSI/AIHA/ASSE, Z10 and others have placed the safety function as part of any design and review team (Occupational Health and Safety Management Systems, 2012).

If a job's steps and tasks are designed to take into account the potential for human error, the tasks will have higher probability for safe completion. Employees may be simply going through the various required steps based on experience but without much attention having been given to how improvements can be made. An opportunity exists to review the existing job design as JHAs are completed.

The JHA should include identifying critical skills and capabilities needed to effectively and safely complete jobs and their series of required steps and tasks.

2.17 ERROR TYPES

The two types of error mentioned earlier can create loss producing events immediately or remain hidden with a long-term potential for loss-producing events.

Active errors are "observable, physical actions that change equipment, system, or facility state, resulting in immediate undesired consequences" (US DOE, 2009a). This type of error can develop from activities where, due to mental and/or physical fatigue, miscommunication, manual require-ments, time, pressure, and stress setup the conditions where an employee makes a decision and receives immediate negative feedback.

Latent errors are those errors that "result in hidden organization-related weakness or equipment flaws"(US DOE, 2009a). By being "latent", they may go for long periods of time before the various factors and conditions come together and result in a tragic loss-producing event.

Many safety rules and regulations currently in place are derived from a long history of design flaws and organizational issues that resulted in such events. Design flaws may be in found in hiring practices and poor work-force skills that allow untrained or inadequate personnel to do tasks beyond their capabilities (Figures 2.3–2.5).

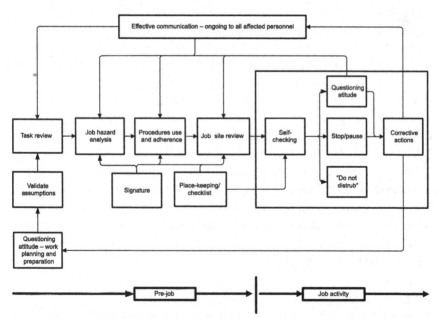

Figure 2.3 *Overview of Human Performance Tools, Example Flow Diagram of Individu-al Tool Use. DOE (2009a).*

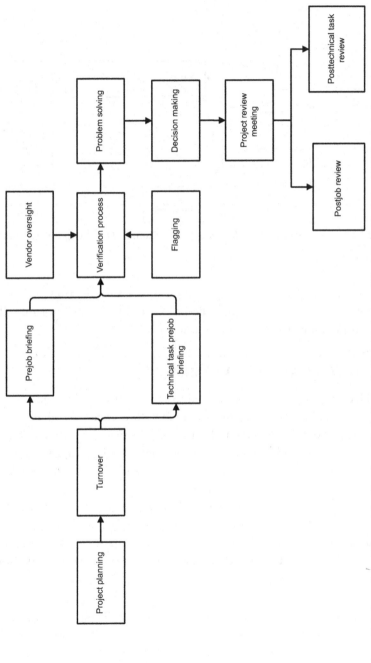

Figure 2.4 *Overview of Human Performance Tools, Example Flow Diagram of Work Team Tool Use. DOE (2009a).*

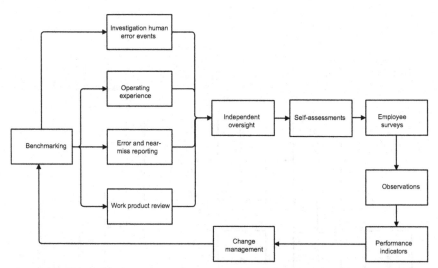

Figure 2.5 *Overview of Human Performance Tools, Example Flow Diagram of Management. DOE (2009a).*

These flow diagrams provide examples of the various tools and techniques that can be used to reduce the potential for human error by individuals, work teams, and the leadership team.

2.18 TECHNOLOGY AS A RISK

JHA must consider the level of automation within a job and the potential impact of the failure of the automation. For example, vehicles with backup or side mirror cameras and other devices may give a false sense of security in backing and lane changing. This becomes more apparent when operating a vehicle without these devices and highlights the loss of basic observational skills acquired through experience.

Dramatic increased use of robotics and computer driven equipment brings addition risk complications into the work place. If the safety system fails, human operators may have to take over. Their lack of experience and expertise puts them at risk that they would not otherwise have had without reliance on the automation.

Several situations indicate that technology designed to improve safety may actually be increasing the potential for errors and tragic mistakes. Over reliance on these mechanism must be taken into account. According to

Nicholas Carr (as cited in Blum, 2014, Chapter 4), "it can be found that technology can take the edge off the ability to make proper decisions during crisis situations" (Blum, 2014).

In addition, the FAA's concern with flight operations data, issued a safety alert to the airlines encouraging "operators to promote manual flight operations when appropriate." The FAA stated that "A recent analysis of flight operations data (including normal flight operations, incidents, and accidents) identified an increase in manual handling errors" (Safety Alert for Operations, 2013).

The FAA further recommended that "Operators are encouraged to take an integrated approach by incorporating emphasis of manual flight operations into both line operations and training (initial/upgrade and recurrent)" (Safety Alert for Operations, 2013).

2.19 POLITICS IN THE ORGANIZATION

An area that receives little attention but is very important is the need to develop an understanding of the politics within an organization. "Politics" or "being political" is considered negative and not looked at favorably by many people due to the media stereotype of "politicians." However, in the true sense of the word, politics is simply being able to present your case for a cause and get other people to buy into what you believe should be accomplished.

Politics is the practice and theory of influencing other people (Politics, n.d.).

Politics is when you know who to approach and when, how to structure a message that has impact and is accepted by the majority of its intended audience (the leadership team, employees, and other departments). In itself, being "political" is not a bad thing. Politics in the best form is an essential part of working with employees and the leadership team who bring their perspectives and experiences into the organization.

By gaining an understanding of the interactions of the organization, objectives have a better chance of being accepted by getting buy-in from people who will work with you to remove obstacles and help move the organization toward the desired goals and objectives.

"To govern a society shared by people of emotion, people of reason, and everybody in between – as well as people who think their actions are shaped by logic but in fact are shaped by feelings and non-empirical philosophies – you need politics. At its best, politics navigates all the minds-states for the sake of the greater good, alert to the rocky shoals of community, identity, and the economy. At its worst, politics thrives on the incomplete disclosure or misrepresentation of data required by an electorate to make informed decisions, whether arrived at logically or emotionally" (Tyson, 2012).

"Getting your message to resonate and stick inside the minds of its recipients is essential" (Heath & Heath, 2007).

2.20 THE ART OF CURATION

The art of curation will be discussed in Chapter 14.

At the beginning of the JHA process, an estimation of the scope and needs for its hard-copy and digital filing system and storage requirements is essential. As JHAs are developed, it is crucial that their administrative and storage needs are addressed. A centralized location in a shared computer internal drive and adequate hardcopy storage should allow ease of access and the capability for updating when necessary. If not properly organized and accessible, these documents may as well not exist. Information that cannot be found is not part of a true or valid knowledge base.

2.21 QUESTIONS TO REVIEW ABOUT THE ORGANIZATION

The goal of hazard control and risk reduction is to achieve stability in process implementation through an efficient safety system. Meanwhile, various internal and external forces are tugging the organization in many directions. As an organization has multiple goals and objectives subject to change, safety criteria must constantly evolve to protect the organization.

To be considered as a core essential part of the leadership team, the safety professional must be politically savvy, develop effective two-way positive communications that ensure risk-related issues move rapidly to key decision makers. In addition, this communication network must be able to identify ways to move around potential organizational obstacles.

Questions to consider should include but not be limited to the following:

- What is the organization's structure, history, general attributes, and culture? What drives the organization – sales/marketing, operations/production, engineering, etc.?
- How diverse is the organization? Multinational, bilingual, multicultural, etc.?
- Who is in charge and what types of "personalities" are in the leadership team?
- What are the primary services and/or products?
- How complex are operations and what technologies are used?
- How were job descriptions developed? Are they centralized or are individual areas developing their own?
- Can jobs be grouped into job families that have similar hazards and associated risk?
- Do any job analyses exist that are similar to the desired JHA?
- What is the history of latent and active human error? Is the current focus on just employee errors (primarily active) or are latent errors (leadership team and administrative, engineering design/development issues) open for discussion?
- What mental and physical skills are required to provide the services and products? What percent of jobs are knowledge based? Rule based? Or Skill based? Does hiring and retention practices match the job requirements?
- Will the organization allow changes to be made in the current job descriptions?
- What part do internal "politics", employee agreements, interdepartmental issues, or other unique organizational features play in job design and leadership?
- Is the organization open to change? As problems or issues are identified, does the support for change exist?
- How does the budget system operate and what are its time frames (fiscal year, planning)?

2.22 ANOTHER AREA FOR CONSIDERATION

2.22.1 Benefits of Behavior-Based Safety

The behavioral approach is a process that provides organizations the opportunity to move to a level higher of safety excellence. An understanding of how antecedents and consequences are designed along with statistically valid data builds ownership, trust, and unity if properly implemented. This behavioral approach provides the leadership team the opportunity to develop and demonstrate core values, improve coaching, and leadership skills.

A properly designed behavioral process involves employees at every level. The atmosphere of trust that results from nonpunitive observation and the feedback process leads to create more employee participation. If a positive approach and communication is developed, employees frequently start asking to be observed and use the feedback given to modify their activity to make themselves and their fellow employees safer. A rapport develops between the observers and the employees being observed leading to more open discussions. As trust increases, the reporting of minor injuries and sources of damage increases allowing root causes to be determined.

Variation is the fluctuations that can occur based on inconsistent environmental, human actions, equipment, tools, etc. Fluctuations of injuries and behaviors occur due to these variations in actions and conditions in the workplace. The statistical process control (SPC) (used in quality management) can aid in the review of injuries and observations, the organization can show the variations in its system. The "SPC" show whether the system is out of control and needs specific issues addressed or if it is "in control" but requires major across the broad safety program improvements (Daniels and Daniels, 2004; Deming, 1986).

2.22.2 Insights on the Human Role in the Safety System

Hazard and associated risk controls and mitigation should be supported by a safety system that incorporates core human behavioral concepts. The following discussion provides an overview of the basic elements of human behavior and how to apply them to the workplace.

Management and business literature go to great lengths to explain and define how humans can work together more effectively. Social norms, laws, rules, procedures are all an attempt to direct and control human activities toward a mutual goal or objective (Roughton & Crutchfield, 2013).

Different techniques and methods are required at different levels from just one individual to work teams and eventually the organization.

Many leaders still believe that changing employee behaviors is all that is necessary. The misconception is that unsafe actions/at-risk behaviors or active human errors only apply to employees with the belief that the employee alone needs to change behavior. In reality, everyone including the leadership team are influenced by the peer pressure and other factors that results in active and latent errors (US DOE, 2009a; Roughton & Crutchfield, 2008).

The leadership team must have an in-depth understanding of the current organizational culture in order to begin the process of what has to change the culture of an organization in order to shape a new culture. Every department in an organization has unique behavioral that include adherence to facility rules, dress codes, etiquette, performance goals, etc.

The control of at-risk events begins with understanding of how specific consequences of exposure may translate into a loss-producing event. For example, are predetermined consequences driving actions toward safe behaviors and use of control methods or toward unsafe behaviors? Does the safety system/culture create an environment that uncovers and analyzes safety issues? Do employees believe that unsafe actions are necessary to keep production schedules?

How are At-Risk Events Developed?

> "The term culture has many definitions: "the ideas, customs, skills, arts, perceptions, pre-judgments, etc. of a given person, in a given period." Dan Peterson said it best "The culture is the way that it is around here" (Petersen, 1993). Every organization develops a unique culture derived from its industry; it is leadership and individuals in the organization" (Roughton & Crutchfield, 2013).

All members of an organization repeat actions that are reinforced directly or indirectly by recognition and/or negative feedback. If actions can be predicted then by changing the work environment and improving the communications regarding hazard recognition, more effective controls can be implemented. Actions become a function of the safety system and driven by the safety culture. "Because of the relatively low probability that any one at-risk event will result in an immediate injury, an employee's perception that risks can be taken and no harm or injury will occur is reinforced. By recognizing that an array of social and other consequences drives our actions and by establishing a process of specific structured quality feedback, an organization can move towards an improved culture" (Roughton & Crutchfield, 2008).

The safety culture in an organization is driven by the leadership team. Management must have a clear understanding of its operations and should make full use of active employee participation in operational hazard identification. With both management and employees, the process of actively involved in identifying and encouraging the practice of safe behavior identifying existing and potential hazards and consequences of exposures is enhanced.

2.23 WHAT CONTRIBUTES TO AN AT-RISK EVENT?

What are at-risk events? How are they different from observations of employees in the safety system? Under the enhanced safety, each employee should be observed and/or coached until a behavior has changed. In both cases, observation data is collected to ensure that the behavior is either changed or an action plan is developed to target specific behaviors. So, the question is, If you do not see this behavior again, has it actually been changed? Or did the employee stop that behavior when an observation was conducted?

For example, when a behavioral observation of an employee is performed and the employee is performing the task under at-risk conditions, this observation would count as one observation. Under a typical behavioral safety process, if an employee is trying to clear a jam from a piece of equipment in an at-risk manner, that observation counts as one at-risk events and the employee would be coached about what should do differently and shown the safe method.

The safety system brings together behavioral science, human performance improvement, and promotes safety as an important value within an organization. It is sometimes forgotten that behavioral observations are only one part of a process. Consideration should be made for latent human errors that build in hidden hazards and associated risk that may not be identified by observation alone.

As employees use an enhanced safety system and make safe behaviors a habit, the potential for loss-producing events decreases. The strength of the safety system is measured by number of "safe behaviors" shown as a percentage of specific defined observed actions. Safety metrics are lagging measures that are recorded after an injury or loss-producing event has occurred, i.e., total case incident rates (TCIR) as offered by OSHA's recordability standard (29 CFR 1904) audit scores, etc (The Department of Energy, Behavior Based Safety Process, 2002). The behavioral approach provides a method to define and establish clear safety criteria as it is being used in real time and addresses actual actions or behaviors.

According to the Department of Energy (DOE), "anecdotal evidence exists to indicate that measurement of "percentage or safe behaviors" is predictive. If used correctly, this means that the employee observation and feedback techniques may be used to predict safety issues that exist in an organization. Intensifying the contact rate (number of employees contacted each month or a given short time frame) can strengthen behaviors and can help to reduce the potential for an injury or loss-producing event" (The Department of Energy, Behavior Based Safety Process, 2002).

In Figure 7.3, engineering and the leadership team approach are designed to counter at-risk events using automated equipment, procedure compliance, administrative controls, and standards. The engineering of hazards from the workplace has been successful in reducing the number of injuries and loss-producing events (The Department of Energy, Behavior Based Safety Process, 2002).

2.24 BEHAVIOR APPROACH

The core philosophies of the behavioral approach complement and are usually integrated into other programs, such as voluntary protection process (VPP), ANSI/AIHA/ASSE, Z10, the Occupational Health and Safety Management System (Occupational Health and Safety Management Systems, 2012). The behavioral approach provides the safety system a systematic approach of identifying and correcting at-risk events and conditions that could can be immediately corrected or provide short-term corrections.

The behavioral approach can be applied across a broad range of safety areas, from the production environment to the office environment and is also applicable in off the job safety. The behavioral approach enhances traditional safety tools, such as management reviews, housekeeping reviews, audits, safety meetings, etc. The behavioral approach provides a method to shift in the focus of safety from theory or just program management to focus on the operational process.

2.25 CHANGING BEHAVIOR

When attempting to implement a behavioral-based system (BBS) process without serious discussions with the leadership team about developing a solid action plan, trying to change behavior can seriously harm the safety system. Attempting to change or modify an individual's behavior is complex. On the surface, there is an appearance of manipulation, if employees are not involved in the planning process. When an employee has performed a task over time, both routinely and nonroutinely, and has been exposed to risk without suffering any negative consequences, the need for change is not apparent and the perception of associated risk is low. This is the case of someone doing something at-risk for so long that the at-risk event has become the right way to doing things. After all, what could happen? We tend to move from one behavior to another in a manner that may limit the ability to assess the impact of the new behavior as we may or may not recognize the change we are undergoing.

A behavioral approach does not identify the interrelationships of specific hazards since it focuses only on individual employee behaviors. The JHA provides the mechanism that helps bridge the gap between how the job is completed and the observation of defined at-risk events using a structured data collection method (Figure 2.6).

2.26 UNDERSTANDING WHY EMPLOYEES PUT THEMSELVES AT RISK

One of the best way to describe behaviors is by using the ABC model (antecedents (activators), behaviors (at-risk events), and consequences (of exposure)). While this model has been around for many years, it is not always fully understood or used properly in assessing the workplace.

All human actions invoke an element of risk. Each day, we, as individuals, are engaged in thousands of at-risk events, many times putting ourselves at risk. Think about what you do on a daily basis? Try to become aware and notice the level and severity of risk that you actually create for yourself and others. A daily example would be driving on a major highway, moving from one lane to another in heavy traffic while on a cell phone, eating, or even reading. What about stopping too close to the car in front of you? Slowing down but not stopping at a stop sign (known as rolling stops), not observing street signs, or learning the dashboard layout of a new car? Then reflect the other drivers that around you who are doing similar things and we wonder why accidents happen.

Safety rules and operating procedures, investigating injuries, conducting safety meetings, training employees are not "behaviors," they are the "antecedents" that should drive the desired safe behavior. Refer to Chapter 12, the development of the JHA addresses the necessary antecedents and combines knowledge of the hazards and associated risk of the job with a structured way to communicate the required knowledge consistently.

Consequences can be stronger then antecedents. To assess behavior, the evaluation of as many consequences to a behavior must be fully assessed. As

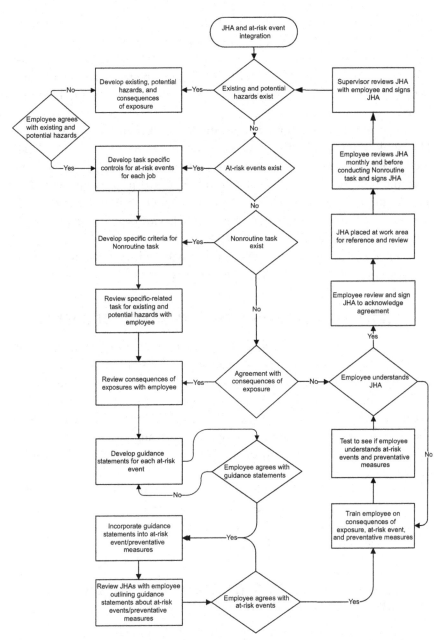

Figure 2.6 *Overview of How the JHA and At-Risk Events can be Integrated into the JHA Process.*

a test, develop a list of your personal behaviors during the day along with a list of potential and existing hazards you encounter. Make an estimate of the potential consequences of those exposures. As you recognize the at-risk events you do without thinking, you create a better awareness of your hazard exposures and can begin to take action to minimize your chance of injury.

For example, think about a motivational speaker that you have heard. The speaker touched on things that you wanted to do and you got all excited about when listening to the speaker. However, what happens after you leave the seminar and try to maintain that enthusiasm on your own? You must begin to routinely practice what you see and hear in order to become successful and to understand that changing behavior begins with your own behavior (Duhigg, 2012; Agnew & Daniels, 2011).

Consequences from your changed behavior will determine whether you stay enthusiastic or drift back into old patterns of thoughts.

2.27 UNDERSTANDING THE OTHER SIDE OF SAFETY

To be successful in program implementation, an understanding of the operational "linking pins" of management commitment, leadership, and employee participation is necessary (Roughton & Crutchfield, 2013). Refer to Chapter 4 for more a more detailed discussion. The workplace is not linear where one action or decision leads directly to another. Having good intentions is not enough as you are surrounded by other professional disciplines that are also demanding attention, time, and budget of management.

These concepts can be addressed through a safety system such as the activity-based safety system (ABSS), one-on-one contacts, preshift safety meetings, etc (Roughton & Crutchfield, 2013). Refer to Chapter 11 for a detailed discussion of how this concept work.

2.28 BEHAVIOR-BASED SAFETY AND INTEGRATED SAFETY MANAGEMENT FUNCTIONS

The Department of Energy (DOE) BBS process outlines "Seven Guiding Principles" of a successful management system and "Five Core Functions." Information that is broadcasted across the entire organization on a day-to-day basis and does not restrict the process to the actual performance of work activities. Many injuries occur when employees are involved in nontask-related activities such as walking from point A to point B, performing nonroutine task, etc. BBS processes also provide the footprints to show that a safety management system is at work around the clock (The Department of Energy, Behavior Based Safety Process, 2002). The following section has been adapted from the DOE public domain manual, "Seven Guiding Principles of a successful management system and Five Core Functions.

2.29 SEVEN GUIDING PRINCIPLES OF INTEGRATED SAFETY MANAGEMENT

- Management commitment and leadership responsibility for safety. The responsibility for safety and the BBS process is led by management with a shared involvement from knowledgeable employees. All levels of the organization are involved in an effective BBS process.
- Clearly defined roles and responsibilities must be in place with job functions defined within the management process. These responsibilities must be performed at the proper level and must be integrated and adapted to fit the organization.
- Competence commensurate with responsibilities. An effective BBS process ensures that the skills needed to perform the tasks and functions associated with the job (steps and task) in a timely manner are present and provides the opportunity to use those skills on a regular basis. It provides for coaching and interaction with other people and organizations.
- Effective use is made of balanced safety data. BBS provides a stream of safety data that enables managers to balance safety effectively within production and other operational needs.
- Safety standards and requirements are identified and followed. Existing safety standards and requirements aid in developing the list of behaviors and definitions used in the BBS process.
- Hazard controls are tailored to work being performed via a JHA. The observation process along with safety data provides ongoing monitoring of processes so that hazard controls reflect the risks associated with work being performed in changing environments and conditions.
- Operations authorization. The BBS process helps provide the behavior-related safety information necessary to make informed decisions prior to initiating operations (The Department of Energy, Behavior Based Safety Process, 2002; US DOE, 2009a).

2.30 FIVE CORE FUNCTIONS OF INTEGRATED SAFETY MANAGEMENT

- Define the project scope. Developing and maintaining a BBS process follows several steps to define the scope of the work:
  - Form assessment team(s).
  - Extract behaviors that were involved in past injuries, damage to product, and/or near misses.
  - Develop definitions that describe the desired safe behaviors.
  - Compile data collection sheets using identified behaviors.
  - Determine observation boundaries.
  - Train observers to understand safety behaviors.
  - Gather data on specific jobs, tasks and their steps.
  - Determine potential barrier removal needs and implementation process.
  - Form barrier removal teams.
  - Follow up on implementation.
- Analyze the hazards. Hazards associated with the work are identified, analyzed, and categorized. Analyzing hazards is built into the BBS process.
  - Hazards are being analyzed during each observation and the worker observed receives immediate feedback on how to minimize the risk.
  - The assessment team and barrier removal team analyzes the data gathered through observations to determine workplace hazards.
  - The teams then develop action plans to remove barriers to safe work.
- Develop and implement hazard controls.
  - Applicable standards and requirements are identified and agreed-upon;
  - Controls to prevent or mitigate hazards are identified;
  - The safety envelope is established; and controls are implemented.
  - Employees tasked with planning or designing work can also use the behavior assessment and data.
  - By studying the definitions and data, barriers that could require a worker to perform at-risk behaviors can be designed-out up front.
- Perform work within controls.
  - Readiness to do the work is confirmed and work is carried out safely.
  - Although work has been designed and training conducted to help the employee know how to work safely, bad habits and shortcuts can introduce at-risk behaviors into the workplace.

- The ongoing observation process encourages the continued use of safe behaviors and reminds workers that one at-risk behavior could cause an accident, injury or even a fatality.
- Provide feedback and continuous improvement.
    - Feedback information on the adequacy of controls is gathered; opportunities for improving how work is defined and planned are identified and implemented;
    - Line and independent oversight is conducted; and,
    - If necessary, regulatory enforcement actions occur.
    - Feedback is provided each time an observation is performed. The feedback process reinforces the use of safe behaviors and helps determine why certain at-risk behaviors were performed.
    - Collecting information about the at-risk behaviors helps the teams determine the root cause of a behavior and develop an action plan to remove the barrier causing the behavior.

Based on and Adapted using The Department of Energy, Behavior Based Safety Process, (2002) and US DOE (2009a).

2.31 WILL A BBS PROCESS WORK FOR YOU?

For a BBS process to succeed, a careful assessment as to whether the organization is ready and the necessary communications, time availability, and budgets are in place. Management leadership commitment and support, effective safety systems, as discussed, the AIHA/ANSI, VPP, and the organization's culture are keys to determining if a organization is ready for BBS (The Department of Energy, Behavior Based Safety Process, 2002).

The BBS process requires learning not just by trial and error, i.e., getting things to work right the first time and other times, not so lucky. To avoid "reinventing the wheel", the safety system must adapt to conditions by providing continuous improvement through the management of risk. By use of the JHA, the foundation for the observation criteria is established. (The Department of Energy, Behavior Based Safety Process, 2002)

The basic concept of behavior change is the systematic use of specific targeted reinforcement. The results of using defined specific reinforcement are improved performance in the area where the reinforcement is connected closely with the behavior (Petersen, 1993). If a person does something and immediately following the act something pleasurable happens, he/she will be more likely to repeat that act (Petersen, 1993). If a person does something and immediately following the act something negative occurs, he/she will be less likely to repeat that act again or will make sure he or she is not being caught in that act (Petersen, 1993). Positive reinforcement may or may not drive safe behavior. In some cases, positive consequences may exist that drive unsafe behavior – the good feeling from accomplishing a task, doing something dangerous and getting away without injury, etc.

SUMMARY

The JHA process requires a strategy that provides for a process administrative structure, employee time, and a resources budget for the implementation of recommended hazard and associated risk controls.

The JHA should be considered more than a tool used to define individual activities. It should be considered part of the overall hazard and associated risk communication process within the safety system. It defines what is to be communicated about ongoing activities and must be viewed as an essential part of the safety system.

The organization may have an established planning process that allows the leadership team to organize, budget, and account for all activities that are considered of value. Projects that are not considered of value are not budgeted and not supported with resources. A major and critical step is ensure that the JHA process follows the same format for project management and budgeting that are used by the organization.

The term "job" seems to have changed over the years from being a specific limited activity to an overall definition as a "job title," which may cover a number of various activities and responsibilities.

The terms "job hazard analysis (JHA)" and "job safety analysis (JSA)" are used somewhat interchangeably. A variety of other terminology such as job task analysis (JTA), activity task analysis (ATA), and others are used depending on the industry and organization.

One of the issues with the structure of the traditional JHA is that it implies that all hazards can be controlled looking only at the job steps (Job Hazard Analysis, 2002). Additional elements must be considered in reviewing a job or families of jobs for its mental and physical requirements, the potential for human error, the impact of technology, and the employee's reliance on technology to complete the required job steps and task.

Potential "error precursors" should be assessed as to their impact on safe job completion. As an example, time pressure to complete a job can result in the employee expected to take short cuts or accept risk as part of the job.

An organization is a series of emerging properties that are the result of its many components of blending together or at the very least colliding together.

The human performance improvement principles provide a new dimension for the JHA process.

An understanding of organizational culture will aid in determining the priorities and values actually held by the organization and provide insights on the best methods to implement the JHA process.

The organizational structure may change the strategy used to implement the JHA process. As part of the review of the organizational culture, how it organizes personnel, assigns responsibilities and authorities, and allocates resources must be reviewed.

Too often that a specific job is "simple" and that it doesn't take a "rocket scientist" to do it. This demeans the employee assigned to do the task as well as establishes a mindset that it is a throwaway job that does not need review.

As a first step in the JHA process, a job inventory is completed with a preliminary review that rank orders jobs by their perceived or known potential hazards and associated risk.

This can provide insights on jobs completed in the same vicinity or work area and how they are coordinated and managed.

Several types of performance must be considered when reviewing jobs for further analysis. The nature of the job performance requirements can impact the nature of the JHA process. Jobs can easily combine elements of each of three performance types – skill based, rule based, and knowledge based.

Organizations are created by humans and as such are subject to errors made at any level and by anyone in the course of everyday operations.

The two error types are latent errors from job and operational design and active errors from actions taken. These errors can create loss-producing events immediately or remain hidden creating a long term potential for loss producing events.

The JHA must consider the level of automation within a job and what is the potential impact of the failure of automation, especially safety-related systems.

An area that receives little attention but is very important is the need to develop an understanding of the politics within an organization.

The maintaining of documents and materials will be covered later in this book. At the beginning of the JHA process, an estimation of the scope and needs for its hard–copy and digital filing system and storage require-ments is essential.

The goal of hazard control and risk reduction is to achieve stability in process implementation through design and efficient structure.

The behavioral approach is a process that provides organizations the op-portunity to move to a level higher of safety excellence. An understanding of how antecedents and consequences are designed along with statistically valid data builds ownership, trust, and unity if properly implemented.

A properly designed behavioral process involves employees at every lev-el. The atmosphere of trust that results from nonpunitive observation and the feedback process leads to creating more employee participation.

CHAPTER REVIEW QUESTIONS

1. What are the main obstacles in implementing a new JHA process?
2. Discuss JHA as a communication tool.
3. What is required to develop a JHA?
4. What questions must be answered about the JHA process implementation?
5. Why is the term "Job" important?
6. How does a parent/child concept apply to the JHA process?
7. Why is an understanding of error precursors important?
8. Are organizations dynamic or static? Discuss and outline your conclusions
9. What are the three levels of an organization's culture
10. Define the three performance types.
11. How can safety technology potentially create rather than reduce risk?
12. What is the impact of not understanding organizational politics on the JHA process?
13. Discuss the core elements of a behavioral–based safety process.
14. Discuss the integrating of BBS with the JHA process.

BIBLIOGRAPHY

Agnew, J., & Daniels, A. (2011, November). Developing High-Impact Leading Indicators for Safety. PM eZine, *Performance Management Magazine*. Retrieved from http://bit.ly/WTK66g

Blum, D. (2014). *The best American science and nature writing 2014*. ADDIN Docear CSL_BIBLIOGRAPHY.

Capra, F., & Luisi, P. L. (2014). *The systems view of life: a unifying vision*. Cambridge CB2 8BS, United Kingdom: Cambridge University Press, University Printing House.

Daniels, A. C., & Daniels, J. E. (2004). *Performance Management: Changing Behavior that Drives Organizational Effectiveness*. Performance Management Publications, Retrieved from https://books.google.com/books?id=5LcHNQAACAAJ

Deming, W. E. (1986). *Out of the crisis*. Cambridge: Massachusetts Institute of Technology, Center for advanced engineering study.

Department of Energy (DOE) (2009a). *Concepts and Principles, Human Performance Improvement Handbook* (Vol. 1). Retrieved from http://bit.ly/1DfdJVU

Department of Energy (DOE) (2009b). *Human performance tools for Individuals, Work teams, and Management, Human Performance Improvement HandBook* (Vol. 2). Retrieved from http://bit.ly/14kc6Lj

Duhigg, C. (2012). *The power of habit: Why we do, what we do in life and business*. Doubleday, Canada.

Espoused Values. (n.d.). Businessdictionary.com. Retrieved from http://bit.ly/1Is3iVJ

Heath, C., & Heath, D. (2007). *Made to stick: Why some ideas survive and others die*. New York: Random House.

Job. (n.d.). Retrieved from http://bit.ly/1C5c2Pb

Job Hazard Analysis, 3071. (2002). *Occupational Safety and Health Administration (OSHA)*. Occupational Safety and Health Administration (OSHA), Public Domain, Modified and/or Adapt as necessary. Retrieved from http://bit.ly/1ZI1Q7y

Occupational Health & Safety Management Systems. (2012). The American Society of Safety Engineers, ANSI/AIHA/ASSE Z10. Retrieved from http://bit.ly/1MsT6MG

Petersen, D. (1993). *The challenge of change: Creating a new safety culture*. Portland, OR: CoreMedia Training Solutions.

Politics. (n.d.). Merriam Webster.com. Retrieved from http://bit.ly/15HqUzF

Risk Assessment Institute. (n.d.). American Society of Safety Engineers, Risk Assessment Institute. Retrieved from http://bit.ly/1GYTij1

Roughton, J., & Crutchfield, N. (2008). *Job Hazard Analysis: A Guide for Voluntary Compliance and Beyond*. MA: Elsevier/Butterworth-Heinemann. Retrieved from http://amzn.to/VrSAq5

Roughton, J., & Crutchfield, N. (2013). *Safety Culture: An Innovative Leadership Approach*. In B. Heinemann (Ed.), MA: Butterworth Heinemann, Retrieved from http://amzn.to/1qoD4oN

Safety Alert for Operations, Manual Flight Operations. (2013).

The Department of Energy, Behavior Based Safety Process, *Summary of behavior based safety* (Vol.1). (2002). Washington, DC. 20585: US Department of Energy, Approved for public release; distribution is unlimited, Public Domain. Retrieved from http://bit.ly/1zgvne8

Tyson, N. deGrasse. (2012). *Space chronicles: Facing the ultimate frontier*.

CHAPTER THREE

Introducing JHA into the Organization

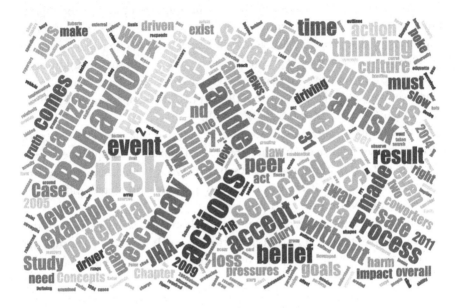

"The culture is the way that it is around here."

— *Dan Petersen*

Chapter Objectives

At the end of the chapter, you should be able to:

- Discuss why safety systems should involve everyone in the organization.
- Discuss how at-risk events develop.
- Describe the ladder of inference.
- Discuss emerging properties of organizations.
- Discuss why employees put themselves at risk.

Job Hazard Analysis. http://dx.doi.org/10.1016/B978-0-12-803441-5.00003-9

3.1 ORGANIZATIONAL AND PEER PRESSURES

As discussed in Chapter 2, a combination of both active and latent errors creates potential loss-producing events. The potential for error is not just at the line employee level but involves all members of the organization. A decision made by a member of senior leadership team can directly impact the acceptance of risk. A purchasing manager may receive praise for reducing expenses but that saving be lost as cost of injuries and maintenance increase.

Organizational and peer pressures may be inherent in the organizational culture creating positive and/or negative feedback. Feedback comes from many sources and in various strengths, depths, and scope, some of which are hidden (Schein, 2004; US DOE, 2009).

The overall organizational norms and industry practices establish patterns of behavior that include adherence to regulatory compliance, effective rule setting, required dress codes, proper work place etiquette, performance goals, etc. All of these impact how jobs are completed and should be understood within the JHA process.

The leadership team determines what it should do each day to reach the overall goals of the organization if it is to survive. It should ensure that the organizational culture shapes the behaviors and actions of employees (US DOE, 2009).

3.2 HOW ARE AT-RISK EVENTS DEVELOPED?

Each organization and its industry respond differently to the challenges faced.

Human actions are driven by an array of leadership decisions, coworkers, personal goals, peer groups, new cultural norms, news and entertainment media, and other social/cultural factors. Social norms can develop that override the actions or behavior necessary for safe completion of a job. A group may act in opposition to training, rules, etc. to make a point with the leadership team, regulators, or society in general. Actions are also driven by the design of the systems that we work within (Senge, 2006; Norm Social, n.d.).

How jobs are completed is a function of the perceived organization culture. The perception that risks can be taken and no injury or damage will occur is reinforced because of the relatively low probability that most at-risk events will result in an immediate injury or damage.

Case Study # 1

Rules and laws are to shape behavior. For example, The State of Georgia implemented a "slow poke" law. The "slow poke" law requires any driver on a divided highway to move to the right when a faster vehicle comes up from behind even if they are driving at the speed limit, or face a misdemeanor charge (Georgia House passes 'Slowpoke' Bill, 2014).

This implies that speeding is an acceptable risk in certain situations.

For example, news reporters and camera operators will knowingly attempt to enter an unsafe area (war zones, hurricanes, riots, crime floods, etc.) in search of a story and consider their actions to be an acceptable risk.

The move should move beyond thinking that recognition and/or disciplinary systems are all that are needed to drive safe behavior. "When it comes to motivation, there is a gap between what science knows and business does. Our current business operating systems – which is built around external, carrot, and stick motivators – does not work and often does harm" (Pink, 2011). Dan Pink demonstrates that there is a new approach that must include autonomy, mastery, and purpose (Pink, 2011).

3.3 LADDER OF INFERENCE – HOW BELIEFS LEAD TO RISK AND HAZARD ACCEPTANCE

The "Ladder of inference" concept describes insights on how we act and is based on the way information is selected and given meaning from our prejudgments, perceptions, and habits. The model outlines how our beliefs affect what we infer about what we observe and therefore become part of how we experience our interaction with other people." As cited in Leadership and Influence, Independent Study (2005).

This is the process that we go through, usually without thinking, to get from an observation to an action. These unconscious-thinking stages can be seen as rungs on a ladder and are demonstrated in Figure 3.1.

"Our ability to achieve the results we truly desire is eroded by our feelings that our beliefs are the truth, the truth is obvious, our beliefs are based on real data, and the data we select are the real data" (Senge et al., 1994).

A series of mental steps leads to how we perform actions and operate. We move up a decision ladder based on our "mental model" without

The Ladder of Inference Concept

I take ACTIONS based on my beliefs.

I adopt BELIEFS about the world.

I draw CONCLUSIONS.

I make ASSUMPTIONS based on the meanings I added.

I add MEANINGS (cultural and personal).

I select DATA from what I observe.

All the information in the world.

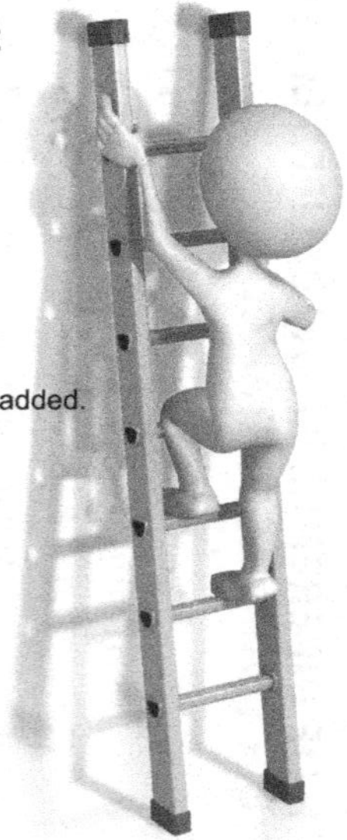

Dr. William Isaacs, Dialogos Institute, Massachusetts Institute of Technology

Belief about Personal Risk Concept

My actions are based on what I believe - Take or avoid risk

I have the belief that I have or do not have to follow set rules, SOP's, etc.

I conclude that even though there is a risk, I will or will not be harmed

I make assumption that I will or will not be harmed while doing the job

I add meaning based on experience; risk/no risk, hazard/no hazard, and easy/simple

I select what I think is important about the Job

Observable data, information, experience about the job

My Personal Beliefs about
Associated Hazards
Leads Me to
Accept or Reject Risks

Figure 3.1 *Overview of the Ladder of Inference Principles. As cited in Leadership and Influence, Independent Study, 2005.*

recognizing or even knowing that we have made the climb (Mental model, n.d.). A leap or jump over sections of the ladder occurs as we draw conclusions without considering how we got to them. For example, the leadership team's perceptions about safety professionals can be based on preconceived beliefs based on selected data, "all safety professions wear hard hats and carry clipboards"; "safety is only regulatory compliance"; "PPE is the only reoccurring problem" and then take actions based on what they believe.

In many cases, as jobs are routinely and habitually completed, thoughtful decisions as to what is happening are not examined. The belief exist that nothing harmful can happen as our observational data has been selected to show that nothing has happened in the past, allowing unsafe actions and conditions to continue to exists. We feel comfortable with our conclusions ("That type of harmful event can't happen here") and we see no need to change behaviors.

A risk guidance card will be discussed in Chapter 8.

> *"There are two primary choices in life: to accept conditions as they exist, or accept the responsibility for changing them."*
>
> — *Dr Denis Waitley*

The following example expands on the ladder of inference and how it impacts the beliefs and acceptance of risk:

- Beginning at the bottom of the ladder of inference, we receive information about our world of work based on observations and past experiences. Injuries and traumatic experiences may or may not be in our history or the organization's history.
- Specific information is selected that appears to be important to properly complete the job.
- Meanings are selected based on the organizational cultures espoused and underlying assumptions, personal experience and perceptions, peer experiences, etc. These meanings include how risk acceptance is viewed by the organization and what level of risk tolerance is expected.
- Assumptions are based on the meanings added. The assumption may be that risk is either acceptable or unacceptable based on the meaning selected. The assumption may be made that risk must be accepted or some form of negative feedback will be received. Alternatively, not accepting a risk and following a procedure may be based on an assumption that a positive feedback is received.

Table 3.1 Self-imposed behavior

Employees attitude, prejudgments, perceptions	Reason for shortcut
Time	
An employee would rather be somewhere else and/or doing other things more important than working.	Taking shortcuts due to a belief that time can be gained to do other things: Increase production; more breaks, or talking to coworkers.
Employee belief	
Low risk: "I am better than anyone else and against them mentally"; "It will not happen to me"; "Nothing has ever happen before." Therefore, I can take as many chances (at-risk events) as I want and I will not get injured." "This is the way that it has always been;" Training without understanding at-risk events and proven safety technology (seatbelts, etc.). Resistance to change; reactive.	Increases "free" time; increases production that increases incentives; low or medium risk; potential at-risk events accepted and/or ignored by management and others, management has "It can't happen to here". "I have done this thousands of times before and have never been hurt."

Source: Adapted from Roughton and Crutchfield (2008).

- Conclusions about risk acceptance are made. It is either okay to accept the risk and the potential for harm or not accept the risk.
- Beliefs about how a job must be completed are adopted.
- Actions based on the selected beliefs. Procedures are followed and at-risk events reported or the hazardous condition and the risk are accepted.

The ladder of inference attempts to explain why the underlying selected data, meanings, assumptions, conclusions, and beliefs impacts the JHA acceptance.

Refer to Table 3.1 for two scenarios outlining this type of thinking, "Self-Imposed Behavior".

3.4 CHANGING BELIEFS

Humans prefer to have a stable, generally predictable environment. As a result when an employee who has performed a task both routinely and nonroutinely over time may have been exposed to risk without suffering any negative consequences. The need for change is not apparent and the perception of associated risk is low. This is the case of someone doing something at-risk for so long, the at-risk event has become the right way to do things. After all, what could happen?

The ladder of inference tells us that we should begin by assessing the beliefs held by an organization if we intend to make change. The change process requires presenting "data" that can be translated into meanings that leads to difference assumptions and conclusions. The belief system may be changed if the positive feedback exceeds the negative feedback.

Case Study # 2

As noted in the "Department of Energy Action Plan; Lessons Learned from the Columbia Space Shuttle Accident and Davis-Besse Reactor Pressure-Vessel Head Corrosion Event " – "When the space shuttle Columbia launched on January 16, 2003, there were 3,233 Criticality 1/1R critical item list hazards that were waived. Hazards that result in Criticality 1/1R component failures are defined as those that will result in loss of the orbiter and crew. In both, the Challenger and Columbia accidents: "The machine was talking to us, but nobody was listening." (US DOE, 2005)

NASA, even though it knew that there was a high probability based on its own determined "Criticality," did not believe that it would suffer a loss. Its underlying assumptions were different from its espoused values even though its own versions of risk assessments and JHAs clearly identified the potential for a catastrophic event.

3.5 WHY EMPLOYEES ACCEPT RISK

All human actions involve some level of risk as they are engaged in thousands of daily at-risk events. Think about what you do on a daily basis? Try to become aware and notice the level and severity of risk that you actually accept for yourself and others. For example, driving on a major highway, moving from one lane to another in heavy traffic while on a cell phone, eating, or engaged in passenger conversation.

One of the authors was once passed by a car on an interstate highway and its driver was reading a newspaper spread across the steering wheel! What could that person have been possibly been thinking!!

Risk is accepted for a wide range of reasons. And its cause is that the consequences of accepting a risk exceed the consequences of avoiding the risk.

Behaviors can be somewhat forecast by using the "ABC" model that stands for Antecedent, Behavior, and Consequences (what happens when the behavior occurs). "An antecedent is something that comes before a behavior, and may trigger that behavior. A behavior is anything an individual does. A consequence is something that follows the behavior" (ABC (Antecedent-Behavior-Consequence) Model, Fact Sheet, n.d.).

Safety rules, operating procedures, beliefs, etc. are antecedents that drive behavior. The JHA addresses antecedents by attempting to communicate the hazards and associated within the job. The strength of the beliefs with regard to what the JHA recommends drives the behavior toward safe completion of the job.

However, consequences are stronger than antecedents. If the belief that the consequences of accepting a risk are stronger than the consequences of following a "safe" course of action, then the behavior would be to take the short cut. To assess potential behavior, the types of consequences should be evaluated (Roughton & Crutchfield, 2008; US DOE, 2002; Wendel, 2014).

SUMMARY

Various levels of activities should be considered when evaluating organizations in order to improve the existing safety system. After decades of research and insights within the safety profession, the misconception still remains that the majority of injuries are due to unsafe actions by employees.

While the quality control movement has been incorporated into general business to a good degree, the safety profession still relies on concepts developed in the early days of manufacturing that in many cases may not be applicable in the current work environment.

Each organization and its industry responds differently to the challenges it faces. The news reporters and camera operators will knowingly attempt to enter an unsafe area (war zones, hurricanes, riots, crime floods, etc.) in search of a story and consider their actions as acceptable risk. An acceptable risk in the construction industry where hazards are constantly changing as trades and crafts rotate onto a site is different from general industry where a process appears unchanging.

The "ladder of inference," provides insights on how we act and is based on the way information is selected and given meaning from our prejudgments, perceptions, and habits. A series of mental steps leads to how we perform actions and operate. We move up a decision ladder based on our "mental model" without recognizing or even knowing that we have made the climb. A leap or jump over sections of the ladder occurs as we draw conclusions without considering how we got to them.

The ladder of inference explains why the underlying workplace selected data, meanings, assumptions, conclusions, and beliefs impacts how the JH process is accepted as it establishes criteria for the control of hazard and associate risk.

Humans prefer to have a stable, generally predictable environment. As a result when an employee who has performed a task both routinely and nonroutinely over time and has been exposed to risk without suffering any negative consequences, the need for change is not apparent and the perception of associated risk is low.

Risk is accepted for a wide range of reasons. At its root cause is that the consequences of accepting a risk exceeds the consequences of avoiding the risk.

Behaviors can be somewhat forecast by using the "ABC" model that stands for antecedent, behavior, and consequences (what happens when the behavior occurs).

The impact of culture, organizational issues, human error potential, and the ladder of inference has made additional considerations for assessing the overall organizational climate and the acceptance of a JHA process necessary. Understanding these concepts provides insights into the development of strategies to use for improving a successful process implementation.

CHAPTER REVIEW QUESTIONS

1. How are the issues found in quality control parallel to those of a safety system?
2. List the various organizational factors that can affect the JHA process. Add to the list others factors you believe can also affect the process.
3. Can social norms impact the way jobs are completed? Discuss the effect of social norms.
4. Outline the ladder of inference. What insights can it provide for JHA process improvement?
5. Make a list of beliefs you have about the JHA. What are your beliefs based on? How did you select your core data?
6. List reasons why a JHA process should understand the underlying beliefs and perceptions of the leadership team and employees.
7. How does the ABC model relate to the ladder of inference and how can it be applied?

BIBLIOGRAPHY

ABC (Antecedent-Behavior-Consequence) Model, Fact Sheet. (n.d.). Indiana Family & Social Services Administration Division of Disability & Rehabilitative Services Bureau of Quality Improvement Services.

Georgia House passes 'Slowpoke' Bill. (2014). Athens Banner-Herald. Retrieved from http://bit.ly/15Gn2mp

Leadership and Influence, Independent Study, Public Domain. (2005, December). Federal Emergency Management Agency (FEMA). Retrieved from http://bit.ly/1GH5VNu

Mental model. (n.d.). Wikipedia, the free encyclopedia. Retrieved from http://bit.ly/124eseh

Norm Social. (n.d.). Wikipedia. Retrieved from http://bit.ly/1I3ckqg

Pink, D.H. (2011). *Drive: The surprising truth about what motivates us.* Penguin Group US. Retrieved from http://bit.ly/VaQStm

Schein, E. H. (2004). Organizational culture and leadership. *The Jossey-Bass business & management series.* John Wiley & Sons.

Senge, P. M. (2006). The fifth discipline: the art & practice of the learning organization. *A currency book.* Rosewood Drive Danvers, MA: Crown Publishing Group.

Senge, P.M., Kleiner, A., Roberts, C., Ross, R., & Smith, B. (1994). In N. Brealy (Ed.), *The fifth discipline field book: strategies and tools for building a learning organization.*

US DOE. (2002). The Department of Energy, Behavior Based Safety Process, *Summary of Behavior Based Safety* (Vol. 1). Washington, D.C. 20585: US Department of Energy, Approved for public release; distribution is unlimited, Public Domain. Retrieved from http://bit.ly/1zgvne8

US DOE. (2005). Columbia Space Shuttle Accident and Davis-Besse Reactor Pressure-Vessel Head Corrosion Event. US Department of Energy Action Plan Lessons Learned, Public Domain. Retrieved from http://1.usa.gov/YOWYft

US DOE. (2009). *Concepts and principles, human performance improvement handbook* (Vol. 1). US Department of Energy. Retrieved from http://bit.ly/1DfdJVU

Wendel, D. S. (2014). *Designing for behavior change.* Gravenstein Highway North Sebastopol, CA: O'Reilly Media, Inc.

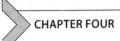

CHAPTER FOUR

Leadership Team and Employee Participation

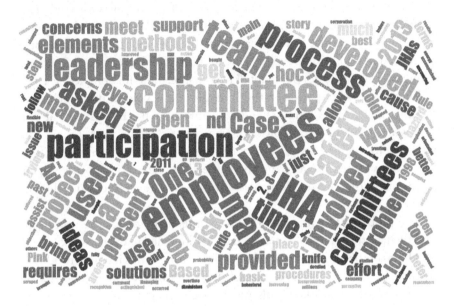

"If someone offers you an amazing opportunity and you not sure you can do it, say yes – then learn how to do it later"

—**Richard Branson**

"Without involvement, there is no commitment. Mark it down, asterisk it, circle it, under line it. No involvement, no commitment."

—**Stephen Covey**

Chapter Objectives

At the end of this chapter, you should be able to:

- Discuss the importance of employee involvement in the JHA process.
- Define methods that can used to increase employee participation.
- Explain why open communication is essential.
- Identify leadership team's role in ensuring employee participation.
- Identify ways to establish a JHA committee.
- Discuss elements of a JHA team charter and its importance.

Job Hazard Analysis. http://dx.doi.org/10.1016/B978-0-12-803441-5.00004-0

4.1 WHY SHOULD EMPLOYEES BE INVOLVED?

As the employees perform assigned duties, they may or may not have developed an understanding of risk depending on the quality of orientation, training, and the probability of a loss-producing event. This understanding is directly based on the quality and effectiveness of the organization's risk and safety communications. As discussed in Chapter 3, the underlying assumptions and espoused value systems may or may not be emphasizing hazard control procedures. Instead, the experience of other employees and the current culture may allow the development of informal methods for completing a job.

Employee participation in the JHA process is vital in uncovering ad hoc informal work method(s) and determining what beliefs exist about how work must be accomplished. The success of the JHA process, as with developing of a strong safety culture, depends on a trusting interaction between employees and the leadership team. With positive open communications, better control solutions can be defined, developed, and implemented.

The problem: The leadership team with its many obligations can overlook the fact that employees have a detailed knowledge of the work.

The main objective of participation is to bring into view where ad hoc methods have been developed for job tasks and may be increasing risk or bypassing desired hazard controls. Alternatively, participation may find these informal methods may be better than what has been designed and have improved the control of inherent hazards. Refer to Chapter 8 for the basic elements as this story emphasizes why it is essential to engage and encourage employees to participant.

One of the authors was told the story of how a large corporation bought a mining operation and designed a very complex process. It was an immediate failure! A management consultant was called in to determine what happened as millions of dollars had been invested. When interviewing the mining employees, he asked what they thought was the cause for the failure. They responded, "We knew the process would not work as soon as we were told about the design." When asked why they didn't speak out about the potential failure, their reply was "We weren't asked."

Seems the new parent company failed to appreciate the experience and expertise that was available and suffered accordingly.

4.2 BENEFITS OF EMPLOYEE PARTICIPATION

Many benefits to employee participation can develop. These reasons can include but not limited to:

- Every employee can be a valuable problem solver based on their past and present experience and expertise.
- Employees are in close contact with existing and/or potential hazards and associated risk and have perceptive insights into how and why things get done.
- Employees who participate in the JHA process are more likely to support changes and continue to use the process.
- If employees are encouraged to offer their ideas and suggestions and if these ideas and suggestions are taken seriously, they will be more apt to become involved (Managing Worker Safety and Health, n.d.; Roughton & Crutchfield, 2013; Pink, 2011).

4.3 REASONS EMPLOYEES ARE NOT INVOLVED IN THE JHA PROCESS

Many reasons may be present that are obstacles to employee participation in the JHA process. These reasons can include but not limited to:

- Time is not made available to participate. The production requirements may not be flexible to allow the involvement of hourly employees.
- No one listens. Concerns, ideas, and suggestions may have been made but no feedback was provided and overtime employees stopped attempting to provide comment. In behavioral terms, the leadership team has extinguished the behavior of making suggestions, as the consequence was resounding silence.
- Too complicated. Participation requires too much effort or has complicated procedures needed to get involved.
- Nothing gets changed. Similar to no one listens in that thoughtful ideas for changes were provided but there is no process in place to get actions moving.
- No feedback from the leadership team. Again, silence stops participation.
- The leadership team does not follow its own written rules. The leadership team can quickly kill participation when expecting others to follow a procedure and then exempting themselves from following what is expected.

- Limited recognition. Participation requires a level of effort beyond the daily work duties. When that effort is not recognized, it diminishes the potential for participation. "Why should I go the extra-mile for nothing"?
- Help and support are not provided. Participation requires resources as questions and issues are brought into the open.

Based on and Adapted from Senge et al. (1999).

Note the theme that runs through this list. Feedback is essential in obtaining employee participation.

Case Study #1

One of the authors remembers a case where an employee reported a piece of dust in an eye. No history existed in this particular plant with regards to eye injuries. However, the leadership team decided to change the entire safety glass policy and program, scraped all safety glasses and replaced them with new types of glasses to solve this perceived problem which was just a piece of dust in the eye (Roughton & Crutchfield, 2013). Little or no employee participation was used to assist in determining if such a total change was necessary

In this case study, no JHA was used, no risk assessment completed, there were no discussions with involved employees or other employees to obtain opinions. Employee participation was minimal at best. The leadership team jumped to a conclusion and made corrective action, which may or may not have been the proper solution. If the JHA process had been effectively in place and employees actively involved, the assessment of whether a true potential problem could have been determined or whether other potential eye injury issues were present.

Case Study #2

An organization was trying to reduce the number of injuries in the workplace. The leadership team implemented a new procedure that each time an injury occurred involving a tool, then that particular tool would be banned from use, regardless of the investigation. In one example, an employee was using a utility knife to cut cardboard. The utility knife slipped from the cardboard cutting the employee's leg. Without conducting an investigation or consulting a JHA to determine the root cause, all utility knives in the organization were immediately banned.

The question is "does banning resolve the immediate issue?" Banning a tool is an easy solution to a problem but where does it end and what are the unintended consequences?

Each case study scenario resulted in actions that made employee task(s) harder to complete without changing how the job was to be completed. The common theme in each of these case studies is that employees were not involved in the process nor asked for their insights. Solutions were selected with little foresight and forced upon them.

This type of authoritarian approach implements a solution without understanding the underlying issues or nature of the task(s) as to why it is being performed. The assumption is made that the higher authority (which is distant from the job) understands how the job task is being performed without consulting employees. By continuing to respond to problems with limited discussions with employees, can employees be expected to seriously participate and remain engaged in solving safety-related issues?

4.4 LISTENING TO EMPLOYEES

"In organizations, real power and energy is generated through relationships. The patterns of relationships and the capacities to form them are more important than tasks, functions, roles, and position."

—Margaret Wheatly

A simple yet effective approach in developing any JHA process is "just listen" to what employees have to say about their job. With positive and open communications, employees will express their concerns. Too often dialog is shut down when employees expressing concern are immediately told their concerns are unwarranted or when ideas are not allowed to be fully developed.

Case Study #3

One of the authors once discussed with a general manager why his employees would not get involved in the safety system. The general manager said he had done everything that he knew to get his employees involved and could not understand why no one wanted to be involved.

After discussing this issue for a few minutes, the author asked a question that shocked him. "Have you just asked them?" His response was "NO!" The author and the general manager then began to walk through the plant talking to as many employees as possible. The general manager was surprised when discussing safety elements with the employees as they provided many suggestions and input that was valuable (Roughton & Crutchfield, 2013).

One of the authors had a similar experience at a facility. The safety committee was being developed and a request for volunteers sent out. The response was answered by a number of retired military safety NCOs who were employees and welcomed the opportunity to be involved. No one knew of this quality of experience as no one had ever asked.

As many employees take pride in their work, they will if asked actively participate.

Rule 1 – Ask and listen to what the employee has to say!

Daniel Pink suggests listening for employee use of "We" and "They" in discussions. He gives credit for this to Robert Reich, former US Labor Secretary. If employees use "we", it indicates they "feel they are part of something significant and meaningful." If "they" is used, it signals that "some amount of disengagement or perhaps even alienation" may be present (Pink, 2011).

4.5 GUIDELINES FOR EMPLOYEE PARTICIPATION IN THE JHA PROCESS

Activities might include assistance during the different phases of establishing, implementing, and evaluating the JHA process. Elements used to guide participation include the following:

- Communicating regularly with employees on the status of the process. An initial information release that communicates the scope of the process can open the line of communication.
- Providing employees with access to relevant information of specific program elements and how it will be of benefit to them.

- Providing assistance to employees with methods to assess and identify hazards, prioritize results, specific training, and program evaluations.
- Providing prompt responses to all communications, reports, and suggested recommendations.
- Using a team to develop the JHAs and assist in reviewing safety-related issues and developing solutions to problems identified.
- Involving employees in developing and revising workplace safety rules.
- Providing training on site-specific safety issues for both newly hired/transferred and experienced employees.
- Presenting completed JHA-related information at safety meetings.
- Providing employees time and resources to participate on the JHA committee.

(Draft Proposed Safety And Health Program Rule: 29 CFR 1900.1, Docket No. S&H-0027, n.d.; Employee Involvement, eTools, n.d.; Managing Worker Safety and Health, n.d.)

4.6 JHA COMMITTEE DEVELOPMENT

Safety committees have been traditionally used as the focal point of employee participation. An effective safety committee can communicate a positive influence for safety-related activities and efforts rapidly through an organization. A JHA committee offers the potential to assess information received about what is actually happening in the workplace.

The JHA committee can develop and review completed JHAs to ensure that they are up to date and meet current operational requirements. The JHA committee is critical to the safety system as it ensures the safety system is maintained and hazards and associated risk are consistently controlled.

It is recommended that a committee charter be used that formalizes its mandate, structure, budget, and training. At the committee's onset, training on the basics of holding a meeting and core training on JHA concepts should be provided. The JHA committee should represent a cross-section of employees as a diversity of group experience and perceptions increases the potential for improving the committee's problem solving skills.

Before developing a JHA committee, a review of how other committees, if any, are being used in the organization. If committee formats and charters are found in other parts of the organization and have been effectively used over time, the JHA committee should be modeled after those committees.

68   Job Hazard Analysis

For example, if a successful quality control committee has been in operation, its meeting structure, charter, and administration may already be familiar to the leadership team and employees. Model it (Godin, 2009). The JHA committee could make minor changes to the charter and not have to reinvent the wheel as to how the committee is organized and managed (Roughton & Crutchfield, 2013).

While the JHA committee is advisory in nature, as it becomes embedded in the network structure of the organization, it can become the conduit for information shared with the leadership team and employees that might otherwise be obstructed or blocked by the nature of the organizational structure.

4.7 ESTABLISHING THE TEAM CHARTER

A JHA committee charter is the document that provides the reasons, authority, and guidance for the establishment of the committee.

"In project management, a project charter or project definition (sometimes called the terms of reference) is a statement of the scope, objectives, and participants in a project. It provides a preliminary delineation of roles and responsibilities, outlines the project objectives, identifies the main stakeholders, and defines the authority of the project manager. It serves as a reference of authority for the future of the project" (Charter, n.d.).

A charter is a living document that should be periodically amended as conditions warrant. A series of questions is used to determine the committee's duties, accountabilities, and authority. These questions should be answered prior to the initial meeting or in revitalizing a JHA committee:
1. What is the purpose of the committee?
2. What authority will the committee have?
3. How will individuals be held accountable?
4. What are its responsibilities?
5. How will the committee measure its success?
6. Who is the committee's leadership team sponsor or champion that will support its efforts and clear organizational obstacles?
7. Who will be the members?
8. How will these members be chosen?
9. How long will each member serve on the committee?
10. How will it create a diverse membership?

11. How will the committee members from the leadership team be determined and rotated?
12. What specific deadlines should the committee maintain?
13. How often is the committee expected to meet?
14. How much time will be allowed for members to participate?
15. When is the best time for the committee to meet?
16. Where will the committee meet?
17. What is the budget for the committee?
18. What resources and advisory expertise will be provided?
19. How will committee reports be communicated to the leadership team and employees?
20. What media will be used?
21. How and where will its records and minutes be maintained?
    (Turner & Turner, 1998; Roughton & Crutchfield, 2013)

After a core charter has been developed, committee members are asked to review, discuss, and question its content, modifying it as warranted.

> "The first step is the most important step in growing a team. The Team Charter specifies the purpose of the team, the boundaries of its scope and authority, and team membership. One of the major reasons that teams fail is that the original charter was too vague. This leads to "mission creep" in which teams spill into areas that were never intended, or teams become confused about how much authority they have and stumble into conflict with supervisors and other teams."
> (Turner & Turner, 1998)

4.8 CHOOSING JHA COMMITTEE MEMBERS

Committee members should have an understanding of how to develop a process and how the organization is structured. A blend of experienced long-term employees and recently hired employees drawn from across departments or divisions can bring a spectrum of perceptions and expertise to the committee. Long-term employees have knowledge of how things are currently done and a history of past problems and issues. Short-term employees bring perceptions from other organizations and questions about why things are done at this location that may challenge the long-term employees.

Having a cross-departmental or divisional blend may find that other areas of the organization may have already developed levels of expertise not present in other departments.

Key functions or roles should be filled which will include members of the leadership team and maintain its structure in order for it to function. These roles can be rotated as warranted to allow mixed types of personalities to be involved. All members are expected to be present at meetings, be active in discussions, and learn the basics of the JHA process.

A basic committee leadership structure includes:

- A committee "Chair" to lead and moderate the meetings to ensure an agenda is developed, followed, and assignments are delegated.
- A secretary keeps notes and records of all discussions at each meeting. Meeting minutes are maintained to track of all projects, activities, and conclusions.
- A time keeper needed to ensure that the meetings begin and end on time. It is critical that members keep the obligation to stay within the defined time constraints for meetings.

(Coble, Taylors, & Jones; Joint Health and Safety Committees: A Practical Guide for Single Employer WorkHealth, n.d.; Roughton & Crutchfield, 2013)

4.9 AD HOC SUB-COMMITTEES

Ad hoc subcommittees can be used to divide the efforts defined by the Charter, review JHAs developed, provide reports for the leadership team and employees, and provide consistency in selecting effective corrective measures (Coble et al., n.d.; Roughton & Crutchfield, 2013).

Refer to Figure 4.1, this fish bone breaks down the various elements that might be useful when trying to increase employee participation. These elements include guidance on the process, use of committees, training, and site review involvement, each with subelements to consider.

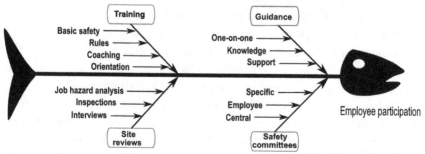

Figure 4.1 *Example Cause and Effect Diagram to Outline Elements of an Effective Employee Participation Process.*

SUMMARY

The main objective of participation is bring into view where methods have been developed for assigned job tasks that may be increasing risk or may be bypassing desired hazard controls.

A busy leadership team with its many obligations can overlook the fact that employees have a detailed knowledge of the work even as it has a basic intuition about that knowledge. A level of trust should be present for open communications between the levels of the organization.

Many reasons may be present that are obstacles to employee involvement in the process with a central theme of no feedback being provided.

A simple yet effective approach in developing any JHA process is "just listen" to what employees have to say about their job. With positive and open communications, employees will express their concerns.

The stage for success should be set by providing employees with the opportunity to become involved. Activities might include assistance during the different phases of establishing, implementing, and evaluating the JHA process.

Safety committees have been traditionally used as the focal point of employee participation. An effective safety committee can communicate a positive influence for safety-related activities and efforts rapidly through an organization. The JHA committee offers the potential to assess information received about what is actually happening in the workplace.

The JHA committee can develop and review completed JHAs to ensure that they are up to date and meet current operational requirements. The JHA committee is critical to the safety system as it ensures the JHA process is maintained and hazards and associated risk are consistently controlled.

A JHA committee charter is the document that provides the reasons, authority, and guidance for the establishment of the committee. A charter is a living document that should be periodically amended as conditions warrant. Its core purpose and structure should be kept as permanent as possible.

Committee members should have an understanding of processes and how the organization is structured. A blend of experienced long-term employees and recently hired employees draw from across departments or divisions can bring a spectrum of perceptions and expertise to the organization.

Depending on the complexity of the event, an ad hoc committee specific to the incident might be established. It would review all reports for consistency and completeness and determine if the basic causes of the event were defined and effective corrective measures taken.

CHAPTER REVIEW QUESTIONS

1. Who might be an untapped valuable source of expertise and knowledge in an organization? Explain why.
2. What is the main objective of employee participation?
3. List the principles of employee participation.
4. Discuss the reasons employees do not want to be involved in the JHA process. What is the underlying theme between these reasons?
5. Why is it important to listen to employees? Discuss.
6. Outline the guidelines that can be used to generate employee participation.
7. What is the benefit of a JHA committee?
8. What is the core purpose of a committee charter?
9. How should JHA Committee members be selected?
10. What are the three JHA committee roles and why are they important?

BIBLIOGRAPHY

Charter. (n.d.). Wikipedia. Retrieved from http://bit.ly/VRaByi

Coble, D., Taylors, B., & Jones, J. (n.d.). Central Safety and Health Management System, Adpated with Permission. CTJ Safety Associates, LLC. Retrieved from http://bit.ly/14Eu85r

Draft Proposed Safety And Health Program Rule: 29 CFR 1900.1, Docket No. S&H-0027. (n.d.). Occupational Safey and Health Administration (OSHA), Public Domain, Based on and Adapted for Use. Retrieved from http://1.usa.gov/TLkITh

Employee Involvement, eTools. (n.d.). Occupational Safety and Health Administration (OSHA), Public Domain, Based on and Adapted for Use. Retrieved from http://1.usa.gov/VIFfdd

Godin, S. (2009). *Define: Brand*. Retrieved from http://bit.ly/XJ6vnX

Joint Health and Safety Committees: *A practical guide for single employer workhealth*. (n.d.). The Canadian Centre for Occupational Health and Safety. Retrieved from http://bit.ly/X4VEqh

Managing Worker Safety and Health. (n.d.). Illinois OSHA Onsite Safety & Health Consultation Program, Public Domain, Based on and Adapted for Use. Retrieved from http://bit.ly/WTsneh

Pink, D.H. (2011). *Drive: The surprising truth about what motivates us*. Penguin Group US. Retrieved from http://bit.ly/VaQStm

Roughton, J., & Crutchfield, N. (2013). *Safety culture: An innovative leadership approach*. MA: Butterworth Heinemann. Retrieved from http://amzn.to/1qoD4oN

Senge, P., Kleiner, A., Roberts, C., Ross, R., Roth, G., & Smith, B. (1999). *Adapted from the dance of change: Mastering the twelve challenges to change in a learning organization*. New York: Doubleday.

Turner, L., & Turner, R. (1998). *How to grow effective teams and run meetings that aren't a waste of time*, Chapter 2. Ends of the Earth Learning Group, Adpated for use. Retrieved from http://bit.ly/UYqQqP

CHAPTER FIVE

Preparing for the Hazard and Risk Assessment

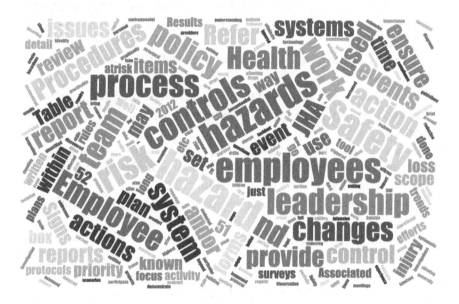

"Think like a wise man but communicate in the language of the people."
—William Butler Yeats

Chapter Objectives

At the end of the chapter, you should be able to:

- Discuss why hazard and risk recognition are foundational to the JHA process
- Conduct a hazard and risk assessment
- Discuss methods to gather information about hazard and risk-related issues
- Discuss recommended controls and an implementation strategy

Job Hazard Analysis. http://dx.doi.org/10.1016/B978-0-12-803441-5.00005-2

5.1 SETTING THE STAGE FOR THE JHA PROCESS

The JHA process begins by establishing how to focus efforts on prioritizing findings of an initial risk assessment and surveys. The following questions provide guidance for the survey development:

- Have existing potential hazards and the consequences of exposures within the organization and specific industry been evaluated? If so, when and by whom?
- Have repeated loss-producing events occurred? What was the scope of these events?
- Have hazards been discovered that were not known to exist during previous investigations of loss-producing event(s)? Why did they remain hidden?
- Have employees reported hazards that were not considered a "priority" and an injury or damage occurred? Did an investigation uncover any warning signs? Why were these ignored?
- Have reviews of loss-producing events identified any of the following situations:
  - Existing hazards that were not associated with any particular event.
  - Employees knew a hazard(s) existed and it was considered "just part of doing the job" and accepted the situation.
  - Received the response: "We have always done it this way," or "I have been doing this way for "X" years and nothing has happened!"

An effective JHA process addresses these situations by building an inventory or portfolio of the activities that should be controlled and monitored.

Loss-Producing Events

A loss-producing event is an incident that causes injury to employees or third parties, property damage, product loss, or any other type of physical damage (Roughton & Crutchfield, 2008).

At-Risk Event

Any activity that has inherent risk but has not triggered any loss-producing event as of yet.

5.2 CONDUCTING A HAZARD AND RISK ASSESSMENT

A formal safety system can provide the structure for an over-all assessment. For example, ANSI/AIHA/ASSE Z10, states that "The organization shall establish a process to set documented objectives, quantified where practicable, based on issues that offer the greatest opportunity for Occupational Health and Safety Management System improvement and risk reduction" (Occupational Health & Safety Management Systems, 2012).

A hazard and risk assessment survey drills down into the details of the organization and identifies specific risk by asking:

- What is currently happening within the organization and its industry? Are major changes ongoing or trends within the industry affecting operations?
- What activities and operations are currently being done that have inherent hazards and risk? Has the potential scope of the loss-potential been assessed?
- Have any organizational changes developed such as administrative/organization structural changes, a high employee and/or leadership turn over, changes in employee and/or leadership experience, skills and expertise, technology shifts or changes in types of tools, equipment, materials, or changes in the workplace environment?
- Are policies, procedures, protocols, rules, and guidelines consistently followed? Are these items kept current with any ongoing change?
- Are potential hazards and increased risk considered prior to any operational change of any process, procedures, facility, etc.?

The hazard and risk assessment survey can be very intensive as well as extensive if it is to be effectively used in developing an overall strategy.

The systematic assessing and analyzing of workplace hazards and risk uses a strategy that includes:

- Conducting a formal hazard and risk assessment of the organization.
- Prioritizing the hazard and risk assessment findings.
- Developing controls to resolve hazard and risk-related.
- Recommending and implementing controls.
- Monitoring the results of the controls.

5.3 PRIORITIZING THE RISK ASSESSMENT

An analysis is made of assessment findings to determine the nature and impact of hazardous conditions, at-risk, and loss-producing events. Jobs and activities with the highest potential for loss are given the first priority for JHA development.

> A process is the "method for doing something, generally, involving a number of steps or operations," (Process, n.d.).

Assessment survey data can graphically present information through process maps and flow diagrams that detail the sequence of actions and components necessary to focus the efforts of the JHA process (Figures 5.1 and 5.2).

5.4 DEVELOPING SOLUTIONS TO RESOLVE HAZARD AND RISK-RELATED ISSUES

The JHA process can be used to determine the sequence of controls necessary for effectively reducing loss-producing events. The leadership team can improve the development of solutions to identified issues by:

- Using a "tool box" of techniques, methods, and concepts that go beyond a regulatory compliance approach. The tool box would include, problem solving techniques, risk and data analysis methods, and effective written communications and presentations.
- Establishing goals and objectives for projects implementing controls.
- Maintaining a clear understanding of the work environment and organizational culture.

5.5 RECOMMENDING AND IMPLEMENTING CONTROLS

The nature and types of controls can range from minor behavioral changes to substantial capital investments necessary to eliminate worst-case scenarios. The selection of solutions should not be taken lightly as any change in a long-standing process can have unintended consequences.

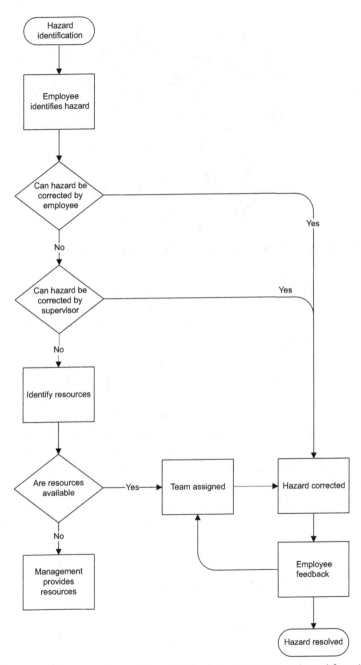

Figure 5.1 *Overview of a Hazard Identification Flow Diagram. Adapted from Hazard Identification Flowchart, Safety and Health Management – Safety Pays Program. (n.d.). Adapted and modified Roughton & Crutchfield (2013).*

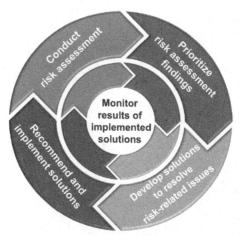

Figure 5.2 *Overview of the Process Elements for Analyzing the Workplace.*

A coordination of all affected departments, employees, and the leadership team is necessary to ensure a full buy-in to changes in the operation. Outside concerns such as the insurance carrier(s) may need to review changes that might create problems within the underwriting contract. Other entities may also need to be involved, for example, equipment providers, human resources, trainers, environmental specialist, and regulatory or legal expertise.

After the appropriate approvals have been made, the desired controls are reviewed for any unintended consequences or organizational issues. Action plans are developed to ensure that controls are implemented, budgets for employee time and expenses and implementation of project is scheduled, and physical changes are completed.

Depending on the complexity of the implementation, a project management approach would be used to ensure all the required elements are scheduled and completed in the desired time frame (Figure 5.3).

5.6 MONITORING THE RESULTS

After hazard and risk controls are implemented, emphasis shifts to ensuring that all controls stay effectively in place and that other hazards and risk do not develop. This is accomplished by continually scanning the organization allowing all employees to participate in the process as discussed in Chapter 4 (Table 5.1).

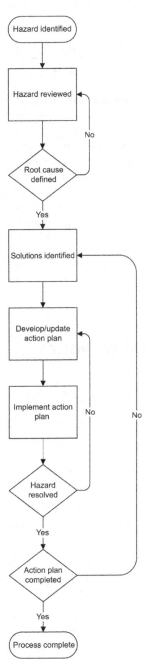

Figure 5.3 *An Overview of Hazard Analysis.* *Based on and adapted using US DOE NE (in press). Based on and Adapted using Roughton and Crutchfield (2013).*

Table 5.1 Scanning the organization for processes, works practices and procedures and warning signs

Processes, works practices and procedures	Warning signs
Review preventive and regular maintenance	Delaying maintenance, deferred repairs.
Review hazard correction procedures and controls.	Items noted from inspections are not corrected and/or remain open for a long period of time.
Determine if employees understand the hazards to which they are exposed.	Limited employee participation, inspections show unguarded equipment unreported by employees; personal protective equipment not being worn, clean, or maintained, etc.
Determine if employees can demonstrate knowledge of safe methods, work rules, procedures, and protocols.	Observation and loss analysis data indicate that administrative controls are bypassed or weakly enforced.

Source: Safety and Health Management, Safety & Health Training, eTools (n.d.); Roughton & Crutchfield (2013).

5.7 COMPANY SAFETY POLICY

"A policy is a statement of intent, and is implemented as a procedure or protocol."
  (Policy, n.d.)

The company safety policies set the tone for leadership's intent as to what is to be accomplished. A safety policy should be brief and clearly written and incorporated into the overall management process. It should be in the same form and style of all other policies used in the organization.

All employees should know of its existence and of its importance. The safety policy is communicated through all types of media used by the organization such as posting on both electronic and hardcopy bulletin boards and/or intranet, newsletters, in-house blogs, emails – any and all methods the organization has found to be effective in disseminating information. It should be emphasized during face-to-face individual discussions, at weekly, monthly meetings, and larger settings such as organizational-wide gatherings. It should be clearly known and understood by all levels and areas of the organization.

A positive safety policy affirms leadership's intentions to protect employees from unsafe conditions. It ensures that no reprisal or negative consequences can be held against employees who bring problems to the leadership team.

As misunderstandings can occur, the document should outline how employee reports will be received in the spirit of improvement of the organization not as a challenge to authority. Refer to Appendix A (Oregon OSHA Workshop Materials, Hazard Identification and Control, n.d.).

5.8 DEVELOPING A SYSTEM TO IDENTIFY AND REPORT HAZARDS

A reliable system for reporting and tracking hazards requires a number of essential elements that include the following:

> Hazards "A condition, a set of circumstances, or inherent property that can cause injury, illnesses, or death" (Occupational Health & Safety Management Systems, 2012). This definition should be expanded to include damage to physical items and the environment.

5.9 EMPLOYEE REPORTING SYSTEMS

Procedures should be provided that allow employees to report hazard through the following:
- Verbal reports: directly talking to supervision.
- Suggestion programs: suggestion box or email systems.
- Use of the risk guidance card. This will be discussed in detail in Chapter 8. (Appendix B)

Refer to Table 5.2 for key points to remember about reporting hazards.

Table 5.2 Important points to remember about reporting hazards

- Develop a policy that encourages employees to report hazards, no matter the scope or nature of the hazard.
- Communicate the policy. Ensure that this policy is known and understood by all employees.
- Build hazard reporting into the safety system."
- Respond to all reported hazards in a timely manner.
- Track all hazard prevention activities to completion.
- Use the information collected to revise JHAs to update the hazard inventory and to improve the hazard recognition program.

Source: Managing Worker Safety and Health (n.d.).

5.10 VERBAL REPORTS

Employees should be able to verbally report hazards directly to the leadership team. When an employee expresses concern(s), the leadership team has the responsibility to assess the situation and immediately correct the concern if possible. It not, a corrective action plan should be developed and a request for assistance made. As with employees, the leadership team should not fear reporting concerns or problems to more senior leadership (Oregon OSHA Workshop Materials, Hazard Identification and Control, n.d.).

On the negative side, verbal reporting does not provide for corrective action tracking, nor does it provide a database for possible trends and patterns of issues that are reported. Verbal reporting does not provide an employee protection from a member of the leadership team who may not understand the issue and does not take the need for response seriously (Overview of System Components, Safety & Health Management Systems eTool, n.d.). One method is to have alternative means for reporting concerns that allow employees to autonomously bypass any communication obstacles. Several of these are discussed below.

5.11 SUGGESTION PROGRAMS

If a suggestion program is used, the leadership team should ensure that collection points, both hardcopy and digital resources are checked frequently. All suggestions and/or comments should be reviewed and feedback provided to employees in a timely manner. Suggestion programs can be just dust collectors or a waste of time without a positive emphasis and routine follow-up (Oregon OSHA Workshop Materials, Hazard Identification and Control, n.d.).

5.12 MAINTENANCE WORK ORDERS

Work order systems that assign special maintenance codes to safety-related items can provide the tracking of corrective actions. These codes require the maintenance department assign a higher priority to safety-related work orders. As specific safety work orders are generated, the list can be posted on safety bulletins or shared electronically so that employees can review the status of the corrective actions.

When complete resolution of a hazard related work order requires ordering parts, materials, involves a lengthy delay, the employees should be provided a periodic status report. This ensures that the perception of employee concerns being overlooked or forgotten does not develop. Alternative or modified control actions should be taken when work orders cannot be immediately be accomplished up to and including a "cease use or activity" mandate (Oregon OSHA Workshop Materials, Hazard Identification and Control, n.d.).

A work order system may go through a help desk that relays request to the safety department, designated leadership team members, human resources, and others to ensure that the safety issues are not lost in the system. The work order system, as with any other aspect of operations, should be reviewed for its reliability. It should clearly provide a way of setting priorities for high hazard and high-risk areas.

5.13 CHECKLIST USED TO REPORT HAZARDS

The hazard reports that work best are a set of customized checklist for a specific workplace and operation. Appendix B provides several sample reporting forms, Sample Forms for Employee Reporting of Hazards, Tracking Hazard Correction, and Follow-Up Documentation.

5.14 ACTION PLANNING

A corrective action plan aids in determining if the JHA process is effective by assessing whether the same or similar hazards reappear. For every hazard identified, an action plan should be developed and tracked until the hazard is eliminated or controlled (Managing Worker Safety and Health, n.d.).

An action plan is important because:
- The leadership team remains informed of the status of long-term corrective actions.
- Benchmarks and status reports can be provided on how well implementation is going.
- A record of actions taken is maintained to determine whether or not the hazard reoccurred again.
- Documents are available on the hazard control history for future use.
- Timely and accurate information is provided for employees who report hazards.
- Alternative controls can be implemented and used until the problem is resolved.

When documenting information about action plans, it is important that all interim preventative measures are listed and include the anticipated date of completion.

Refer to Appendix C for an example of several basic action planning forms (Managing Worker Safety and Health, n.d.).

5.15 FOLLOW-UP REVIEWS

Follow-up reviews assess the effectiveness of controls that have been implemented. The frequency of follow-up surveys depends on the complexity of the hazards. They can determine if additional hazards or unintended consequences have developed.

SUMMARY

This chapter highlights the important points of hazard recognition and control.

A point of beginning is to establish what is to be accomplished by a JHA Process and how to best focus its efforts by prioritizing the findings of the initial assessment.

The systematic assessing and analyzing of workplace hazards and risk uses a strategy that includes (1) Conducting a formal hazard and risk assessment of the organization. (2) Prioritizing the hazard and risk assessment findings. (3) Developing controls to resolve hazard and risk-related issues. (4) Recommending and implementing controls.

Use of an accepted safety management system can provide the structure for an overall assessment. As example, the American Nationals Standards Institute's Z10-2012, Occupational Health and Safety Management Systems, a voluntary standard states "The organization shall establish a process to set documented objectives, quantified where practicable, based on issues that offer the greatest opportunity for Occupational Health and Safety Management System improvement and risk reduction."

An analysis is made of assessment findings to determine the nature and impact of hazardous conditions, unsafe practices, past history of losses, and at-risk events involved in the operation.

As the scope and location of hazards and risks are identified, the JHA process is used to determine the sequence of controls necessary for effectively reducing loss potential.

The nature and types of controls can range from minor behavioral changes to substantial capital investments necessary to eliminate worst-case scenarios. The selection of solutions to identified issues should not be taken lightly as any change in a long standing process can have unintended consequences.

A coordination of all affected departments, employees, and leadership is necessary to ensure that full buy-in to change is present. In addition, outside parties such as the insurance carriers may need to review changes that might create problems within the underwriter contract. Equipment providers, human resources, trainers, environmental specialist, and regulatory legal expertise may be needed.

After hazards and risk controls are implemented, emphasis shifts ensuring that all controls stay effectively in place and that other hazards and risk do not develop. This is accomplished by continually scanning the organization using employee involvement as discussed in Chapter 4.

Developing a reliable system for reporting and tracking hazards is an essential element of a safety system.

A safety policy sets the tone for what is to be accomplished. It should be brief and clearly written, and incorporated into the safety system. All employees should know it exist and its importance.

The primary method used to identify workplace hazards remains the comprehensive workplace inspection. The hazard assessment identifies the overall scope of hazards and risk. At the operational level, inspections are used ranging from simple observations to customized checklists for high-hazard operations.

It is better to have employees' erring on the side of caution with occasional nonhazards issue reported than to overlook even one real hazard because an employee failed to report it believing that the leadership team would not respond.

Employees should be able to verbally report hazards directly to the leadership team. When an employee expresses concern(s), leadership has the responsibility to assess the situation and immediately correct the concern if warranted.

If a suggestion program is used, the leadership team should ensure that collection points, both hardcopy and digital are checked frequently with suggestion comments reviewed and feedback provided to employees in a timely manner.

Work order systems that assign special maintenance codes to safety-related items can provide the tracking of corrective actions. These codes require the maintenance department to assign a higher priority to safety-related work orders.

The hazard reports that work best are those customized for a specific workplace and operation.

For every hazard identified, an action plan should be developed and tracked until the hazard is eliminated or controlled. Some hazards can be quickly corrected and may not present a safety issue. Corrections that are complicated with capital budget requirements or time-consuming criteria require placement in a tracking system.

Follow-up reviews assess the effectiveness of controls that have been implemented. The frequency of follow-up surveys depends on the complexity of the hazards.

CHAPTER REVIEW QUESTIONS

1. What questions setup the parameters for a hazard and risk assessment?
2. List possible questions that can begin the hazard and risk assessment.
3. What are the three essentials skills for a safety professional to be successful?
4. What coordination is essential when recommending and implementing controls?
5. Why is monitoring changes made important?
6. What activities accompany a reporting system?
7. What does a safety policy do and who should know about it?
8. What are some of the reliable methods to developing a system to identify and report hazards?
9. What is a company safety policy and why is it necessary?
10. List the types of methods used to report hazards. Rank these methods in the order you believe is most effective and be able to discuss why you ranked them in this order.

BIBLIOGRAPHY

Managing Worker Safety and Health. (n.d.). Missouri Occupational Safety and Health Administration (OSHA), Office of Cooperative Programs, Public Domain, Adapted for Use. Retrieved from http://on.mo.gov/15C4FyS

Managing Worker Safety and Health, Appendix 9–4 Hazard Analysis Flow Charts. (n.d.). Missouri Safety & Health Consultation Program (OSHA), Public Domain, Adapted for Use. Retrieved from http://on.mo.gov/XVZ6BD

Occupational Health & Safety Management Systems. (2012). The American Society of Safety Engineers, ANSI/AIHA/ASSE Z10. Retrieved from http://bit.ly/1MsT6MG

Oregon OSHA Workshop Materials, Hazard Identification and Control. (n.d.). Oregon Occupational Safety and Health Division (Oregon OSHA), Public Domain, Permission to Reprint, Modify, and/or Adapt as necessary. Retrieved from http://bit.ly/1tg4a8A and http://bit.ly/1yIBKVk

OSHA Handbook for small businesses, safety management series. (1996) (Revised). US Department of Labor, Occupational Safety Administration, OSHA 2209. Appendix C, pp. 51, Public Domain.

Overview of System Components, Safety & Health Management Systems eTool. (n.d.). Occupational Safety and Health Administration (OSHA), Public Domain, Based on and Adapted for Use. Retrieved from http://1.usa.gov/U5Zr5R

Policy. (n.d.). Wikipedia, the free encyclopedia. Retrieved from http://bit.ly/16LNDyX
Process. (n.d.). Dictionary.com. Retrieved from http://bit.ly/1z25ERd
Roughton, J., & Crutchfield, N. (2008). Job hazard analysis: A guide for voluntary compliance and beyond. *Chemical petrochemical & process.* MA: Elsevier/Butterworth-Heinemann, Retrieved from http://amzn.to/VrSAq5.
Roughton, J., & Crutchfield, N. (2013). In B. Heinemann (Ed.), *Safety culture: An innovative leadership approach.* MA: Butterworth Heinemann, Retrieved from http://amzn.to/1qoD4oN.
Roughton, J., & Mercurio, J. (2002). *Developing an effective safety culture: A leadership approach.* MA: Butterworth-Heinemann, Appendix A, pp. 389–392.
Safety and Health Management, Safety & Health Training, eTools. (n.d.). Occupational Safety and Health Adminstration (OSHA), Public Domain, Based on and Adapted for Use. Retrieved from http://1.usa.gov/Ute9q5
US Department of Energy Office of Nuclear Energy. Developing a Solution to Solve the Problem DOE-NE-STD-1004-92.

Appendix A Sample Guidance in Writing a Policy Statement: Sample Policy Safety Statements

A.1 Introduction

Generally, a written safety policy statement will run 6–12 sentences in length. It includes some or all of the five elements:

- An introductory statement
- A statement of the purpose or philosophy of the policy
- A summary of management responsibilities
- A summary of employee responsibilities
- A closing statement.

A.2 Introductory statement

The written policy statement generally starts with a clear, simple expression of your concern for and attitude about employee safety. Examples of introductions to policy statements include:

- This company considers no phase of its operation or administration more important than the safety of our employees. We will provide and maintain safe working conditions, and establish and insist on safe work methods and practices at all times.
- Injury prevention is a primary job of management, and management is responsible for establishing safe working conditions.
- This company has always believed that our employees are our most important assets. We will always place the highest value on safe operations and on the safety of our employees.
- The company will, at all times and at every level of management, attempt to provide and maintain a safe working environment for all employees.

All safety protection programs are aimed at preventing injuries and exposures to harmful atmospheric contaminants.
- All members of management and all employees must make safety protection a part of their daily concerns.

A.3 Purpose/philosophy

An effective safety program will have a stated purpose or philosophy. This is included in a written policy statement so that both you and your employees are reminded of the purpose and value of the program. You may wish to incorporate the purpose/philosophy into your policy. Examples of purpose and philosophy include:
- We have established our safety program to eliminate work-related injuries and damage. We expect it to improve operations and reduce personal and financial losses.
- Safety protection shall be an integral part of all operations, including planning, procurement, development, production, administration, sales, and transportation. Injuries have no place in our company.
- We want to make our safety protection efforts so successful that we make elimination of injuries a way of life.
- We aim to resolve safety problems through prevention.
- We will involve both management and employees in planning, developing, and implementing safety protection.

A.4 Management responsibilities

A safety action plan will describe in detail who is to develop the program and make it work, as well as who is assigned specific responsibilities, duties, and authority. The policy statement may include a summary of the following responsibilities:
- Each level of management must reflect an interest in company safety and must set a good example by complying with company rules for safety protection. Management interest must be vocal, visible, and continuous from top management to departmental supervisors.
- The company management is responsible for developing an effective safety and program.
- Plant superintendents are responsible for maintaining safe and healthful working conditions and practices in areas under their jurisdiction.
- Department heads and supervisors are responsible for preventing injuries.
- Supervisors are responsible for preventing exposures to hazard in their specific work areas. Supervisors will be accountable for the safety of all employees working under their supervision.

- The safety director has the authority and responsibility to provide guidance to supervisors and to help management prevent injuries.
- Management representatives who have been assigned safety responsibilities will be held accountable for meeting those responsibilities.

A.5 Employee responsibilities

Many companies acknowledge the vital role of their employees in the operation of a successful safety process by developing specific employee roles and contributions in the policy statement. Employees have the unique responsibility to assist management with all injury prevention efforts through active participation in all risk-control activities, especially providing direct feedback regarding the effectiveness of these efforts.

The following are examples of employee responsibilities:
- All employees are expected to follow safe practices, obey rules and regulations, and work in a way that maintains the high safety standards developed and sanctioned by the company.
- All employees are expected to give full support to risk control activities.
- Every employee must observe established safety regulations, procedures, and protocols.
- All employees are expected to take an active interest in the safety process, participate in program activities, and abide by the rules and regulations of this company.
- All employees must recognize their responsibility to prevent injuries and must take necessary actions. Their performance in this regard will be measured as part of their overall job performance.

A.6 Closing statement

The closing statement is often a reaffirmation of your commitment to provide a safe workplace. It appeals for the cooperation of all company employees in support of the safety program.
- I urge all employees to make this safety process an integral part of your daily job tasks and activities.
- By accepting our individual responsibilities to operate safely, we will all contribute to the well being of one another and consequently the company.
- We must be successful in our efforts for the elimination of injuries and for safety management to become a way of life.

Source: Adapted from Roughton & Mercurio, 2002.

A.7 Sample model policy statements

The following are some samples of model policy statements. Some may have been presented earlier. These states are general in nature and inclusive of many types of business activities. These statements are intended as a model only and should be adapted to describe your own site-specific work environment.

A.7.1 Sample #1
"The Occupational Safety and Health Act (OSHA) of 1970 clearly require that the company shall provide a workplace with safe and healthful working conditions. The Safety of our employees continues to be the first consideration in the operation of this business."

A.7.2 Sample #2
"Safety in our business must be a part of every operation. Without question it must be every employee's responsibility at all levels of the organization."

A.7.3 Sample #3
"It is the intent of our organization to comply with all rules and applicable laws. To do this, we must constantly be aware of conditions in all work areas that can produce injuries. No employee is required to work at a job that is not safe. Your cooperation in detecting hazards is part of your job. You must inform your supervisor immediately of any situation beyond your ability or authority to correct."

A.7.4 Sample #4
"The personal Safety of each employee of this company is of primary importance. The prevention of occupationally-induced injuries is of such consequence that it will be given precedence over operating productivity. To the greatest degree possible, management will provide the resources required for personal safety in keeping with the highest standards."

A.7.5 Sample #5
"We will maintain a safety process conforming to the best practices we can achieve. To be successful, our program will embody the proper attitudes toward injury prevention on the part of supervision and employees. It requires cooperation in all Safety matters, not only between supervisor and employee, but between each employee and their coworkers. Only through such a cooperative effort can a safety program in the best interest of all be established and preserved."

A.7.6 Sample #6
"Our objective is a safety process that will reduce the number of injuries to an absolute minimum, not merely in keeping with, but surpassing, the best experience of operations similar to ours. Our goal is zero injuries."
    "Our safety process will include the following elements:
- Providing mechanical and physical safeguards to the maximum extent possible.

- Conducting a program of safety inspections to find and eliminate unsafe working conditions or at-risk events, to control safety hazards, and to comply fully with all safety standards for every job.
- Training all employees in good safety practices.
- Providing necessary PPE and instructions for its proper use and care.
- Developing and enforcing safety rules and requiring that employees cooperate with all rules as a condition of employment.
- Investigating, promptly and thoroughly, every injury to find out what caused it and to correct the problem so that it will not happen again.
- Setting up a system of recognition and awards for outstanding safety service or performance."

A.7.7 Sample #7

"We recognize that the responsibilities for safety must be shared by everyone as such:
- As a corporation, we will accept the responsibility for management and leadership of the safety program, for its effectiveness and improvement, and for providing the safeguards required to ensure safe conditions.
- Supervisors are responsible for developing the proper attitudes toward safety in themselves and in those they supervise, and for ensuring that all operations are performed with the utmost regard for the Safety of all personnel involved, including them.
- Employees are responsible for wholehearted, genuine operation with all aspects of the safety program including compliance with all rules and regulations and for continuously practicing safety while performing their duties."
Adapted from OSHA, 1996.

A.8 Summary

Policy statements can vary in length and content. The briefest are typically basic statements of policy only. Longer statements may include company philosophy. Others will address the safety responsibilities of management and other employees.

Policy statements can cover in detail items such as specific assignment of safety duties, description of specific duties, delegation of authority, safety rules and procedures, and encouragement of employee involvement. While some companies may wish to include these additional items in the policy statement, we believe it usually is best to leave these details for later discussion.

These are examples that may give you an idea for a policy statement that can be written in your style, expressing your attitudes and value to the safety process (Managing Worker Safety and Health, Appendix 9–4 Hazard Analysis Flow Charts, n.d.; Roughton & Crutchfield, 2008, 2013).

Appendix B Sample Forms for Employee Reporting of Hazards Tracking Hazard Corrections Follow-Up Documentation

B.1 Example #1
Form for employees to report hazards
Part 1

Hazard or safety problem

Department where hazard or problem is observed

Date: Time:

Suggested action:

Employee's signature (optional)

Employee: Completes Part 1 and gives to supervisor
Part 2

Action taken:

Department:

Date:

Supervisors signature:

Supervisor: Completes and gives to manager
Part 3

Date:

Review/comments:

Managers signature:

B.2 Example #2
Reporting safety or health problem

Date

Description of problem (include exact location, if applicable)

Note any previous attempts to notify management of this problem and provide name of person notified:

Date

Optional: Submitted by: Name

Safety department findings:

Actions taken

Safety committee review comments:

All actions completed by: Date

B.2.1 Sample #3

Employee report of hazard

This form is provided to assist employees in reporting hazards.

I believe that a condition or practice at the following location is a hazard or safety problem.

Is there an immediate   Yes   No
threat of serious
physical harm?

Provide information that will help locate the hazard, such as building or area of building or the supervisor's name.

Describe briefly the hazard you believe exists and the approximate number of employees exposed to it.

If this hazard has been called to anyone's attention, as far as you know, please provide the name of the person or committee member notified and the approximate date.

Signature (optional)

Type or print name (optional)

Date

Management evaluation of reported hazard

Final action taken

All actions completed by initials   Date

B.2.2 Sample

Follow-up review

This form can be used as part of sample forms 1, 2, or 3 or separately

Hazard

Possible injury or damage

Exposure   Frequency of exposure

Duration

Interim protection provided

Corrective action taken

Follow-up review made on   Date

Any additional action taken?

Signature of manager or supervisor   Date

Is corrective action still in place?   Yes   No

Three month follow-up check made on   Date

Sources: Managing Worker Safety and Health, Appendix 9–4 Hazard Analysis Flow Charts (n.d.); Roughton and Crutchfield (2008, 2013).

Appendix C Three Sample Basic Action Planning Forms

C.1 Sample action plan #1

Activity	Responsibility	Target date	Status
Management leadership			
Employee participation			
Job hazard analysis to be completed			
Hazard reduction and control measures			
Training			

C.2 Sample #2

C.2.1 Tracking Hazard Corrective Actions Form

Instructions: Under the column heading "System", note how the hazard was found. Enter Insp. for inspection, ERH and name of employee reporting hazard, or INC. for incident investigation.

Under the column Hazard Description (column 2), use as many lines needed to describe the hazard. In the third column, provide the name of the person who has been assigned responsibility for corrective actions (column 3). In column 4, list any interim corrective actions to correct the hazard and the date performed. In the last column, enter the completed corrective action and the date that final correction was made.[1]

1	2	3	4	5
System	Hazard description	Responsibility: Assigned	Interim completed action	Action with date

[1]Place activities to be completed on Gantt Chart, calendar, and/or individual performance objectives.

C.3 Sample Action Plan #3

Activity	Conduct monthly employee safety meetings	Establish procedures for management and employee participation in inspections and injury investigations	Provide hazard recognition and injury investigation training to management and employees
Time commitment	Begin by June	Inspections and investigations begin by September 30	Complete by December 31
Responsible employees	Plant manager	Plant/safety manager	Safety manager
Resources needed	1-h safety meeting each month for all employees. audio-visual equipment	Time spent by employees on inspections and investigations	Time for developing training materials, possibly outside professional/trainer
Results expected	Employee input on safety matters; volunteers for participation programs	Inspections and investigations being performed	Inspections that ID all hazards; investigations that uncover root causes; fewer injuries
Possible roadblocks	Employee mistrust at first; limited knowledge about all potential hazards	Lack of employee interest	Cost of reduced production; unwillingness to spend funds for improvements
Status/ evaluation	Monthly reports to plant manager; assessment annually	Quarterly reports to CEO, look for patterns or trends	Keep training records; retrain periodically

Sources: Managing Worker Safety and Health (n.d.); Roughton & Crutchfield (2008, 2013).

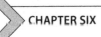

CHAPTER SIX

Hazard Analysis and Review of Associated Risk

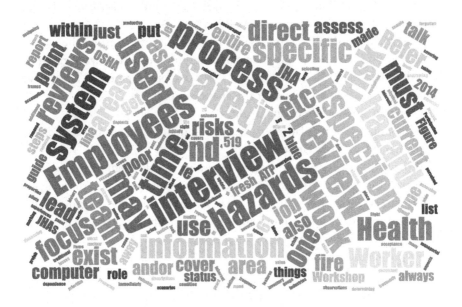

"Hope is not a Strategy"

—*Rick Page*

Chapter Objectives

At the end of the chapter, you should be able to:

- Identify the use of audits and inspections.
- Discuss the tools used to gather information for the workplace review.
- Discuss the differences between an audit and an inspection.
- Define the roles played by outside specialist, supervisors, employees.
- Determine who should be involved in the review.
- Identify sources for risk and hazard data.

6.1 HAZARD REVIEW AND ANALYSIS OF THE WORKPLACE

Hazard reviews and analysis provide the foundational information and data used to further enhance the effectiveness of the safety system (Oregon OSHA Workshop Materials, Hazard Identification and Control, n.d.). Refer to Figure 6.1 (Risk Management, ATP 5-19, 2014).

The starting point in hazard review and analysis is to consider the workplace as a system of cause and effects or emerging properties with inherent hazards and associated risk built into the work environment. The review and analysis has features that are critical and should:

- Cover all areas of the organization.
- Be conducted at regular intervals. The frequency depends on the potential hazards and severity of risks.
- Provide the necessary guidance for reviewers to help them recognize hazards and associated risk and encouraged to bring fresh ideas to the analysis.
- Provide information from the analysis to expand the organization's hazard inventory and used to modify and/or update JHAs and/or improve the safety system.

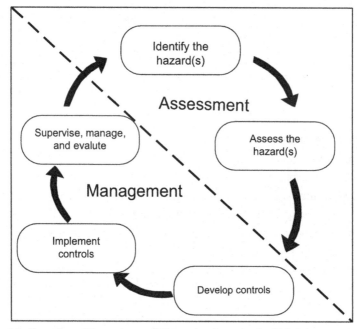

Figure 6.1 *Overview of Assessing and Managing Steps in the Risk Assessment Process. Based on and adapted from Risk Management, ATP 5-19 (2014).*

The following actions assist in selecting the methods or tools that can be used to identify and analyze the work environment. They include:

- Reviewing job descriptions and protocols that identify what employees are expected to accomplish or tasks they are assigned.
- Identifying specific jobs known to have hazards and associated risks.
- Reviewing appropriate standards, procedures, regulations, etc. that guide the operations.
- Reviewing and discussing planned, new, modified or relocated facilities, processes, materials, and equipment.
- Reviewing similar industries and past workplace experience history.

Oregon OSHA Workshop Materials, Hazard Identification and Control (n.d.)

Actions should include interviewing experienced employees who have knowledge of the operation. As discussed in Chapter 4, employees are valuable resources of experiences and perceptions that can lead to the discovery of additional hazards or potential risks not initially considered in an assessment.

6.2 INSPECTIONS AND AUDITS

Inspections and audits are similar to "tactics" and "strategy." Inspections are "tactics" used as part of a process to review specific tasks or areas. An audit, like "strategy," covers the overall process and reviews the entire organization for function and effectiveness; i.e., are the specific safety programs being utilized as designed and are they effective? (Risk Management, ATP 5-19, 2014)

6.3 INSPECTIONS

Inspections are the most frequently recommended activity used to assess hazards. They have been the traditional method used in regulatory and organizational safety programs. The "inspection" is usually a general "walk-around" to identify conditions that do not comply with defined safety procedures, protocols, and requirements. They can range from informal to highly complex as found in extremely high risk operations such as space flight, aircraft, nuclear power plants, etc.

Inspections remain a key component as they offset the natural tendency to lose sight of changes in activities that can lead to a long-term scope drift and acceptance of current conditions. For example, a guard is removed from a piece of equipment and not immediately replaced as maintenance personnel are called away to a more important crisis. The inspection is necessary to get things back on track and the hazardous condition into the work order system (Chapter 5).

Inspections are also the worst implemented part of a safety system. They can be perceived as time consuming, taking individuals away from "productive" work, and in many cases not adding any value to the operation. Inspections are not always utilized effectively because the organization has not experienced severe losses and a low perception of risk exists.

6.4 AUDITS

Audit is a process that attempts to determine overall safety program element status by assigning a rating to its findings. The audit is a comprehensive review of all aspects of an organizational safety system and is performed over specific time frames. The audit involves a very thorough review of the administrative, physical, and managerial requirements of a safety system. This also involves employee interviews and observations of work activities. Its findings are made in a formal report that is presented and reviewed with the leadership team.

> If organizations look at the audit process in a positive method they can use it as a benchmarking opportunity. Audits provide the leadership team with a control panel to gauge process status and prioritize area(s) for improvement.

6.5 CHECKLIST

The checklist is essential in ensuring that a comprehensive review is completed. Checklists are the starting point and should be based on the experience and knowledge of employees and the leadership team.

Generic inspection checklists can be used to save time in covering areas of universal concern such as basic life safety, housekeeping, or fire protection. However, generic checklists need to be customized for the specific operational needs that may exist.

The use of a customized checklist provides a consistent approach for determining where changes are occurring or where problems may be developing within an area or job. They provide a memory aid that reduces the chance of critical items or steps from being forgotten when used for preshift and prejob briefings. For example, aircraft pilots and crews have extensive checklists that cover a wide array of possible scenarios. No matter what type of project (a grocery list or a surgical procedure,) without a checklist, dependence is on the memory and the mood of the individual conducting the review (Gawande, 2009)(Appendix D).

6.6 CONSULTANTS AND OUTSIDE SPECIALISTS

A variety of outside services may be needed to assess the organization using independent consultants, engineers, or other specialist to supplement internal resources. One source for possible assistance is with the property and casualty insurance carriers who may provide consulting services, such as general hazard surveys, workers' compensation guidance, property protection surveys and other specialty loss control reviews. These services must be managed and all recommendations defined and discussed, as they become part of the underwriting for insurance premium development.

Industry experts and specialist with extensive knowledge of specific disciplines may be needed to review complex engineering, safety-related issues. These consultants and outside specialists may include specific trades such as industrial hygienist, ergonomist, environmental/civil/electrical/sanitary engineers, machinist/millwrights, fire protection engineers, architects, computer specialist to name, etc.

This professional assistance from outside brings a depth of expertise as well as a fresh set of eyes and insights. A combination of outside specialists and internal expertise used as a team has potential greater impact for identifying and analyzing targeted hazardous operations (Managing Worker Safety and Health, n.d.).

6.7 EMPLOYEE INTERVIEWS AND SURVEYS

Interviewing employees is one of the most important part of the organizational review. These interviews can range from informal conversations to gain insights on current perceptions, group discussions, response sessions, hardcopy survey questionnaires, and online computer surveys.

6.8 SURVEYS

Types of surveys range from employee opinion, attitude, satisfaction, engagement, and performance to name several. If a questionnaire is to be used, the development of the survey instrument requires special expertise so that it is not skewed toward conscious or unconsciously desired results. How questions are asked has a major impact on what response is received (Kahneman, 2011). Implementing a survey must take into account the reading skills, language, writing, and comprehension of its recipients. The time requirements and its scope must be determined as it can create a negative response and not taken seriously if too lengthy or complicated. Surveys are used for gathering responses from large groups where direct interviews are not feasible or a statistical analysis is desired.

6.9 INTERVIEWS

Completing a direct one-on-one employee interview can tap into the current levels of expertise and knowledge about how things are actually being done. The direct employee interview provides more than just a method for gathering information. The body language, tone of voice, attitudes, and general response to the interview may tell much about the actual work environment and perceptions about the organization.

Interviewing is somewhat of an art form in that it attempts to draw out from an individual what they really know and opens up a line of trusting communications that a computer or paper survey cannot achieve. Refer to Table 6.1 for general guidelines for conducting employee interviews.

Lesson Learned #1
Interviews almost always result in one or more surprise. In one situation, a safety director was asked by an employee, "if the blue stuff in the boiler room can hurt you?" When the safety director ask why he was asking, the employee stated, he and coworkers had found the "blue" chemical to be a good laxative and he just wanted to know if it was OK to drink. Needless to say, the safety director was appalled and began an immediate review. Establishing a trusting relationship during interviews and even conversations, can lead to interesting dialogs. Stay open and alert for opportunities to learn.

Lesson Learned #2

The following is advice to consider when conducting any interview:

A rule of thumb is to listen approximately 80% of the time and only talk 20% of the time. For example, when an employee is constantly interrupted during an interview, the employee may shut down and not see the discussion of benefit. They may begin to revise what they intended to say just to get the interview over with. Your interruptions send the signal that you are more interested in your opinion than their opinion.

When someone is talking, do not interrupt them until they have completed their statement. Breaking in reduces the chance of getting their perception of the facts into the open.

Table 6.1 General guidelines for conducting employee interviews

- Put employee(s) at ease: Keep the interview informal. If possible, know in advance a little background information, name, job, etc. Be friendly, understanding, and open-minded. Explain the purpose of the interview and your role in the process, i.e., JHA development, injury review, change analysis, etc.
- Keep focused on the purpose of the interview: The intent of an interview is to open and maintain a line of communication with employees. As the interview develops, information not pertinent to your inquiry may develop. You must be prepared to direct this information to other resources for the appropriate response.
- Be calm, do not rush the interview: Ensure that you have scheduled your time and have flexibility with your schedule. If you are having issues or problems that will impact your ability to listen, reschedule the interview.
- Use active listening: Let the employee(s) talk! Put your ego aside. It is an interview, not your opportunity to discuss what you think. Repeat the information given to you. If you are conducting a group interview, talk with the employee(s) until you understand what they are trying to convey.
- Ask open-ended questions. One effective question is: "Tell me about the procedures for......" "Help me understand how it ....." Ask the employee(s) to tell you about potential hazards they think or know exist.
- At the end of the interview, ask the employee(s) if they have any questions for you. Answer these questions as best as you can or tell them that you will get an answer back to them as soon as possible.
- Notes should be taken very carefully, and as casually as possible. Offer to let the employees read the notes if they desire.
- Provide feedback: Conclude the interview with a statement of appreciation for their contribution. Thank the employees for their time and insight. Advise the employee(s) of the outcome of the interview as soon as possible.
- Be available: Ask the employee(s) to contact you if they think of anything else that may be of interest or concern.

Based and adapted from Managing Worker Safety and Health (n.d.)

6.10 TYPES OF INSPECTIONS

6.10.1 General Walk-Around Inspections

"Walk-arounds" are used to conduct ongoing daily safety inspections of the workplace. This type of inspection identifies obvious or observable blatant hazards or visible risk that may be related to unsafe work practices or conditions. If properly conducted, it is effective in identifying active error potential but is not as effective in identifying latent error potential (US DOE, 2009).

A walk-around inspection assesses only conditions that exist at that point in time. To improve effectiveness, the time during the work day or shift for the inspection should be varied to see if hazardous conditions develop throughout the shift. For example, housekeeping may deteriorate and increase the number of unsafe conditions (fire hazards, tripping/slips/falls, lifting, etc.). Conditions may be totally different at the beginning of a work day from its ending as well as between shifts. The walk-around must be varied and cover all work time periods.

The walk-around inspection should routinely include a member of the leadership team as part of the designated inspection team. A checklist should be used to guide the inspection and, as discussed, be customized to the specific area under review (Managing Worker Safety and Health, n.d.).

6.10.2 Focus Reviews

A form of inspection is the focus review that is conducted in conjunction with a comprehensive or verification review. This type of review is usually as result of a significant risk or hazard finding, an insurance/risk management project or an enforcement action by a regulatory agency.

The purpose of a focus review is to concentrate on a particular process or audit component that requires a specialized team that is experienced in the category of focus required. For example, the focus review inspection of an electrical power generating plant required a team of millwrights, pipefitters, electricians, plumbers, and other trades when a property fire protection insurance visit was made to the plant.

6.10.3 Document Review

As the JHA process begins to unfold, the why, where, and how its documents are to be stored is very important. Documents and records are reviewed to verify that what was to be collected and recorded has been properly completed and curated, i.e., correctly filed and is retrievable within a reasonable amount of time.

> The document review is not a hazard assessment. It is only the determination that policy statements, safety policies and/or procedures, training, recordkeeping, JHAs, etc. are being used as intended, kept up to date and current within the organization. If it can't be found, then it doesn't exist (Occupational Health & Safety Management Systems, 2012).

Lesson Learned #3
One problem found is the lack of developing an organized filing system, either hardcopy or electronic that allows desired documents to be properly stored for use and retrieval. If documents are not completely filled out, missing or do not meet program guidelines and standards, a strong probability exist that your system is improperly functioning. Curation will be discussed in more detail in Chapter 15.

6.10.4 Verification Reviews

Verification is an essential action that must be included in the overall inspection process. It is performed to ensure that problems, concerns, or issues identified in previous reviews have been corrected and no further action is needed. Verification includes reviewing whether corrective actions remain effective or need to be modified. Verification also includes ensuring that all the types of reviews undertaken actually were completed and "confirms" (authenticates) conditions are as stated by the documentation (Figure 6.2).

6.11 WRITTEN INSPECTION REPORTS

Written inspection reports document hazards identified, the assignment of responsibility for correction, and when corrective actions were completed. A well-designed format will help to ensure that:
- Responsible individuals are assigned responsibility so that the hazard(s) is corrected in a timely manner.
- Methods of tracking corrective actions to completion are implemented.

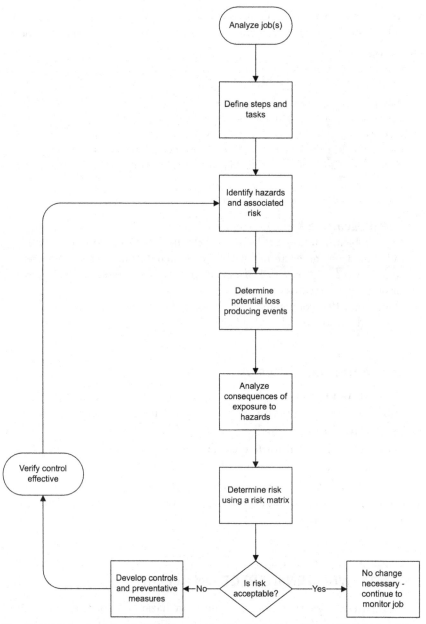

Figure 6.2 Overview of a Risk Assessment Toolkit. *Based on and adapted from Cox & Cox (1996) and Roughton & Crutchfield (2008).*

- Problems in the hazard control system are identified when the same type(s) of hazard continue to occur after an action plan is completed and verified.
- Problems are identified in the accountability system.
- Hazards where no prevention or controls have been planned are identified.

The administrative process must ensure that documented records are read, analyzed and put into the action planning process. Documenting hazards or risks and not following through on their correction may lead to charges of negligence, regulatory fines and lawsuit should a severe loss event occur (Managing Worker Safety and Health, n.d.; Roughton & Crutchfield, 2013; Roughton, n.d.).

6.12 WHO SHOULD REVIEW THE WORKPLACE?

Cross-functional or interdepartmental teams provide the specific skills and perspectives needed in reviewing the workplace (Managing Worker Safety and Health, n.d.). Who reviews the workplace varies depending on the nature and scope of what is being reviewed. The most obvious is that the various levels of leadership team have a direct responsibility for the entire operation and their assigned areas of responsibility. Employees have the responsibility to review their work area and report issues. In general, everyone should be trained in the review of both their assigned area as well as have an understanding of the entire operation.

For complex situations, the outside specialists as discussed earlier are brought in to assess complex processes and equipment beyond the expertise of in-house reviewers.

6.13 PREVENTIVE MAINTENANCE PROGRAMS

Preventive maintenance plays a major role in ensuring that hazard controls continue to function effectively. Preventive maintenance records assist in targeting areas of potential high risk. Records concerning equipment or facilities that have recurring problems, delayed repair, bypassed systems, etc. are an excellent source for identifying jobs to analyze and for special focus review. Paralleling inspections with scheduled preventive maintenance activity combines knowledge of safety criteria and related maintenance expertise (Managing Worker Safety and Health, n.d.; Roughton & Crutchfield, 2008, 2013).

Maintenance records should be periodically reviewed for reactive maintenance repair or replacement of defective parts after failure (breakdown maintenance) has been completed. Poor maintenance and poor housekeeping are direct indicators that the quality of the work environment is poor with hazards and risk having a high probability of creating loss-producing events.

To be effective, maintenance should be performed on a routine basis and as recommended by the process designer and equipment manufacturers (Safety et al., n.d.; Roughton & Crutchfield, 2008, 2013). Reviewing and comparing the work order list, maintenance records, and inspections/reviews gives a strong indicator about actual facility and operational conditions.

6.14 INCIDENT INVESTIGATIONS

Incident investigations are used to identify and uncover the underlying causes of hazards that were missed or created when a process or operation has slipped out of control. The focus of an incident investigation is to determine the combination of factors that came together at a point in time to create the event. It attempts to determine what actually triggered the event.

Loss-producing events are complex situations and a thorough discussion is beyond the scope of this book. However, the use of JHA can provide insights that locate the primary elements and potentially pinpoint where the event began in the course of completing the job.

The investigation process used should be presented as a positive problem-solving tool and focuses on finding the root cause, not placing blame per se. The process of gathering information on "near-misses" should be considered. It attempts to gather information on those disruptive events that can occur but did not cause damage or injury, but could have under slightly different circumstances.

SUMMARY

The JHA process begins with the development of an understanding of all aspects of the organization – many jobs requirements, specific elements, and activities necessary, on down into the required steps and tasks required within each step. The starting point in hazard review and analysis is to consider the workplace as a system of cause and effects or emerging properties with inherent hazards and associated risk built into the work environment.

Inspections and audits as similar to "tactics" and "strategy". Inspections are "tactics" used as part of a process to review specific tasks or areas. An audit, like "strategy", covers the overall process and reviews the entire organization for function and effectiveness. Inspections are the most frequently recommended activity used to assess hazards. They have been the traditional method used in regulatory and organizational safety programs

A variety of outside services may be needed from independent consultants, engineers, or other specialists to supplement internal resources. As the JHA process and the overall hazard and risk assessment findings are analyzed, the complexity of most operations requires specialists with in-depth expertise necessary to provide specific solutions.

Interviewing employees is one of the most important part of the organizational review. These interviews can range from informal conversations to gain insights on current perceptions, group discussion response sessions, hardcopy survey questionnaires, and online computer surveys.

Types of surveys range from employee opinion, attitude, satisfaction, engagement, and performance to name several. If a questionnaire is to be used, the development of the survey instrument requires special expertise so that it is not skewed toward conscious or unconsciously desired results.

Completing a direct one-on-one employee interview can tap into the current levels of expertise and knowledge about how things are actually being done. The direct employee interview provides more than just a method for gathering information. The body language, tone of voice, attitudes and general response to the interview may tell much about the actual work environment and perceptions about the organization.

"Walk-rounds" are used to conduct ongoing daily safety inspections of the workplace. This type of inspection identifies obvious or observable blatant hazards or visible risk that related to unsafe work practices or conditions.

The purpose of a focus review is to concentrate on a particular process or audit component that needs greater assistance in implementing a sustainable hazard control. It requires a specialized team that is experienced in the category of focus required.

As the JHA process begins to unfold, the why, where, and how its documents are to be stored is very important. Documents and records are reviewed to verify that what was to be documented has been properly completed and curated.

Written inspection reports record hazards identified, whose responsibility has been assigned for correction, and when corrective actions were completed.

Cross-functional or interdepartmental reviews conducted provide the specific skills and perspectives needed in reviewing the workplace.

CHAPTER REVIEW QUESTIONS

1. What does JHA provide and why is it important?
2. What is the starting point for a hazard review and analysis
3. What actions assist in selecting methods and tools to be used?
4. What are the tools that can be used to analyse the workplace?
5. Name four main features of a worksite analysis.
6. Contrast between inspections and audits.
7. Discuss the reasons inspections not effectively utilized in organizations?
8. Why are checklists important?
9. Why is it necessary to use consultant and outside specialist surveys?
10. Brainstorm a list of the types of specialist expertise that might be needed in an organization. How comprehensive is your list?
11. Why is it important to know and be skilled with interviewing techniques?
12. List the types of inspections and why they are important?
13. Discuss who and what types of expertise should review the workplace.

BIBLIOGRAPHY

Adapted from Checklists. (n.d.). Oregon Occupational Safety and Health Division (Oregon OSHA), Public Domain. Retrieved from http://bit.ly/1UvLiNm

Cox, S., & Cox, T. (1996). Safety systems, and people, MA: Butterworth-Heinemann, pp. 41.

Gawande, A. (2009). In Holt. Henry (Ed.), The checklist manifesto: how to get things right. New York: Henry Holt and Company.

Kahneman, D. (2011). Thinking, fast and slow. Farrar, Straus and Giroux.

Managing Worker Safety and Health. (n.d.). Missouri Occupational Safety and Health Administration (OSHA), Office of Cooperative Programs, Public Domain, Adapted for Use. Retrieved from http://on.mo.gov/15C4FyS

Occupational Health & Safety Management Systems. (2012). The American Society of Safety Engineers, ANSI/AIHA/ASSE Z10. Retrieved from http://bit.ly/1MsT6MG

Oregon OSHA Workshop Materials, Hazard Identification and Control. (n.d.). Oregon Occupational Safety and Health Division (Oregon OSHA), Public Domain, Permission to Reprint, Modify, and/or Adapt as necessary. Retrieved from http://bit.ly/1tg4a8A and http://bit.ly/1yIBKVk

Risk Management, ATP 5-19. (2014). Department of the Army, Public Domain.

Roughton, J. (n.d.). Safety culture – Management leadership and employee participation. Ezine Articles. Retrieved from http://bit.ly/14EuXeo

Roughton, J., & Crutchfield, N. (2008). Job hazard analysis: a guide for voluntary compliance and beyond. (Elsevier/Butterworth-Heinemann, Ed.) Chemical, Petrochemical & Process. MA: Elsevier/Butterworth-Heinemann. Retrieved from http://amzn.to/VrSAq5.

Roughton, J., & Crutchfield, N. (2013). In B. Heinemann (Ed.), Safety culture: An innovative leadership approach. Butterworth Heinemann, Retrieved from http://amzn.to/1qoD4oN.

Safety and health program management: Fact sheets. (n.d.). Safety and Health Program Management Systems eTool (OSHA), Public Domain, Based on and Adapted for Use. Retrieved from http://1.usa.gov/1A9D85S

Safety Management System (SMS) Audit. (n.d.). OTN Safety Management System Audit. Retrieved from http://bit.ly/1KK1Az8, PDF version http://bit.ly/1H6VK4M

Small Business Safety and Health Management Series, OSHA 2209-02R. (2005). Occupational Safety and Health Administration (OSHA), Public Domain. Retrieved from http://1.usa.gov/16Yv4r7

US DOE. (2009). *Concepts and principles, human performance improvement handbook* (Vol. 1). US Department of Energy. Retrieved from http://bit.ly/1DfdJVU

Appendix D Self-Inspection Checklist

This checklist is by no means all-inclusive. There are number of checklists offered by various Occupational Safety and Health Administration (OSHA), federal and state. The idea of this checklist is to add or delete items that apply to your facility; however, carefully consider each item as you come to it and then make your decision. You also will need to refer to OSHA standards for complete and specific standards that may apply to your work condition. (Note: This checklist is typical for general industry but not intended for construction or maritime.) (Small Business Safety and Health Management Series, OSHA 2209-02R, 2005)

Other Resources

We have identified several other useful resources that may help.

Safety Management System (SMS) Audit (Safety Management System (SMS) Audit, n.d.)

Oregon OSHA various checklist (Checklists, n.d.)

D.1 Sample checklist

Employer posting	Yes	No
Is the required OSHA workplace poster displayed in a prominent location where all employees are likely to see it?		
Are emergency telephone numbers posted where they can be readily found in case of emergency?		
Where employees may be exposed to any toxic substances or harmful physical agents, has appropriate information concerning employee access to medical and exposure records and "Material Safety Data Sheets" been posted or otherwise made readily available to affected employees?		
Are signs concerning "Exiting from buildings," room capacities, floor loading, biohazards, exposures to X-ray, microwave, or other harmful radiation or substances posted where appropriate?		
Is the Summary of Occupational Illnesses and Injuries (OSHA Form 200) posted in the month of February?		

Recordkeeping   Yes   No

Is all occupational injury or illnesses, except minor injuries
requiring only first aid, being recorded as required on
the OSHA log?

Are employee medical records and records of employee
exposure to hazardous substances or harmful physical agents up-to-date and in compliance with current
OSHA standards?

Are employee training records kept and accessible for review by employees, when required by OSHA standards?

Have arrangements been made to maintain required records
for the legal period of time for each specific type record?
(Some records must be maintained for at least 40 years.)

Are operating permits and records up-to-date for such items
as elevators, air pressure tanks, and liquefied petroleum
gas tanks?

Safety and health program   Yes   No

Do you have an active safety and health program in operation that deals with general safety and health program
elements as well as the management of hazards specific
to your worksite?

Is one person clearly responsible for the overall activities
of the safety and health program? Do you have a safety
committee or group made up of management and labor
representatives that meets regularly and report in writing on its activities?

Do you have a working procedure for handling in-house
employee complaints regarding safety and health?

Are you keeping your employees advised of the successful effort and accomplishments you and/or your safety
committee have made in assuring they will have a
workplace that is safe and healthful?

Have you considered incentives for employees or work-
groups who have excelled in reducing workplace
injury/illnesses?

Medical services and first aid   Yes   No

Is there a hospital, clinic, or infirmary for medical care in
proximity of your workplace?

If medical and first aid facilities are not in proximity of
your workplace, is at least one employee on each shift
currently qualified to render first aid?

Medical services and first aid	Yes	No

Have all employees who are expected to respond to medical emergencies as part of their work (1) received first-aid training; (2) had hepatitis B vaccination made available to them; (3) had appropriate training on procedures to protect them from bloodborne pathogens, including universal precautions; and (4) have available and understand how to use appropriate personal protective equipment to protect against exposure to bloodborne diseases?

Where employees have had an exposure incident involving bloodborne pathogens, did you provide an immediate post-exposure medical evaluation and follow-up?

Are medical personnel readily available for advice and consultation on matters of employees' health?

Are emergency phone numbers posted?

Are first-aid kits easily accessible to each work area, with necessary supplies available, periodically inspected and replenished as needed?

Have first-aid kit supplies been approved by a physician, indicating that they are adequate for a particular area or operation?

Are means provided for quick drenching or flushing of the eyes and body in areas where corrosive liquids or materials are handled?

Fire protection	Yes	No

Is your local fire department well acquainted with your facilities, its location and specific hazards

If you have a fire alarm system, is it certified as required?

If you have a fire alarm system, is it tested at least annually?

If you have interior standpipes and valves, are they inspected regularly?

If you have outside private fire hydrants, are they flushed at least once a year and on a routine preventive maintenance schedule?

Are fire doors and shutters in good operating condition?

Are fire doors and shutters unobstructed and protected against obstructions, including their counterweights?

Are fire door and shutter fusible links in place?

Are automatic sprinkler system water control valves, air and water pressure checked weekly/periodically as required?

Fire protection	Yes	No

Is the maintenance of automatic sprinkler systems assigned
to responsible persons or to a sprinkler contractor?

Are sprinkler heads protected by metal guards, when
exposed to physical damage?

Is proper clearance maintained below sprinkler heads?

Are portable fire extinguishers provided in adequate
number and type?

Are fire extinguishers mounted in readily accessible locations?

Are fire extinguishers recharged regularly and noted on
the inspection tag?

Are employees periodically instructed in the use of
extinguishers and fire protection procedures?

Personal protective equipment and clothing	Yes	No

Are employers assessing the workplace to determine if
hazards that require the use of personal protective
equipment (e.g., head, eye, face, hand, or foot protection) are present or are likely to be present?

Pursuant to an OSHA memorandum of July 1, 1992, employees who render first aid only as a collateral duty do
not have to be offered pre-exposure hepatitis B vaccine
only if the employer puts the following requirements into
his/her exposure control plan and implements them: (1)
the employer must record all first-aid incidents involving the presence of blood or other potentially infectious
materials before the end of the work shift during which
the first-aid incident occurred; (2) the employer must
comply with post-exposure evaluation, prophylaxis, and
follow-up requirements of the standard with respect to
"exposure incidents," as defined by the standard; (3) the
employer must train designated first-aid providers about
the reporting procedure; and (4) the employer must offer
to initiate the hepatitis B vaccination series within 24 h
to all unvaccinated first-aid providers who have rendered
assistance in any situation involving the presence of blood
or other potentially infectious materials.

If hazards or the likelihood of hazards are found, are
employers selecting and having affected employees use
properly fitted personal protective equipment suitable
for protection from these hazards?

Personal protective equipment and clothing	Yes	No

Has the employer been trained on PPE procedures, i.e., what PPE is necessary for a job tasks, when they need it, and how to properly adjust it?

Are protective goggles or face shields provided and worn where there is any danger of flying particles or corrosive materials?

Are approved safety glasses required to be worn at all times in areas where there is a risk of eye injuries such as punctures, abrasions, contusions, or burns?

Are employees who need corrective lenses (glasses or contacts) in working environments having harmful exposures, required to wear *only* approved safety glasses, protective goggles, or use other medically approved precautionary procedures?

Are protective gloves, aprons, shields, or other means provided and required where employees could be cut or where there is reasonably anticipated exposure to corrosive liquids, chemicals, blood, or other potentially infectious materials? See 29 CFR 1910.1030(b) for the definition of "other potentially infectious materials."

Are hard hats provided and worn where danger of falling objects exists?

Are hard hats inspected periodically for damage to the shell and suspension system?

Is appropriate foot protection required where there is the risk of foot injuries from hot, corrosive, poisonous substances, falling objects, crushing, or penetrating actions?

Are approved respirators provided for regular or emergency use where needed?

Is all protective equipment maintained in a sanitary condition and ready for use?

Do you have eye wash facilities and a quick Drench Shower within the work area where employees are exposed to injurious corrosive materials?

Where special equipment is needed for electrical workers, is it available?

Where food or beverages are consumed on the premises, are they consumed in areas where there is no exposure to toxic material, blood, or other potentially infectious materials?

Personal protective equipment and clothing   Yes   No

Is protection against the effects of occupational noise exposure provided when sound levels exceed those of the
OSHA noise standard?

Are adequate work procedures, protective clothing and
equipment provided and used when cleaning up spilled
toxic or otherwise hazardous materials or liquids?

Are there appropriate procedures in place for disposing
of or decontaminating personal protective equipment
contaminated with, or reasonably anticipated to be
contaminated with, blood or other potentially infectious materials?

General work environment   Yes   No

Are all worksites clean, sanitary, and orderly?

Are work surfaces kept dry or appropriate means taken to
assure the surfaces are slip-resistant?

Are all spilled hazardous materials or liquids, including
blood and other potentially infectious materials,
cleaned up immediately and according to proper
procedures?

Is combustible scrap, debris, and waste stored safely and
removed from the worksite promptly? Is all regulated
waste, as defined in the OSHA blood borne pathogens
standard (29 CFR 1910.1030), discarded according to
federal, state, and local regulations?

Are accumulations of combustible dust routinely removed
from elevated surfaces including the overhead structure
of buildings, etc.?

Is combustible dust cleaned up with a vacuum system to
prevent the dust going into suspension?

Is metallic or conductive dust prevented from entering
or accumulating on or around electrical enclosures or
equipment?

Are covered metal waste cans used for oily and paint
soaked waste?

Are all oil and gas fired devices equipped with flame
failure controls that will prevent flow of fuel if pilots or
main burners are not working?

Are paint spray booths, dip tanks, etc., cleaned regularly?

Are the minimum number of toilets and washing facilities
provided?

General work environment	**Yes**	**No**

Are all toilets and washing facilities clean and sanitary?

Are all work areas adequately illuminated?

Are pits and floor openings covered or otherwise guarded?

Have all confined spaces been evaluated for compliance
with 29 CFR 1910.146?

Walkways	**Yes**	**No**

Are aisles and passageways kept clear?

Are aisles and walkways marked as appropriate?

Are wet surfaces covered with non-slip materials?

Are holes in the floor, sidewalk or other walking surface
repaired properly, covered or otherwise made safe?

Is there safe clearance for walking in aisles where motorized or mechanical handling equipment is operating?

Are materials or equipment stored in such a way that sharp
projectives will not interfere with the walkway?

Are spilled materials cleaned up immediately?

Are changes of direction or elevations readily identifiable?

Are aisles or walkways that pass near moving or operating machinery, welding operations or similar operations
arranged so employees will not be subjected to potential
hazards?

Is adequate headroom provided for the entire length of
any aisle or walkway?

Are standard guardrails provided wherever aisle or walkway
surfaces are elevated more than 30 in. (76.20 cm) above
any adjacent floor or the ground?

Are bridges provided over conveyors and similar hazards?

Floor and wall openings	**Yes**	**No**

Are floor openings guarded by a cover, a guardrail, or
equivalent on all sides (except at entrance to stairways or
ladders)?

Are toeboards installed around the edges of permanent floor
opening (where persons may pass below the opening)?

Are skylight screens of such construction and mounting that
they will withstand a load of at least 200 pounds (90 kg)?

Is the glass in the windows, doors, glass walls, etc., which
are subject to human impact, of sufficient thickness and
type for the condition of use?

Floor and wall openings   **Yes   No**

Are grates or similar type covers over floor openings such
   as floor drains of such design that foot traffic or rolling
   equipment will not be affected by the grate spacing?

Are unused portions of service pits and pits not actually in use either covered or protected by guardrails or
   equivalent?

Are manhole covers, trench covers and similar covers, plus
   their supports designed to carry a truck rear axle load
   of at least 20,000 pounds (9,000 kg) when located in
   roadways and subject to vehicle traffic?

Are floor or wall openings in fire resistive construction
   provided with doors or covers compatible with the fire
   rating of the structure and provided with a self-closing
   feature when appropriate?

Stairs and stairways   **Yes   No**

Are standard stair rails or handrails on all stairways having
   four or more risers?

Are all stairways at least 22 in. (55.88 cm) wide?

Do stairs have landing platforms not less than 30 in.
   (76.20 cm) in the direction of travel and extend 22 in.
   (55.88 cm) in width at every 12 ft. (3.6576 m) or less of
   vertical rise?

Do stairs angle no more than 50 and no less than 30°?

Are stairs of hollow-pan type treads and landings filled to
   the top edge of the pan with solid material?

Are step risers on stairs uniform from top to bottom?

Are steps on stairs and stairways designed or provided with
   a surface that renders them slip resistant?

Are stairway handrails located between 30 (76.20 cm) and
   34 in. (86.36 cm) above the leading edge of stair treads?

Do stairway handrails have at least 3 in. (7.62 cm) of clearance between the handrails and the wall or surface they
   are mounted on?

Where doors or gates open directly on a stairway, is there
   a platform provided so the swing of the door does not
   reduce the width of the platform to less than 21 in.
   (53.34 cm)?

Are stairway handrails capable of withstanding a load of
   200 pounds (90 kg), applied within 2 in. (5.08 cm) of
   the top edge, in any downward or outward direction?

Stairs and stairways	Yes	No

Where stairs or stairways exit directly into any area where vehicles may be operated, are adequate barriers and warnings provided to prevent employees stepping into the path of traffic?

Do stairway landings have a dimension measured in the direction of travel, at least equal to the width of the stairway?

Is the vertical distance between stairway landings limited to 12 ft. (3.6576 cm) or less?

Elevated surfaces	Yes	No

Are signs posted, when appropriate, showing the elevated surface load capacity?

Are surfaces elevated more than 30 in. (76.20 cm) above the floor or ground provided with standard guardrails?

Are all elevated surfaces (beneath which people or machinery could be exposed to falling objects) provided with standard 4-in. (10.16 cm) toe boards?

Is a permanent means of access and egress provided to elevated storage and work surfaces?

Is required headroom provided where necessary?

Is material on elevated surfaces piled, stacked or racked in a manner to prevent it from tipping, falling, collapsing, rolling, or spreading?

Are dock boards or bridge plates used when transferring materials between docks and trucks or rail cars?

Exiting or egress	Yes	No

Are all exits marked with an exit sign and illuminated by a reliable light source?

Are the directions to exits, when not immediately apparent, marked with visible signs?

Are doors, passageways or stairways, that are neither exits nor access to exits, and which could be mistaken for exits, appropriately marked "NOT AN EXIT," "TO BASEMENT," "STOREROOM," etc.?

Are exit signs provided with the word "EXIT" in lettering at least 5 in. (12.70 cm) high and the stroke of the lettering at least 1/2-in. (1.2700 cm) wide?

Are exit doors side-hinged?

Are all exits kept free of obstructions?

Exiting or egress   Yes   No

Are at least two means of egress provided from elevated
platforms, pits or rooms where the absence of a second
exit would increase the risk of injury from hot, poisonous, corrosive, suffocating, flammable, or explosive
substances?

Are there sufficient exits to permit prompt escape in case
of emergency?

Are special precautions taken to protect employees during
construction and repair operations?

Is the number of exits from each floor of a building and
the number of exits from the building itself, appropriate
for the building occupancy load?

Are exit stairways that are required to be separated from
other parts of a building enclosed by at least 2-h
fire-resistive construction in buildings more than four
stories in height, and not less than 1-h fire-resistive
constructive elsewhere?

Where ramps are used as part of required exiting from a
building is the ramp slope limited to 1 ft. (0.3048 m)
vertical and 12 ft. (3.6576 m) horizontal?

Where exiting will be through frame less glass doors,
glass exit doors, or storm doors are the doors fully
tempered and meet the safety requirements for human impact?

Exit doors   Yes   No

Are doors that are required to serve as exits designed and
constructed so that the way of exit travel is obvious and
direct?

Are windows that could be mistaken for exit doors, made
inaccessible by means of barriers or railings?

Can exit doors be opened from the direction of exit travel
without the use of a key or any special knowledge or
effort when the building is occupied?

Is a revolving, sliding, or overhead door prohibited from
serving as a required exit door?

Where panic hardware is installed on a required exit door,
will it allow the door to open by applying a force of
15 pounds (6.75 kg) or less in the direction of the exit
traffic?

Exit doors	Yes	No

Are doors on cold storage rooms provided with an inside release mechanism that will release the latch and open the door even if it's padlocked or otherwise locked on the outside?

Where exit doors open directly onto any street, alley or other area where vehicles may be operated, are adequate barriers and warnings provided to prevent employees from stepping into the path of traffic?

Are doors that swing in both directions and are located between rooms where there is frequent traffic, provided with viewing panels in each door?

Portable ladders	Yes	No

Are all ladders maintained in good condition, joints between steps and side rails tight, all hardware and fittings securely attached and moveable parts operating freely without binding or undue play?

Are nonslip safety feet provided on each ladder?

Are nonslip safety feet provided on each metal or rung ladder?

Are ladder rungs and steps free of grease and oil?

Is it prohibited to place a ladder in front of doors opening toward the ladder except when the door is blocked open, locked or guarded?

Is it prohibited to place ladders on boxes, barrels, or other unstable bases to obtain additional height?

Are employees instructed to face the ladder when ascending or descending?

Are employees prohibited from using ladders that are broken, missing steps, rungs, or cleats, broken side rails or other faulty equipment?

Are employees instructed not to use the top step of ordinary stepladders as a step?

When portable rung ladders are used to gain access to elevated platforms, roofs, etc., does the ladder always extend at least 3 ft. (0.9144 m) above the elevated surface?

Is it required that when portable rung or cleat type ladders are used, the base is so placed that slipping will not occur, or it is lashed or otherwise held in place?

Portable ladders   Yes   No

Are portable metal ladders legibly marked with signs reading "CAUTION" – Do Not Use Around Electrical
   Equipment" or equivalent wording?

Are employees prohibited from using ladders as guys,
   braces, skids, gin poles, or for other than their intended
   purposes?

Are employees instructed to only adjust extension ladders
   while standing at a base (not while standing on the ladder or from a position above the ladder)?

Are metal ladders inspected for damage

Are the rungs of ladders uniformly spaced at 12 in.,
   (30.48 cm) center to center?

Hand tools and equipment   Yes   No

Are all tools and equipment (both company and employee
   owned) used by employees at their workplace in good
   condition?

Are hand tools such as chisels and punches, which develop
   mushroomed heads during use, reconditioned or replaced as necessary?

Are broken or fractured handles on hammers, axes and
   similar equipment replaced promptly?

Are worn or bent wrenches replaced regularly?

Are appropriate handles used on files and similar tools?

Are employees made aware of the hazards caused by faulty
   or improperly used hand tools?

Are appropriate safety glasses, face shields, etc., used while
   using hand tools or equipment, which might produce
   flying materials or be subject to breakage?

Are jacks checked periodically to ensure they are in good
   operating condition?

Are tool handles wedged tightly in the head of all tools?

Are tool cutting edges kept sharp so the tool will move
   smoothly without binding or skipping?

Are tools stored in dry, secure location where they won't
   be tampered with?

Is eye and face protection used when driving hardened or
   tempered spuds or nails?

Portable (power operated) tools and equipment	Yes	No

Are grinders, saws, and similar equipment provided with appropriate safety guards?

Are power tools used with the correct shield, guard, or attachment, recommended by the manufacturer?

Are portable circular saws equipped with guards above and below the base shoe?

Are circular saw guards checked to assure they are not wedged up, thus leaving the lower portion of the blade unguarded?

Are rotating or moving parts of equipment guarded to prevent physical contact?

Are all cord-connected, electrically operated tools, and equipment effectively grounded or of the approved double insulated type?

Are effective guards in place over belts, pulleys, chains, sprockets, on equipment such as concrete mixers, and air compressors?

Are portable fans provided with full guards or screens having openings 1/2 in. (1.2700 cm) or less?

Is hoisting equipment available and used for lifting heavy objects, and are hoist ratings and characteristics appropriate for the task?

Are ground-fault circuit interrupters provided on all temporary electrical 15 and 20-ampere circuits, used during periods of construction?

Are pneumatic and hydraulic hoses on power-operated tools checked regularly for deterioration or damage?

Abrasive wheel equipment grinders	Yes	No

Is the work rest used and kept adjusted to within 1/8 in. (0.3175 cm) of the wheel?

Is the adjustable tongue on the topside of the grinder used and kept adjusted to within 1/4 in. (0.6350 cm) of the wheel?

Do side guards cover the spindle, nut, and flange and 75% of the wheel diameter?

Are bench and pedestal grinders permanently mounted?

Are goggles or face shields always worn when grinding?

Is the maximum RPM rating of each abrasive wheel compatible with the RPM rating of the grinder motor?

Abrasive wheel equipment grinders	Yes	No
Are fixed or permanently mounted grinders connected to their electrical supply system with metallic conduit or other permanent wiring method?		
Does each grinder have an individual on and off control switch?		
Is each electrically operated grinder effectively grounded?		
Before new abrasive wheels are mounted, are they visually inspected and ring tested?		
Are dust collectors and powered exhausts provided on grinders used in operations that produce large amounts of dust?		
Are splashguards mounted on grinders that use coolant to prevent the coolant-reaching employees?		
Is cleanliness maintained around grinders?		

Powder-actuated tools	Yes	No
Are employees who operate powder-actuated tools trained in their use and carry a valid operator's card?		
Is each powder-actuated tool stored in its own locked container when not being used?		
Is a sign at least 7 in. (17.78 cm) by 10 in. (25.40 cm) with bold face type reading "POWDER-ACTUATED TOOL IN USE" conspicuously posted when the tool is being used		
Are powder-actuated tools left unloaded until they are actually ready to be used?		
Are powder-actuated tools inspected for obstructions or defects each day before use?		
Do powder-actuated tool operators have and use appropriate personal protective equipment such as hard hats, safety goggles, safety shoes and ear protectors?		

Machine guarding	Yes	No
Is there a training program to instruct employees on safe methods of machine operation?		
Is there adequate supervision to ensure that employees are following safe machine operating procedures?		
Is there a regular program of safety inspection of machinery and equipment?		
Is all machinery and equipment kept clean and properly maintained?		

Machine guarding	Yes	No

Is sufficient clearance provided around and between machines to allow for safe operations, set up and servicing, material handling, and waste removal?

Is equipment and machinery securely placed and anchored, when necessary to prevent tipping or other movement that could result in personal injury?

Is there a power shut-off switch within reach of the operator's position at each machine?

Can electric power to each machine be locked out for maintenance, repair, or security?

Are the noncurrent-carrying metal parts of electrically operated machines bonded and grounded? Are foot-operated switches guarded or arranged to prevent accidental actuation by personnel or falling objects?

Are manually operated valves and switches controlling the operation of equipment and machines clearly identified and readily accessible?

Are all emergency stop buttons colored red?

Are all pulleys and belts that are within 7 ft. (2.1336 m) of the floor or working level properly guarded?

Are all moving chains and gears properly guarded?

Are splashguards mounted on machines that use coolant to prevent the coolant from reaching employees?

Are methods provided to protect the operator and other employees in the machine area from hazards created at the point of operation, ingoing nip points, rotating parts, flying chips, and sparks?

Are machinery guards secure and so arranged that they do not offer a hazard in their use?

If special hand tools are used for placing and removing material, do they protect the operator's hands?

Are revolving drums, barrels, and containers required to be guarded by an enclosure that is interlocked with the drive mechanism, so that revolution cannot occur unless the guard enclosures is in place, so guarded?

Do arbors and mandrels have firm and secure bearings and are they free from play?

Are provisions made to prevent machines from automatically starting when power is restored after a power failure or shutdown?

Machine guarding	Yes	No

Are machines constructed so as to be free from excessive vibration when the largest size tool is mounted and run at full speed?

If machinery is cleaned with compressed air, is air pressure controlled and personal protective equipment or other safeguards utilized to protect operators and other workers from eye and body injury?

Are fan blades protected with a guard having openings no larger than 1/2 in. (1.2700 cm), when operating within 7 ft. (2.1336 m) of the floor?

Are saws used for ripping, equipped with antikick back devices and spreaders?

Are radial arm saws so arranged that the cutting head will gently return to the back of the table when released?

Lockout/tagout procedures	Yes	No

Is all machinery or equipment capable of movement, required to be de-energized or disengaged and locked-out during cleaning, servicing, adjusting, or setting up operations, whenever required?

Where the power disconnecting means for equipment does not also disconnect the electrical control circuit:

Are the appropriate electrical enclosures identified?

Is means provided to assure the control circuit can also be disconnected and locked-out?

Is the locking-out of control circuits in lieu of locking-out main power disconnects prohibited?

Are all equipment control valve handles provided with a means for locking-out?

Does the lockout procedure require that stored energy (mechanical, hydraulic, air, etc.) be released or blocked before equipment is locked-out for repairs?

Are appropriate employees provided with individually keyed personal safety locks?

Are employees required to keep personal control of their key(s) while they have safety locks in use?

Is it required that only the employee exposed to the hazard, place or remove the safety lock?

Is it required that employees check the safety of the lockout by attempting a startup after making sure no one is exposed?

Lockout/tagout procedures   Yes   No

Are employees instructed to always push the control circuit
stop button immediately after checking the safety of the
lockout?

Is there a means provided to identify any or all employees
who are working on locked-out equipment by their
locks or accompanying tags?

Are a sufficient number of accident preventive signs or tags
and safety padlocks provided for any reasonably foreseeable repair emergency?

When machine operations, configuration or size requires
the operator to leave his or her control station to install
tools or perform other operations, and that part of the
machine could move if accidentally activated, is such element required to be separately locked or blocked out?

In the event that equipment or lines cannot be shut down,
locked-out and tagged, is a safe job procedure established and rigidly followed?

Welding, cutting, and brazing   Yes   No

Are only authorized and trained personnel permitted to
use welding, cutting or brazing equipment?

Does each operator have a copy of the appropriate operating instructions and are they directed to follow them?

Are compressed gas cylinders regularly examined for obvious signs of defects, deep rusting, or leakage?

Is care used in handling and storing cylinders, safety valves,
and relief valves to prevent damage?

Are precautions taken to prevent the mixture of air or
oxygen with flammable gases, except at a burner or in a
standard torch?

Are only approved apparatus (torches, regulators, pressure
reducing valves, acetylene generators, and manifolds)
used?

Are cylinders kept away from sources of heat?

Are the cylinders kept away from elevators, stairs, or
gangways?

Is it prohibited to use cylinders as rollers or supports?

Are empty cylinders appropriately marked and their valves
closed?

Are signs reading: DANGER—NO SMOKING, MATCHES,
OR OPENLIGHTS, or the equivalent, posted?

Welding, cutting, and brazing   Yes   No

Are cylinders, cylinder valves, couplings, regulators, hoses, and apparatus kept free of oily or greasy substances?

Is care taken not to drop or strike cylinders?

Unless secured on special trucks, are regulators removed and valve-protection caps put in place before moving cylinders?

Do cylinders without fixed hand wheels have keys, handles, or nonadjustable wrenches on stem valves when in service?

Are liquefied gases stored and shipped valve-end up with valve covers in place?

Are provisions made to never crack a fuel gas cylinder valve near sources of ignition?

Before a regulator is removed, is the valve closed and gas released from the regulator?

Is red used to identify the acetylene (and other fuel gas) hose, green for oxygen hose, and black for inert gas and air hose?

Are pressure-reducing regulators used only for the gas and pressures for which they are intended?

Is open circuit (No Load) voltage of arc welding and cutting machines as low as possible and not in excess of the recommended limits?

Under wet conditions, are automatic controls for reducing no load voltage used?

Is grounding of the machine frame and safety ground connections of portable machines checked periodically?

Are electrodes removed from the holders when not in use?

Is it required that electric power to the welder be shut off when no one is in attendance?

Is suitable fire extinguishing equipment available for immediate use?

Is the welder forbidden to coil or loop welding electrode cable around his body?

Are wet machines thoroughly dried and tested before being used?

Are work and electrode lead cables frequently inspected for wear and damage, and replaced when needed?

Do means for connecting cable lengths have adequate insulation?

Welding, cutting, and brazing	Yes	No

When the object to be welded cannot be moved and fire hazards cannot be removed, are shields used to confine heat, sparks, and slag?

Are firewatchers assigned when welding or cutting is performed in locations where a serious fire might develop?

Are combustible floors kept wet, covered by damp sand, or protected by fire-resistant shields?

When floors are wet down, are personnel protected from possible electrical shock?

When welding is done on metal walls, are precautions taken to protect combustibles on the other side?

Before hot work is begun, are used drums, barrels, tanks, and other containers so thoroughly cleaned that no substances remain that could explode, ignite, or produce toxic vapors?

Is it required that eye protection helmets, hand shields and goggles meet appropriate standards?

Are employees exposed to the hazards created by welding, cutting, or brazing operations protected with personal protective equipment and clothing?

Is a check made for adequate ventilation in and where welding or cutting is performed?

When working in confined places, are environmental monitoring tests taken and means provided for quick removal of welders in case of an emergency?

Compressors and compressed air	Yes	No

Are compressors equipped with pressure relief valves, and pressure gauges?

Are compressor air intakes installed and equipped so as to ensure that only clean uncontaminated air enters the compressor?

Are air filters installed on the compressor intake?

Are compressors operated and lubricated in accordance with the manufacturer's recommendations?

Are safety devices on compressed air systems checked frequently?

Before any repair work is done on the pressure system of a compressor, is the pressure bled off and the system locked-out?

Compressors and compressed air	Yes	No

Are signs posted to warn of the automatic starting feature of the compressors?

Is the belt drive system totally enclosed to provide protection for the front, back, top, and sides?

Is it strictly prohibited to direct compressed air towards a person?

Are employees prohibited from using highly compressed air for cleaning purposes?

If compressed air is used for cleaning off clothing, is the pressure reduced to less than 10 psi?

When using compressed air for cleaning, do employees wear protective chip guarding and personal protective equipment?

Are safety chains or other suitable locking devices used at couplings of high-pressure hose lines where a connection failure would create a hazard?

Before compressed air is used to empty containers of liquid, is the safe working pressure of the container checked?

When compressed air is used with abrasive blast cleaning equipment, is the operating valve a type that must be held open manually?

When compressed air is used to inflate auto ties, is a clip-on chuck and an inline regulator preset to 40 psi required?

Is it prohibited to use compressed air to clean up or move combustible dust if such action could cause the dust to be suspended in the air and cause a fire or explosion hazard?

Compressors air receivers	Yes	No

Is every receiver equipped with a pressure gauge and with one or more automatic, spring-loaded safety valves?

Is the total relieving capacity of the safety valve capable of preventing pressure in the receiver from exceeding the maximum allowable working pressure of the receiver by more than 10%?

Is every air receiver provided with a drainpipe and valve at the lowest point for the removal of accumulated oil and water?

Compressors air receivers	Yes	No

Are compressed air receivers periodically drained of moisture and oil?

Are all safety valves tested frequently and at regular intervals to determine whether they are in good operating condition?

Is there a current operating permit used by the Division of Occupational Safety and Health?

Is the inlet of air receivers and piping systems kept free of accumulated oil and carbonaceous materials?

Compressed gas cylinders	Yes	No

Are cylinders with water weight capacity over 30 pounds (13.5 kg), equipped with means for connecting a valve protector device, or with a collar or recess to protect the valve?

Are cylinders legibly marked to clearly identify the gas contained?

Are compressed gas cylinders stored in areas which are protected from external heat sources such as flame impingement, intense radiant heat, electric arcs, or high-temperature lines

Are cylinders located or stored in areas where they will not be damaged by passing or falling objects or subject to tampering by unauthorized persons

Are cylinders stored or transported in a manner to prevent them from creating a hazard by tipping, falling, or rolling?

Are cylinders containing liquefied fuel gas, stored or transported in a position so that the safety relief device is always in direct contact with the vapor space in the cylinder?

Are valve protectors always placed on cylinders when the cylinders are not in use or connected for use?

Are all valves closed off before a cylinder is moved, when the cylinder is empty, and at the completion of each job?

Are low-pressure fuel-gas cylinders checked periodically for corrosion, general distortion, cracks, or any other defect that might indicate a weakness or render it unfit for service?

Compressed gas cylinders	Yes	No

Does the periodic check of low-pressure fuel-gas cylinders
include a close inspection of the cylinders' bottom?

Hoist and auxillary equipment	Yes	No

Is each overhead electric hoist equipped with a limit
device to stop the hook travel at its highest and lowest
point of safe travel?

Will each hoist automatically stop and hold any load up to
125% of its rated load if its actuating force is removed?

Is the rated load of each hoist legibly marked and visible to
the operator?

Are stops provided at the safe limits of travel for trolley
hoist?

Are the controls of hoist plainly marked to indicate the
direction of travel or motion?

Is each cage-controlled hoist equipped with an effective
warning device?

Are close-fitting guards or other suitable devices installed
on hoist to assure hoist ropes will be maintained in the
sheave groves?

Are all hoist chains or ropes of sufficient length to handle
the full range of movement of the application while still
maintaining two full wraps on the drum at all times?

Are nip points or contact points between hoist ropes
and sheaves, which are permanently located within 7 ft.
(2.1336 m) of the floor, ground or working platform,
guarded?

Is it prohibited to use chains or rope slings that are kinked
or twisted?

Is it prohibited to use the hoist rope or chain wrapped
around the load as a substitute, for a sling?

Is the operator instructed to avoid carrying loads over
people?

Industrial trucks – forklifts	Yes	No

Are only employees who have been trained in the proper
use of hoists allowed to operate them? Are only trained
personnel allowed to operate industrial trucks?

Is substantial overhead protective equipment provided on
high lift rider equipment? Are the required lift trucks
operating rules posted and enforced?

Industrial trucks – forklifts	Yes	No

Is directional lighting provided on each industrial truck that operates in an area with less than 2 ft.-candles per square foot of general lighting?

Does each industrial truck have a warning horn, whistle, gong, or other device which can be clearly heard above the normal noise in the areas where operated?

Are the brakes on each industrial truck capable of bringing the vehicle to a complete and safe stop when fully loaded?

Will the industrial trucks' parking brake effectively prevent the vehicle from moving when unattended?

Are industrial trucks operating in areas where flammable gases or vapors, or combustible dust or ignitable fibers may be present in the atmosphere, approved for such locations?

Are motorized hands and hand/rider trucks so designed that the brakes are applied, and power to the drive motor shuts off when the operator releases his or her grip on the device that controls the travel?

Are industrial trucks with internal combustion engine, operated in buildings or enclosed areas, carefully checked to ensure such operations do not cause harmful concentration of dangerous gases or fumes?

Are powered industrial trucks being safely operated?

Spraying operations	Yes	No

Is adequate ventilation assured before spray operations are started?

Is mechanical ventilation provided when spraying operations are done in enclosed areas?

When mechanical ventilation is provided during spraying operations, is it so arranged that it will not circulate the contaminated air?

Is the spray area free of hot surfaces?

Is the spray area at least 20 ft. (6.096 m) from flames, sparks, operating electrical motors and other ignition sources?

Are portable lamps used to illuminate spray areas suitable for use in a hazardous location?

Is approved respiratory equipment provided and used when appropriate during spraying operations?

Spraying operations   Yes   No

Do solvents used for cleaning have a flash point to 100°F
  or more?

Are fire control sprinkler heads kept clean?

Are "NO SMOKING" signs posted in spray areas, paint
  rooms, paint booths, and paint storage areas?

Is the spray area kept clean of combustible residue?

Are spray booths constructed of metal, masonry, or other
  substantial noncombustible material?

Are spray booth floors and baffles noncombustible and
  easily cleaned?

Is infrared drying apparatus kept out of the spray area during spraying operations?

Is the spray booth completely ventilated before using the
  drying apparatus?

Is the electric drying apparatus properly grounded?

Are lighting fixtures for spray booths located outside of the
  booth and the interior lighted through sealed clear panels?

Are the electric motors for exhaust fans placed outside
  booths or ducts?

Are belts and pulleys inside the booth fully enclosed?

Do ducts have access doors to allow cleaning?

Do all drying spaces have adequate ventilation

Entering confined spaces   Yes   No

Are confined spaces thoroughly emptied of any corrosive
  or hazardous substances, such as acids or caustics, before
  entry?

Are all lines to a confined space, containing inert, toxic,
  flammable, or corrosive materials valved off and blanked
  or disconnected and separated before entry?

Are all impellers, agitators, or other moving parts and
  equipment inside confined spaces locked-out if they
  present a hazard?

Is either natural or mechanical ventilation provided prior
  to confined space entry?

Are appropriate atmospheric tests performed to check for
  oxygen deficiency, toxic substances and explosive con-
  centrations in the confined space before entry?

Is adequate illumination provided for the work to be performed in the confined space?

Entering confined spaces	Yes	No

Is the atmosphere inside the confined space frequently tested or continuously monitored during conduct of work?

Is there an assigned safety standby employee outside of the confined space, when required, whose sole responsibility is to watch the work in progress, sound an alarm if necessary, and render assistance?

Is the standby employee appropriately trained and equipped to handle an emergency?

Is the standby employee or other employees prohibited from entering the confined space without lifelines and respiratory equipment if there is any question as to the cause of an emergency?

Is approved respiratory equipment required if the atmosphere inside the confined space cannot be made acceptable?

Is all portable electrical equipment used inside confined spaces either grounded and insulated, or equipped with ground fault protection?

Before gas welding or burning is started in a confined space, are hoses checked for leaks, compressed gas bottles forbidden inside of the confined space, torches lightly only outside of the confined area and the confined area tested for an explosive atmosphere each time before a lighted torch is to be taken into the confined space?

If employees will be using oxygen-consuming equipment – such as salamanders, torches, and furnaces, in a confined space – is sufficient air provided to assure combustion without reducing the oxygen concentration of the atmosphere below 19.5% by volume?

Whenever combustion-type equipment is used in a confined space, are provisions made to ensure the exhaust gases are vented outside of the enclosure?

Is each confined space checked for decaying vegetation or animal matter that may produce methane?

Is the confined space checked for possible industrial waste that could contain toxic properties?

If the confined space is below the ground and near areas where motor vehicles will be operating, is it possible for vehicle exhaust or carbon monoxide to enter the space?

Environmental controls   **Yes   No**

Are all work areas properly illuminated?

Are employees instructed in proper first aid and other emergency procedures?

Are hazardous substances, blood, and other potentially infectious materials identified, which may cause harm by inhalation, ingestion, or skin absorption or contact?

Are employees aware of the hazards involved with the various chemicals they may be exposed to in their work environment, such as ammonia, chlorine, epoxies, caustics, etc.?

Is employee exposure to chemicals in the workplace kept within acceptable levels?

Can a less harmful method or process be used?

Is the work area's ventilation system appropriate for the work being performed?

Are spray-painting operations done in spray rooms or booths equipped with an appropriate exhaust system?

Is employee exposure to welding fumes controlled by ventilation, use of respirators, exposure time, or other means?

Are welders and other workers nearby provided with flash shields during welding operations?

If forklifts and other vehicles are used in buildings or other enclosed areas, are the carbon monoxide levels kept below maximum acceptable concentration?

Has there been a determination that noise levels in the facilities are within acceptable levels?

Are steps being taken to use engineering controls to reduce excessive noise levels?

Are proper precautions being taken when handling asbestos and other fibrous materials?

Are caution labels and signs used to warn of hazardous substances (e.g., asbestos) and biohazards (e.g., bloodborne pathogens)?

Are wet methods used, when practicable, to prevent the emission of airborne asbestos fibers, silica dust and similar hazardous materials?

Are engineering controls examined and maintained or replaced on a scheduled basis?

Is vacuuming with appropriate equipment used whenever possible rather than blowing or sweeping dust?

Are grinders, saws, and other machines that produce respirable dusts vented to an industrial collector or central exhaust system?

Environmental controls   Yes   No

Are all local exhaust ventilation systems designed and operating properly such as airflow and volume necessary for the
application, ducts not plugged or belts slipping?

Is personal protective equipment provided, used and maintained wherever required?

Are there written standard operating procedures for the selection and use of respirators where needed?

Are restrooms and washrooms kept clean and sanitary?

Is all water provided for drinking, washing, and cooking potable?

Are all outlets for water not suitable for drinking clearly
identified?

Are employees' physical capacities assessed before being assigned to jobs requiring heavy work?

Are employees instructed in the proper manner of lifting
heavy objects?

Where heat is a problem, have all fixed work areas been provided with spot cooling or air conditioning?

Are employees screened before assignment to areas of high
heat to determine if their health condition might make
them more susceptible to having an adverse reaction?

Are employees working on streets and roadways where they
are exposed to the hazards of traffic, required to wear
bright colored (traffic orange) warning vests?

Are exhaust stacks and air intakes so located that contaminated air will not be recirculated within a building or other
enclosed area?

Is equipment producing ultraviolet radiation properly shielded?

Are universal precautions observed where occupational exposure to blood or other potentially infectious materials can
occur and in all instances where differentiation of types of
body fluids or potentially infectious materials is difficult or
impossible?

Flammable and combustible materials   Yes   No

Are combustible scrap, debris, and waste materials (oily rags,
etc.) stored in covered metal receptacles and removed from
the worksite promptly?

Is proper storage practiced to minimize the risk of fire including spontaneous combustion?

Are approved containers and tanks used for the storage and
handling of flammable and combustible liquids?

Flammable and combustible materials   Yes   No

Are all connections on drums and combustible liquid piping, vapor and liquid tight?

Are all flammable liquids kept in closed containers when not in use (e.g., parts cleaning tanks, pans, etc.)?

Are bulk drums of flammable liquids grounded and bonded to containers during dispensing?

Do storage rooms for flammable and combustible liquids have explosion-proof lights?

Do storage rooms for flammable and combustible liquids have mechanical or gravity ventilation?

Is liquefied petroleum gas stored, handled, and used in accordance with safe practices and standards?

Are "NO SMOKING" signs posted on liquefied petroleum gas tanks?

Are liquefied petroleum storage tanks guarded to prevent damage from vehicles?

Are all solvent wastes, and flammable liquids kept in fire-resistant, covered containers until they are removed from the worksite?

Is vacuuming used whenever possible rather than blowing or sweeping combustible dust?

Are firm separators placed between containers of combustibles or flammables, when stacked one upon another, to assure their support and stability?

Are fuel gas cylinders and oxygen cylinders separated by distance, and fire-resistant barriers, while in storage?

Are fire extinguishers selected and provided for the types of materials in areas where they are to be used?
• Class A Ordinary combustible material fires.
• Class B Flammable liquid, gas or grease fires.
• Class C Energized-electrical equipment fires.

Are appropriate fire extinguishers mounted within 75 ft. (2286 m) of outside areas containing flammable liquids, and within 10 ft. (3.048 m) of any inside storage area for such materials?

Are extinguishers free from obstructions or blockage?

Are all extinguishers serviced, maintained and tagged at intervals not to exceed 1 year?

Are all extinguishers fully charged and in their designated places?

Flammable and combustible materials	Yes	No

Where sprinkler systems are permanently installed, are the nozzle heads so directed or arranged that water will not be sprayed into operating electrical switchboards and equipment?

Are "NO SMOKING" signs posted where appropriate in areas where flammable or combustible materials are used or stored?

Are safety cans used for dispensing flammable or combustible liquids at a point of use?

Are all spills of flammable or combustible liquids cleaned up promptly?

Are storage tanks adequately vented to prevent the development of excessive vacuum or pressure as a result of filling, emptying, or atmosphere temperature changes?

Are storage tanks equipped with emergency venting that will relieve excessive internal pressure caused by fire exposure?

Are "NO SMOKING" rules enforced in areas involving storage and use of hazardous materials?

Hazardous chemical exposure	Yes	No

Are employees trained in the safe handling practices of hazardous chemicals such as acids, caustics, etc.?

Are employees aware of the potential hazards involving various chemicals stored or used in the workplace such as acids, bases, caustics, epoxies, and phenols?

Is employee exposure to chemicals kept within acceptable levels?

Are eye wash fountains and safety showers provided in areas where corrosive chemicals are handled?

Are all containers, such as vats, and storage tanks labeled as to their contents, e.g., "CAUSTICS"?

Are all employees required to use personal protective clothing and equipment when handling chemicals (gloves, eye protection, and respirators)?

Are flammable or toxic chemicals kept in closed containers when not in use?

Are chemical piping systems clearly marked as to their content?

Where corrosive liquids are frequently handled in open containers or drawn from storage vessels or pipelines, are adequate means readily available for neutralizing or disposing of spills or overflows and performed properly and safely?

Hazardous chemical exposure	Yes	No

Have standard operating procedures been established, and are they being followed when cleaning up chemical spills?

Where needed for emergency use, are respirators stored in a convenient, clean, and sanitary location?

Are respirators intended for emergency use adequate for the various uses for which they may be needed?

Are employees prohibited from eating in areas where hazardous chemicals are present?

Is personal protective equipment provided, used, and maintained whenever necessary?

Are there written standard operating procedures for the selection and use of respirators where needed?

If you have a respirator protection program, are your employees instructed on the correct usage and limitations of the respirators? Are the respirators NIOSH–approved for this particular application?

Are they regularly inspected and cleaned, sanitized and maintained?

If hazardous substances are used in your processes, do you have a medical or biological monitoring system in operation?

Are you familiar with the threshold limit values or permissible exposure limits of airborne contaminants and physical agents used in your workplace?

Have control procedures been instituted for hazardous materials, where appropriate, such as respirators, ventilation systems, and handling practices?

Whenever possible, are hazardous substances handled in properly designed and exhausted booths or similar locations?

Do you use general dilution or local exhaust ventilation systems to control dusts, vapors, gases, fumes, smoke, solvents or mists which may be generated in your workplace?

Is ventilation equipment provided for removal of contaminants from such operations as production grinding, buffing, spray painting, and/or vapor degreasing, and is it operating properly?

Do employees complain about dizziness, headaches, nausea, irritation, or other factors of discomfort when they use solvents or other chemicals?

Hazardous chemical exposure   Yes   No

Is there a dermatitis problem? Do employees complain about dryness, irritation, or sensitization of the skin?

Have you considered the use of an industrial hygienist or environmental health specialist to evaluate your operation?

If internal combustion engines are used, is carbon monoxide kept within acceptable levels?

Is vacuuming used, rather than blowing or sweeping dusts whenever possible for clean up?

Are materials that give off toxic asphyxiant, suffocating or anesthetic fumes, stored in remote or isolated locations when not in use?

Hazardous substances communication   Yes   No

Is there a list of hazardous substances used in your workplace?

Is there a current written exposure control plan for occupational exposure to bloodborne pathogens and other potentially infectious materials, where applicable?

Is there a written hazard communication program dealing with material safety data sheets (MSDS), labeling, and employee training?

Is each container for a hazardous substance (i.e., vats, bottles, storage tanks, etc.) labeled with product identity and a hazard warning (communication of the specific health hazards and physical hazards)?

Is there a material safety data sheet readily available for each hazardous substance used?

Is there an employee-training program for hazardous substances?

Does this program include:

• An explanation of what an MSDS is and how to use and obtain one?

• MSDS contents for each hazardous substance or class of substances?

• Explanation of "Right to Know?"

• Identification of where an employee can see the employers written hazard communication program and where hazardous substances are present in their work areas?

• The physical and health hazards of substances in the work area, and specific protective measures to be used?

• Details of the hazard communication program, including how to use the labeling system and MSDS's?

Hazardous substances communication	Yes	No

Does the employee training program on the bloodborne pathogens standard contain the following elements:
- An accessible copy of the standard and an explanation of its contents
- A general explanation of the epidemiology and symptoms of bloodborne diseases
- An explanation of the modes of transmission of bloodborne pathogens
- An explanation of the employer's exposure control plan and the means by which employees can obtain a copy of the written plan
- An explanation of the appropriate methods for recognizing tasks and the other activities that may involve exposure to blood and other potentially infectious materials
- An explanation of the use and limitations of methods that will prevent or reduce exposure including appropriate engineering controls, work practices, and personal protective equipment
- Information on the types, proper use, location, removal, handling, decontamination, and disposal of personal protective equipment
- An explanation of the basis for selection of personal protective equipment
- Information on the hepatitis B vaccine
- Information on the appropriate actions to take and persons to contact in an emergency involving blood or other potentially infectious materials
- An explanation of the procedure to follow if an exposure incident occurs, including the methods of reporting the incident and the medical follow-up that will be made available Information on post exposure evaluations and follow-up
- An explanation of signs, labels, and color-coding?

Are employees trained in the following:
- How to recognize tasks that might result in occupational exposure?
- How to use work practice and engineering controls and personal protective equipment and to know their limitations?
- How to obtain information on the types, selection, proper use, location, removal, handling, decontamination, and disposal of personal protective equipment?
- Who to contact and what to do in an emergency?

Electrical	Yes	No

Do you specify compliance with OSHA for all contract electrical work?

Are all employees required to report as soon as practicable any obvious hazard to life or property observed in connection with electrical equipment or lines?

Are employees instructed to make preliminary inspections and/or appropriate tests to determine what conditions exist before starting work on electrical equipment or lines?

When electrical equipment or lines are to be serviced, maintained or adjusted, are necessary switches opened, locked-out and tagged whenever possible?

Are portable electrical tools and equipment grounded or of the double insulated type?

Are electrical appliances such as vacuum cleaners, polishers, and vending machines grounded?

Do extension cords being used have a grounding conductor?

Are multiple plug adaptors prohibited?

Are ground-fault circuit interrupters installed on each temporary 15 or 20 A, 120 V AC circuit at locations where construction, demolition, modifications, alterations, or excavations are being performed?

Are all temporary circuits protected by suitable disconnecting switches or plug connectors at the junction with permanent wiring?

Do you have electrical installations in hazardous dust or vapor areas? If so, do they meet the National Electrical Code (NEC) for hazardous locations?

Is exposed wiring and cords with frayed or deteriorated insulation repaired or replaced promptly?

Are flexible cords and cables free of splices or taps?

Are clamps or other securing means provided on flexible cords or cables at plugs, receptacles, tools, equipment, etc., and is the cord jacket securely held in place?

Are all cord, cable and raceway connections intact and secure?

In wet or damp locations, are electrical tools and equipment appropriate for the use or location or otherwise protected?

Electrical	Yes	No

Is the location of electrical power lines and cables (overhead, underground, underfloor, other side of walls)
determined before digging, drilling or similar work is
begun?

Are metal measuring tapes, ropes, handlines or similar devices
with metallic thread woven into the fabric prohibited
where they could come in contact with energized parts of
equipment or circuit conductors?

Is the use of metal ladders prohibited in areas where the ladder
or the person using the ladder could come in contact with
energized parts of equipment, fixtures or circuit conductors?

Are all disconnecting switches and circuit breakers labeled to
indicate their use or equipment served?

Are disconnecting means always opened before fuses are
replaced?

Do all interior wiring systems include provisions for
grounding metal parts of electrical raceways, equipment
and enclosures?

Are all electrical raceways and enclosures securely fastened
in place?

Are all energized parts of electrical circuits and equipment
guarded against accidental contact by approved cabinets or
enclosures?

Is sufficient access and working space provided and maintained about all electrical equipment to permit ready and
safe operations and maintenance?

Are all unused openings (including conduit knockouts) in
electrical enclosures and fittings closed with appropriate
covers, plugs or plates?

Are electrical enclosures such as switches, receptacles, and
junction boxes, provided with tight fitting covers or plates?

Are disconnecting switches for electrical motors in excess
of two horsepower, capable of opening the circuit when
the motor is in a stalled condition, without exploding?
(Switches must be horsepower rated equal to or in excess
of the motor hp rating.)

Is low voltage protection provided in the control device of
motors driving machines or equipment that could cause
probable injury from inadvertent starting?

Is each motor disconnecting switch or circuit breaker located
within sight of the motor control device?

Electrical   Yes   No

Is each motor located within sight of its controller or the
  controller disconnecting means capable of being locked
  in the open position or is a separate disconnecting
  means installed in the circuit within sight of the motor?

Is the controller for each motor in excess of two horsepower, rated in horsepower equal to or in excess of the
  rating of the motor it serves?

Are employees who regularly work on or around energized electrical equipment or lines instructed in the
  cardiopulmonary resuscitation (CPR) methods?

Are employees prohibited from working alone on energized lines or equipment over 600 V?

Noise   Yes   No

Are there areas in the workplace where continuous noise
  levels exceed 85 dBA?

Is there an ongoing preventive health program to educate
  employees in: safe levels of noise, exposures; effects of
  noise on their health; and the use of personal protection?

Have work areas where noise levels make voice communication between employees difficult been identified and
  posted?

Are noise levels being measured using a sound level meter
  or an octave band analyzer and are records being kept?

Have engineering controls been used to reduce excessive
  noise levels? Where engineering controls are determined
  not feasible, are administrative controls (i.e., worker
  rotation) being used to minimize individual employee
  exposure to noise?

Is approved hearing protective equipment (noise attenuating
  devices) available to every employee working in noisy
  areas?

Have you tried isolating noisy machinery from the rest of
  your operation?

If you use ear protectors, are employees properly fitted and
  instructed in their use?

Are employees in high noise areas given periodic audio-
  metric testing to ensure that you have an effective hearing protection system?

Fueling   Yes   No

Is it prohibited to fuel an internal combustion engine with a
flammable liquid while the engine is running?

Are fueling operations done in such a manner that likelihood
of spillage will be minimal?

When spillage occurs during fueling operations, is the spilled
fuel washed away completely, evaporated, or other measures
taken to control vapors before restarting the engine?

Are fuel tank caps replaced and secured before starting the
engine?

In fueling operations, is there always metal contact between
the container and the fuel tank?

Are fueling hoses of a type designed to handle the specific
type of fuel?

Is it prohibited to handle or transfer gasoline in open containers?

Are open lights, open flames, sparking, or arcing equipment
prohibited near fueling or transfer of fuel operations?

Is smoking prohibited in the vicinity of fueling operations?

Are fueling operators prohibited in buildings or other enclosed
areas that are not specifically ventilated for this purpose?

Where fueling or transfer of fuel is done through a gravity
flow system, are the nozzles of the self closing type?

Identification of piping systems   Yes   No

When nonpotable water is piped through a facility, are outlets
or taps posted to alert employees that it is unsafe and not
to be used for drinking, washing or other personal use?

When hazardous substances are transported through above
ground piping, is each pipeline identified at points
where confusion could introduce hazards to employees?

When pipelines are identified by color painting, are all visible parts of the line so identified?

When pipelines are identified by color painted bands or
tapes, are the bands or tapes located at reasonable intervals and at each outlet, valve or connection?

When pipelines are identified by color, is the color code
posted at all locations where confusion could introduce
hazards to employees?

When the contents of pipelines are identified by name or
name abbreviation, is the information readily visible on
the pipe near each valve or outlet?

Identification of piping systems	Yes	No

When pipelines carrying hazardous substances are identified by tags, are the tags constructed of durable materials, the message carried clearly and permanently distinguishable and are tags installed at each valve or outlet?

When pipelines are heated by electricity, steam or other external source, are suitable warning signs or tags placed at unions, valves, or other serviceable parts of the system?

Material handling	Yes	No

Is there safe clearance for equipment through aisles and doorways?

Are aisleways designated, permanently marked, and kept clear to allow unhindered passage?

Are motorized vehicles and mechanized equipment inspected daily or prior to use?

Are vehicles shut off and brakes set prior to loading or unloading?

Are containers of combustibles or flammables, when stacked while being moved, always separated by dunnage sufficient to provide stability?

Are dock boards (bridge plates) used when loading or unloading operations are taking place between vehicles and docks?

Are trucks and trailers secured from movement during loading and unloading operations?

Are dock plates and loading ramps constructed and maintained with sufficient strength to support imposed loading?

Are hand trucks maintained in safe operating condition?

Are chutes equipped with sideboards of sufficient height to prevent the materials being handled from falling off?

Are chutes and gravity roller sections firmly placed or secured to prevent displacement?

At the delivery end of the rollers or chutes, are provisions made to brake the movement of the handled materials?

Are pallets usually inspected before being loaded or moved

Material handling	Yes	No

Are hooks with safety latches or other arrangements used
when hoisting materials so that slings or load attachments won't accidentally slip off the hoist hooks?

Are securing chains, ropes, chockers, or slings adequate
for the job to be performed?

When hoisting material or equipment, are provisions
made to assure no one will be passing under the suspended loads?

Are material safety data sheets available to employees
handling hazardous substances?

Transporting employees and materials	Yes	No

Do employees who operate vehicles on public thorough-
fares have valid operator's licenses?

When seven or more employees are regularly transported
in a van, bus or truck, is the operator's license appropriate for the class of vehicle being driven?

Is each van, bus or truck used regularly to transport
employees equipped with an adequate number of
seats?

When employees are transported by truck, are provisions
provided to prevent their falling from the vehicle?

Are vehicles used to transport employees equipped with
lamps, brakes, horns, mirrors, windshields and turn
signals and are they in good repair?

Are transport vehicles provided with handrails, steps, stir-
rups or similar devices, so placed and arranged that
employees can safely mount or dismount?

Are employee transport vehicles equipped at all times with
at least two reflective type flares?

Is a full charged fire extinguisher, in good condition, with
at least 4 BC rating maintained in each employee transport vehicle?

When cutting tools or tools with sharp edges are carried in passenger compartments of employee transport
vehicles, are they placed in closed boxes or containers,
which are secured in place?

Are employees prohibited from riding on top of any load,
which can shift, topple, or otherwise become unstable?

Control of harmful substances by ventilation	Yes	No

Is the volume and velocity of air in each exhaust system sufficient to gather the dusts, fumes, mists, vapors or gases to be controlled, and to convey them to a suitable point of disposal?

Are exhaust inlets, ducts, and plenums designed, constructed, and supported to prevent collapse or failure of any part of the system?

Are clean-out ports or doors provided at intervals not to exceed 12 ft. (3.6576 m) in all horizontal runs of exhaust ducts?

Where two or more different type of operations are being controlled through the same exhaust system, will the combination of substances being controlled, constitute a fire, explosion or chemical reaction hazard in the duct?

Is adequate makeup air provided to areas where exhaust systems are operating?

Is the source point for makeup air located so that only clean, fresh air, which is free of contaminates, will enter the work environment?

Where two or more ventilation systems are serving a work area, is their operation such that one will not offset the functions of the other?

Sanitizing equipment and clothing	Yes	No

Is personal protective clothing or equipment that employees are required to wear or use, of a type capable of being cleaned easily and disinfected?

Are employees prohibited from interchanging personal protective clothing or equipment, unless it has been properly cleaned?

Are machines and equipment, which process, handle or apply materials that could be injurious to employees, cleaned and/or decontaminated before being overhauled or placed in storage?

Are employees prohibited from smoking or eating in any area where contaminates that could be injurious if ingested are present?

Sanitizing equipment and clothing	Yes	No

When employees are required to change from street clothing into protective clothing, is a clean change room
with separate storage facility for street and protective
clothing provided?

Are employees required to shower and wash their hair as
soon as possible after a known contact has occurred
with a carcinogen?

When equipment, materials, or other items are taken into
or removed from a carcinogen regulated area, is it done
in a manner that will contaminate nonregulated areas or
the external environment?

Tire inflation	Yes	No

Where tires are mounted and/or inflated on drop center
wheels is a safe practice procedure posted and enforced?

Where tires are mounted and/or inflated on wheels with
split rims and/or retainer rings, is a safe practice procedure posted and enforced?

Does each tire inflation hose have a clip-on chuck with at
least 24 in. (6.9 cm) of hose between the chuck and an
in-line hand valve and gauge?

Does the tire inflation control valve automatically shutoff
the airflow when the valve is released?

Is a tire-restraining device such as a cage, rack or other
effective means used while inflating tires mounted on
split rims, or rims using retainer rings?

Are employees strictly forbidden from taking a position directly over or in front of a tire while it's being inflated?

CHAPTER SEVEN

Enhancing the Safety Management System in Managing Risk

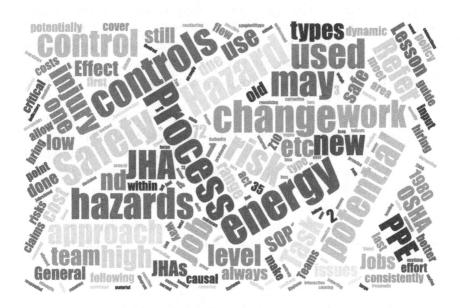

"Any policy or rule ignored is a policy or rule rewritten"

—Anon

Chapter Objectives

At the end of the chapter, you should be able to:

- Discuss the nature of organization as being dynamic and not static
- Discuss why the JHA can be considered the centerpiece and link between the elements of the safety process
- Outline and discuss the hierarchy of controls and how it is used for determining the actions necessary to control hazards
- Outline and discuss Haddon's countermeasures for the control of hazards
- Discuss the differences between the hierarchy of controls and Haddon's countermeasures and why each should be considered in a safety process
- Discuss various organizational traits and activities that impact the safety process and that should be considered in the JHA process.

Job Hazard Analysis. http://dx.doi.org/10.1016/B978-0-12-803441-5.00007-6

7.1 ORGANIZATIONS ARE DYNAMIC AND NOT STATIC

As discussed earlier, organizations are dynamic and are always in a state of flux, ever changing. This change is due to many types of internal and external influences, which are always present and do not always act consistently. Change can range from the daily variations in human performance to shifts in production and can impact many areas from general maintenance of facilities and equipment to administrative practice, training, and hiring. Influences are not just internal to the organization but are impacted by the environment of regulatory, market, industry, and other factors.

The leadership team may or may not be sensitive to these influences and allow the creation of conditions that effect the safety of employees, the environment, and the overall organization. Implementing a safety system helps to provide a structure that monitors a full range of activities from risk assessment, hazard identification, and correction tracking to develop consistent rules, procedures, and safe work practices.

When used in conjunction with a safety system, the JHA process can provide indicators that loss potential is increasing or not being effectively control.

7.2 THE CENTERPIECE AND CRITICAL LINK

The premise is that the JHA should be considered the centerpiece for a safety system to operate effectively. JHA provides the critical linkage between all aspects of a safety management system. The following are examples using several ANSI/AIHA/ASSE, Z10 elements:

- Hierarchy of controls: Without an understanding of a job's hazards and associated risk, assumption are made on selecting the hazard control level potentially leaving a high risk still uncontrolled.
- Feedback to the planning process: Without the JHA input, planning may focus on low risk and not adequately budget or establish corrective action criteria.
- OHSMS policy: Without the JHA, the policy may focus on issues of low risk.
- Responsibilities and authority: This area may not be strongly defined as the details of the actual activities with their hazards and associated risk remaining vague and/or unknown.

A causal loop concept can be used to better understand the linkage between the JHA process and the safety system. "Interactions are not linear as system components do not flow along one path from "A to B to C, etc" (Senge, 2006) (Figure 7.1). Each component may have multiple connections with consequences that should be considered. Refer to Figure 7.2 for

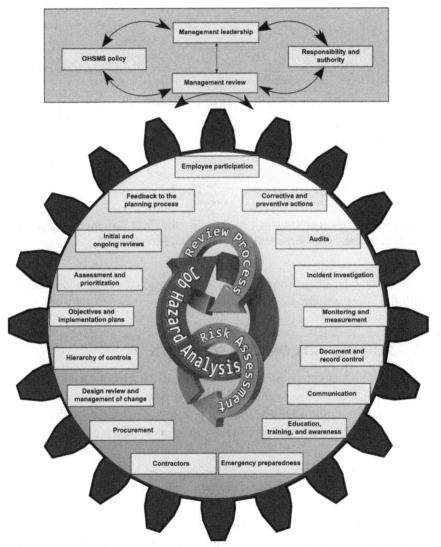

Figure 7.1 *Overview of ANSI/AIHA/ASSE Safety Management System Interactions with the Job Hazard Analysis. Based on and adapted using the ANSI/AIHA/ASSE, Z10-2012 as a model.*

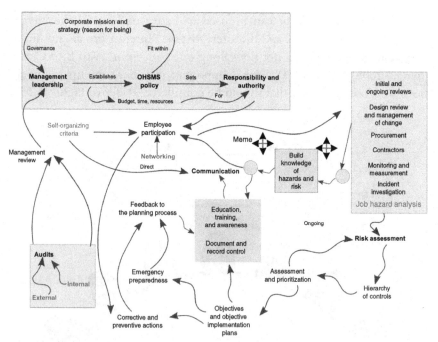

Figure 7.2 *Visualization of Various Component Interaction with the Safety System.* *Based on and adapted using the ANSI/AIHA/ASSE, Z10-2012 as a model.*

a "spaghetti-type" diagram will allow the user a way to visualize interactions with the safety system.

7.3 HAZARD CONTROL CONCEPTS

This linkage can be used to provide essential information for the leadership team and employees about the scope and severity of hazards and risk exposure. With this linkage, the leadership team can better weigh the impact of changes in job related tasks with a more informed decision approach.

> A great hazard control program is worthless if the individual will not or cannot follow the desired hazard and risk control criteria.

After job-related hazards have been identified by JHAs, determining the control methods and types begins. Two primary tools can be used in the development of controls within a job's tasks and steps – The Hierarchy of Controls and Haddon's countermeasures.

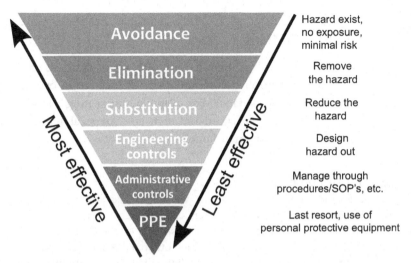

Figure 7.3 *Overview of the Hierarchy of Controls. Based on and adapted using the Center for Disease Control and Prevention (CDC) Hierarchy of Controls, Workplace Safety and Health Topics.*

7.4 HIERARCHY OF CONTROLS

The "Hierarchy of Controls" as defined by the ANSI/AIHA/ASSE, Z10 "provides a systemic way to determine the most effective feasible method to reduce risk associated with the hazard" (Occupational Health & Safety Management Systems, 2012)(Figure 7.3). The Hierarchy of Controls follows a tiered approach that begins with total hazard avoidance and ends with personal protection if the hazard(s) cannot be eliminated.

7.5 AVOIDANCE

No exposure to a hazard(s) is allowed. Risk of injury or damage is zero, as no exposure exist. This is accomplished by eliminating or removing exposure to the hazard(s) by changing work methods, tools, material, equipment, and the environment, anything that is a potential hazard is removed so there is no exposure. The risk is entirely eliminated.

When conducting the assessment of an operation, the first question to be asked is: Does this activity or task have to do to be done? Is the activity or task essential to the operation or job? If not essential or no purpose is served, can the hazard(s) be removed, avoided, or completely eliminated from the operation? No possible exposure translates into no risk.

7.6 SUBSTITUTION

Substitution is replacing a high hazard with a less hazardous element or activity that can be controlled. A hazard may still exist but its overall risk is at an acceptable level of tolerance. For example, substituting a low or no hazardous chemical for a high hazard and high-risk chemical, removes the higher hazard from the work environment.

Lesson Learned #1

During an industrial hygiene study, it was found that an operation was using a large quantity of a harmful chemical to the extent that it was causing employee illnesses. The question was asked: "Do you have to use this much?" The leadership team looked at each other and responded by saying: "We have never been asked that question before!!" The chemical blend was changed and a study confirmed that they only needed to use a minimal amount at a time. The change in process eliminated the hazard and in turn saved them considerable money.

7.7 ENGINEERING AND DESIGN

Engineering controls design the environment, the process, equipment, and/or materials to directly eliminate or control the hazard(s). The hazard may be completely removed or if it still exists, mechanisms are in place to contain it. This level attempts to remove latent human error potential from the process as well as control the scope and nature of hazards and associated risks (Prevention through Design, 2012).

"The initial cost of engineering controls can be higher than the cost of administrative controls or PPE, but over the longer term, operating costs are frequently lower, and in some instances, can provide a cost savings in other areas of the process" (Prevention through Design, 2012).

Engineering controls focus on the direct source of the hazard(s). The basic concept of engineering control(s) is that the work environment and required activity should be designed in such a manner that eliminates hazards or at least reduces the exposure. Potential solutions for example may be adding a guard to cover moving parts, adding an interlock to shut down the equipment when a guard is open, improving ventilation controls, changing work flow, using new technology, etc (Oregon OSHA Workshop Materials, Hazard Identification and Control, n.d.).

7.8 ADMINISTRATIVE

Administrative control(s) are used to communicate actions necessary to minimize any exposure to hazards. Administrative methods are used to advise, warn, train, alert, etc., that a hazard(s) exist and the protocols and procedures are to be used. Administrative methods attempt to reduce active human error potential by behavioral controls.

Administrative control(s) is a "paper work" function that tells what to do to be safe but does not monitor activities nor eliminate or reduce the hazard and the associated risk. Employees are most likely to forget written administrative procedure(s) unless an ongoing refresher is provided.

7.9 PERSONAL PROTECTIVE EQUIPMENT

Personal protective equipment (PPE) is the last line of defense against job related hazards (Safety and Health Program Management: Fact Sheets, n.d.). PPE reduces the risk of injury through head, eye, arm/hand, body, leg, foot, hearing, and respiratory protective gear.

A PPE risk assessment is used to ensure the PPE is properly selected for both the hazard and to the employee exposed to the hazard (Managing Worker Safety and Health, n.d.). The JHA provides the information and starting point for the PPE risk assessment. Do not assume that the purchasing department or the leadership team understands PPE selection.

Refer to Appendix E for resources that can help you to develop a successful personal protective equipment (PPE) assessment for inclusion into the JHA form (PPE Assessment, n.d.).

Lesson Learned #2

In one company, a military CS (riot gas) mask was found for use for emergencies. The recommendation was for a specific respirator for a certain area and the purchasing manager thought that "one mask was the same as any other." Unfortunately, linking the purchase to the hazard was not a part of their buying process.

Lesson Learned #3

A conflict can easily develop when the administrative controls demand the use of PPE without understanding all of the considerations necessary for PPE selection, fitting, use, etc. *"One size does not fit all"*.

7.10 HADDON'S ENERGY APPROACH

A classic strategy to reduce the potential for injury was developed by William Haddon and provides a systematic approach to controlling hazards. His concept list a series of actions that reduce the consequences of what he termed "energy transfer."

Energy was categorized in the forms of kinetic, thermal, chemical, electrical, biological, acoustic, and radiation (Haddon, 1980).

The approach can be used in conjunction with the hierarchy of controls to review or revise workplace hazard control measures. Haddon's approach can be integrated into the JHA process as it focuses on eliminating, controlling, modifying, and mitigating various energy types and reducing their potential harmful effects.

Energy Release Theory

"... an accident is caused by energy out of control. The theory states that various techniques can be employed to reduce accidents, including preventing the buildup of energy, reducing the initial amount of energy, preventing the release of energy, carefully controlling the release of energy, and separating the energy being released from the living or nonliving object" (Energy Release Theory, n.d.).

These strategies included:

1. Preventing the initial energy buildup. Can the energy type be avoided?
2. Reducing the amount of energy. Can the energy level be reduced?
3. Preventing the release of the energy. How can the energy be contained?
4. Modifying the rate of release of energy from its source. How can the energy release be limited, slowed or reduced so that its harm is reduced?
5. Separating in space or time the energy being released. How can the energy be kept separated from potentially exposed individuals?
6. Separating the energy being released from the susceptible individuals or structures or barriers. Can adequate barriers (guards) be placed between potential target persons and/or objects?

7. Modifying the contact surface, subsurface, or basic structure, which can be impacted. What can be done to modify the exposed individuals and or structures?

8. Strengthening the structure, which might be damaged by an energy release. What can be done to harden individuals or structures against the hazardous effects of the energy release?

9. Rapid detection and evaluation of damage and countermeasures to reduce energy release continuation and extension. What countermeasures or emergency response plans are immediately needed should the energy release or contact made with the target individuals or objects?

Based on and adapted from (Haddon, 1980).

These energy-related measures cover the time between the damaging energy release or transfer and the final stabilization of the situation (Collins, n.d.). Different energy types have different hazards and potential risk severity. Overlapping energy types will require specific controls based on the nature of the hazard(s) scope and the nature of the targets of the hazard (Haddon, 1980).

Case Study #1

A technician climbs a ladder (kinetic energy), uses a bug spray (chemical energy) to kill a wasp nest (biological energy), then proceeds to complete a task of working with electrical equipment (electrical energy) and tools that may have a high noise level (acoustic energy). The technician may be working on a hot, humid day (thermal energy) and in the sun (radiation energy). Each of these energy types as identified by Haddon will require a different approach to their control for hazards and risk that would be present.

7.11 OTHER AREAS FOR CONSIDERATION

7.11.1 Work Practice Controls

Work practice controls are administrative controls that define the methods used to perform a task in order to reduce potential hazards. They are integrated into job procedures and general safety work rules. A comprehensive JHA is used to develop work practices controls and the implementing of specific training. Work practices are used in conjunction with and not as a substitute for engineering controls.

7.12 GENERAL SAFETY RULES

Safety rules define what behaviors are expected while jobs are being completed. Safety rules are used to establish and guide employees when undertaking any activity or task. Rules are most effective when clearly written, communicated, and discussed with all employees. A combination of individual one-on-one, small groups or work teams, department and organization-wide meetings are used (Appendix F) (Small Business Safety and Health Management Series OSHA 2209-02R 2005).

Lesson Learned #4

One of the authors observed in one organization a process of turning injury-related causal factors into rules that were incorporated into a comprehensive *"Book of Safety Rules."* This book had grown to 35 pages of mandated rules over the years, along with many documented causes of injuries. Every time a new injury occurred, the *Book of Safety Rules* would be reviewed to identify what "violation" may have transpired. If a rule was found in the book based on a past injury, then that rule would be applied to the current injury and disciplinary action would be taken against the injured employee. As employees were expected to know the 35 or so pages of rules, the ever-growing book was used as primarily as a disciplinary tool and its original intent was lost (Roughton & Crutchfield, 2013).

7.13 STANDARD OPERATING PROCEDURES

The JHA has the potential to provide the overall foundation for standard operating procedures (SOP). The JHA's primary focus is on the control, reduction, or removal of hazards and identifying the consequences of exposure. The SOP details the quality control requirements, criteria for the service or specific product production or delivery, the time requirements, employee requirements, and all other details necessary to do the job. Refer to Table 7.1 for an overview of areas where the JHA can assist the SOP process

Table 7.1 Overview of areas where the JHA can assists the SOP process

- Job orientation criteria.
- Enhances training criteria.
- Aligns steps/tasks, tools/equipment/materials, job environment, current policies/procedures, people doing the job.
- Points out potential gaps in efficient job completion.
- Allows updating of inspection forms, checklist, guidelines and job observation criteria.

7.14 EMPLOYEE CHANGES

Employee changes can be divided into three basic areas:
- Changes in staffing
- Individual change
- Temporary workers

7.15 CHANGES IN STAFFING

New or recently transferred employees do not bring job experience or expertise to their new assignments nor do they have an understanding of the hazards and risks inherent in the new or different work environment. Without in-depth training (based on findings of JHAs), mentoring, and supervision, the potential for injury and/or damage is greatly increased. From experience with injury claims analysis, a surge in injuries appears in the first six months of employment. Nonroutine tasks even by experienced employees fall into this category.

A worksite having a high turnover of employees can be expected to have a high potential for injuries unless the job activity or task are of very low hazard or that the hazards are engineered totally out of the production process which is not 100% feasible.

Paralleling turnover as an issue is not having enough employees to adequately staff a production or service process. For example, longer work hours might be required and the accompanying physical and mental stress may increase the potential for human errors and the resulting loss-producing event (US DOE, 2009a,b).

7.16 INDIVIDUAL CHANGE

Physical and mental variations can occur due to temporary or chronic medical problems, partially disabling conditions, stress from family responsibilities, personal crisis, and other life changing issues. Alcohol or drug abuse can directly impact on the potential for error resulting in injury. An aging workforce may be unable to meet the demands and stress of the workplace.

The analysis of personal change can provide a perspective on the level of the hierarchy of controls to use while Haddon's energy approach provides insights on addressing the control of energy forces. Physical and/or administrative methods can then be designed to ensure that workplace conditions remain consistently safe.

Administrative controls should be fully coordinated within the organization to ensure individual mental and physical skills and expected changes overtime are factored into hiring practices as well as meet safety and labor law compliance.

7.17 TEMPORARY WORKERS

The last category is temporary workers that have increased as organizations search for ways to reduce costs, avoid regulatory issues, increase flexibility as market conditions change, etc. This group is usually not treated the same as regular employees as they are under separate temporary service company leadership. Depending on the contracts, they may not be as trained or experienced appropriately for the task being performed.

With this increase in temporary workers, the Occupational Safety and Health Administration (OSHA) has implemented a major effort to provide guidance and mandates to employers who use temporary workers (Policy Background on the Temporary Worker Initiative, 2014). The JHA process is no different for permanent or temporary workers.

7.14 ADAPTING TO CHANGE

Change analysis provides a side-by-side comparison of an older process against changes made necessary by a proposed new process. A change analysis may include:
- Developing a process map detailing and overlaying the old process versus the new process, noting the differences.
- Developing cause and effect diagrams of the current versus proposed changes.
- Comparing JHA's steps and task currently being performed against the proposed change. Jobs viewed at a high level may appear to have the same requirements and only after comparing the required steps and tasks will the differences be made visible.
- Comparing the old work environment against the proposed changes to determine what environmental elements may change, that is, ventilation, lighting, air quality, temperatures, environmental, etc.?
- Comparing old policies, procedures, and protocols against new requirements to determine what is no longer relevant and what

needs to be updated or modified. New regulatory requirements may be introduced and new technology may make current administrative controls obsolete.

- Comparing the current organizational changes to determine if the leadership team is still adequate and if additional or different employees will be needed due to changing physical and mental skill needs
- Completing a comprehensive risk assessment using the process maps and JHA comparisons.

Any change to a process is a crucial step and should consider the potential effect on all areas of an operation. All affected employees should be consulted on what is being changed to gather their input. Once the change is complete, employees should be provided the appropriate education and training and attention given to the employee responses with the change monitored until everyone has adapted.

Management of Change

"OSHA believes that contemplated changes to a process must be thoroughly evaluated to fully assess their impact on employee safety and health and to determine needed changes to operating procedures. To this end, the standard contains a section on procedures for managing changes to processes. Written procedures to manage changes (except for "replacements in kind") to process chemicals, technology, equipment, and procedures, and change to facilities that affect a covered process, must be established and implemented. These written procedures must ensure that the following considerations are addressed prior to any change:

The technical basis for the proposed change,
- Impact of the change on employee safety and health,
- Modifications to operating procedures,
- Necessary time period for the change, and
- Authorization requirements for the proposed change.
- Employees who operate a process and maintenance and contract employees whose job tasks will be affected by a change in the process must be informed of, and trained in, the change prior to startup of the process or startup of the affected part of the process. If a change covered by these procedures results in a change in the required process safety information, such information also must be updated accordingly. If a change covered by these procedures changes the required operating procedures or practices, they also must be updated (Process Safety Management OSHA 3132, 2000).

Refer to Appendix G for an "Example of Safety Review of New/Relocated Equipment Major Modification Sign-Off Form" have been used by the authors with some success. This sign-off procedure can apply to any type of installation, whether it is new modified, relocated equipment, a chemical process, etc.

7.19 PREDICTIVE VERSUS REACTIVE

The immediate urgency of injury reduction by its nature draws any time and budget away from a focus on the true underlying causes of any loss-producing event. A safety professional can easily be drawn into (or required) to act as the lead person in claims management, which is reactive to an already developed situation. This approach can be alluring as it can be very active and even exciting involving legal and financial elements that give the appearance that problems are being resolved. As a result, the organization responds to the past and drifts away from focus on predictive actions to reduce system failures and human error potential. Establishing intent to shift to a predictive mode is the ideal goal but does require a constant effort to bring a risk assessment approach into the organization (Figure 7.4) (Task Analysis Tools Used Throughout Development, Human Error Analysis, n.d.).

The safety system should identify activity that can be defined as reactive, proactive, or predictive. The structure of a safety system provides organizations greater insight into their operational environment, generating process

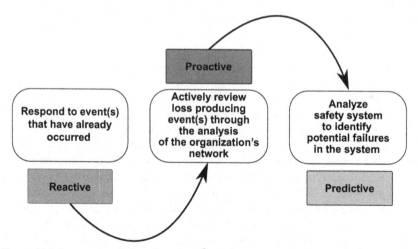

Figure 7.4 *Integrating Safety Concepts into the Reactive, Proactive, and Predictive System.* *Based on and adapted from Safety Management System Basis, Federal Aviation Administration (FAA).*

efficiencies and cost avoidance (Safety Management System Basis Public Domain, 2014).

7.20 OTHER ANALYTICAL TOOLS FOR CONSIDERATION

Various analytical tools can be used in conjunction with the JHA process. These are used for specific purposes or conditions depending on the industry and range widely complexity. Examples would include – Process Hazard Analysis, "What-If" Analysis and Checklists for scenario development, Hazard and Operability Studies (HAZOP), Failure Mode and Effect Analysis (FMEA), "Fault-tree" Analysis, Activity Hazard Analysis (Appendix H).

SUMMARY

A safety process should be able to balance and coordinate its many elements to be effective. When implemented within the safety process, the JHA becomes the centerpiece that provides the critical linkage between process elements and the risk assessment.

Organizations are dynamic and are always in some state of flux. They are subject to ongoing changes some of which occur over time and many that can without warning (Roughton & Crutchfield, 2013). Organizations change due to many types of internal and external influences. These influences are always present and do not always act consistently.

The premise is that the JHA when considered the centerpiece for a safety process provides the critical linkage between all aspects of a safety management system.

The view of the JHA as the linkage is used to provide essential information for the leadership team and employees about the scope and severity of hazards and risk exposure. With this information the leadership team can then better weigh the impact of changes in job related tasks and select more informed decisions as loss producing consequences are made visible.

The "hierarchy of controls" follows a tiered approach that begins with total hazard avoidance and ends with personal protection if the hazard(s) cannot be eliminated.

Personal protective equipment (PPE) is the last line of defense against job related hazards. The nature of the work and other factors may prevent the use of engineering, avoidance, or substitution leaving the need for a combination of administrative and PPE as the primary controls remaining.

A classic strategy to reduce the potential for injury was developed by William Haddon and provides a systematic approach to controlling hazards.

His concepts list a series of actions that reduce the consequences of what he termed "energy transfer."

Energy was categorized in the forms of kinetic, thermal, chemical, electrical, biological, acoustic, and radiation.

Work practice controls are administrative controls that define the methods used to perform a task in order to reduce potential hazards.

Safety rules define what behaviors are expected while jobs are being completed. They are to establish and guide employees and what flexibility is allowed when undertaking tasks.

The SOP details the quality control requirements, criteria for the service or specific product production or delivery, the time requirements, personnel requirements, and all other details necessary to do the job.

Employee changes can be divided into three basic areas: Changes in staffing, individual change, and temporary workers

Change analysis provides a side-by-side comparison of an older process against changes made necessary by a proposed new process.

The immediate urgency of injury reduction by its nature draws any time and budget away from a focus on the true underlying causes of any loss-producing events.

Various analytical tools can be used in conjunction with the JHA process. Examples include – Process hazard analysis, "What-If" analysis and Checklists for scenario development, Hazard and Operability Studies (HAZOP), Failure Mode and Effect Analysis (FMEA), "Fault-tree" Analysis, Activity Hazard Analysis.

CHAPTER REVIEW QUESTIONS

1. When should a hazard identification and assessment analysis be conducted?
2. Define the hierarchy of controls
3. What is the underlying concept of Haddon's Countermeasures and why are they important?
4. How are engineering controls used to minimize hazards and risk?
5. What are examples of administrative controls?
6. Why is PPE considered the last resort to controlling hazards?
7. What are the limitations of work practices?
8. What are the three types of employee changes that can occur?

9. In a changing work environment, does employee education and training become more important? Why

10. Discuss why a safety system is predictive and not reactive?

BIBLIOGRAPHY

Collins, D. (n.d.). *Haddon's countermeasures – A better alternative to the hierarchy of hazard control?* Retrieved from http://bit.ly/1HQnO24

EM 385-1-1, *Safety and health requirements manual.* (2014). US Army Corps of engineers, Public Domain. Retrieved from http://1.usa.gov/1Fu8Yfo

Energy Release Theory. (n.d.). International Risk Management Institute, Inc. (IRMI). Retrieved from http://bit.ly/1DH7Foo

Google Advance Search. (n.d.). Google. Retrieved from http://bit.ly/15lPe8Y

Haddon, W. (1980). *The basic strategies for reducing damage from hazards of all kinds* (pp. 8–12). Systems Safety Society.

Hazard Assessment for PPE. (n.d.).Washington State Department of Labor and Industries, Public Domain, Based on and Adapted for Use. Retrieved from http://1.usa.gov/1DJTwtA

Job Hazard Analysis, 3071. (2002). Occupational Safety and Health Administration (OSHA). Public Domain, Modified and/or Adapt as necessary. Retrieved from http://1.usa.gov/11zbazr

Managing Worker Safety and Health. (n.d.). Missouri Occupational Safety and Health Administration (OSHA), Office of Cooperative Programs, Public Domain, Adapted for Use. Retrieved from http://on.mo.gov/15C4FyS

Occupational Health & Safety Management Systems. (2012). The American Society of Safety Engineers, ANSI/AIHA/ASSE Z10. Retrieved from http://bit.ly/1MsT6MG

Oregon OSHA Workshop Materials, Hazard Identification and Control. (n.d.). Oregon Occupational Safety and Health Division (Oregon OSHA), Public Domain, Permission to Reprint, Modify, and/or Adapt as necessary. Retrieved from http://bit.ly/1tg4a8A and http://bit.ly/1yIBKVk

Oregon OSHA's Quick Guide to the PPE Hazard Assessment. (n.d.). Oregon OSHA, Public domain. Retrieved from http://bit.ly/1LOiQDC

Personal Protective Equipment, 1915 Subpart I App A, Non-mandatory Guidelines for Hazard Assessment, Personal Protective Equipment (PPE) Selection, and PPE Training Program. (n.d.). Occupational Safety & Health Administration (OSHA), Public Domain. Retrieved from http://1.usa.gov/1CdxSxu

Personal Protective Equipment, OSHA 3151-12R 2003. (2003). Occupational Safety and Health Administration (OSHA), Public Domain. Retrieved from http://bit.ly/1LOi75q

Policy Background on the Temporary Worker Initiative. (2014). Occupational Safety and Health Administration (OSHA). Retrieved from http://1.usa.gov/1xqcJ33

PPE Assessment. (n.d.). Occupational Safety and Health Administration (OSHA), Public Domain, Based on and Adapted for Use. Retrieved from http://1.usa.gov/14LzifU

Preventing chemical accidents, introduction to process hazard analysis, (1st ed.). (n.d.). NJ Work Environment Council, Public Domain. Retrieved from http://bit.ly/1HaJIHw, http://1.usa.gov/1fnhL8J Word Document.

Prevention through Design. (2012). Centers for Disease Control and Prevention (CDC), National Institute for Occupational Safety and Health (NIOSH), Public Domain. Retrieved from http://1.usa.gov/11f7iTQ

Process Safety Management, OSHA 3132. (2000). Occupational Safety and Health Administration (OSHA), Public Domain, Modified and/or Adapt as necessary. Retrieved from http://1.usa.gov/1BHmiMw

Roughton, J., & Crutchfield, N. (2013). In B. Heinemann (Ed.), *Safety culture: An innovative leadership approach.* MA: Butterworth Heinemann, Retrieved from http://amzn.to/1qoD4oN.

Safety and Health Program Management: Fact Sheets. (n.d.). Safety and Health Program Management Systems eTool (OSHA), Public Domain, Based on and Adapted for Use. Retrieved from http://1.usa.gov/1A9D85S

Safety Management System Basis, Public Domain. (2014). Federal Aviation Administration. Retrieved from http://1.usa.gov/1dbnehT

Senge, P. M. (2006). *The fifth discipline: The art & practice of the learning organization. A currency book.* MA: Crown Publishing Group.

Small Business Safety and Health Management Series, OSHA 2209-02R. (2005). Occupational Safety and Health Administration (OSHA), Public Domain. Retrieved from http://1.usa.gov/16Yv4r7

Task Analysis Tools Used Throughout Development, Human Error Analysis. (n.d.). Federal Aviation Administration, FAA Human Factors, Public Domain. Retrieved from http://1.usa.gov/1Dbg0DR

US DOE. (2009a). *Concepts and principles, human performance improvement handbook* (Vol. 1). US Department of Energy. Retrieved from http://bit.ly/1DfdJVU

US DOE. (2009a). *Human performance tools for individuals, work teams, and management, human performance improvement handbook* (Vol. 2). US Department of Energy. Retrieved from http://bit.ly/14kc6Lj

Appendix E Resources for a Successful Personal Protective Equipment (PPE) Assessment

One of the best resources that we have found to help you prepare for the required PPE assessment is the Washington State Department of Labor and Industries, which includes the following documents:

Guidelines for complying with PPE requirements

Hazard assessment for PPE, Option 1

Job hazard analysis assessment for PPE, Option 2

PPE training certificate form

PPE training quiz

Sample PPE policies (PPE Assessment, n.d.)

Additional Resources

We have included these additional resources for your convenience. Please bear in mind that web links are always subject to change. Please compare these documents to the actual documents based on the resource(s) provided to verify accuracy.

Assessing the Need for Personal Protective Equipment (PPE) (Hazard Assessment for PPE, n.d.)

Personal Protective Equipment (Personal Protective Equipment OSHA 3151-12R 2003, 2003)

Nonmandatory Guidelines for Hazard Assessment, Personal Protective Equipment (PPE) Selection, and PPE Training Program (Personal Protective Equipment, 1915 Subpart I App A, Non-mandatory Guidelines for Hazard Assessment, Personal Protective Equipment (PPE) Selection, and PPE Training Program, n.d.)

PPE hazard assessment quick guide – Oregon OSHA (Oregon OSHA's Quick Guide to the PPE Hazard Assessment, n.d.)

Note: Web links are subject to change. If any web links do not work as provided, you can use the Google advanced search by searching for the title of what is presented in this appendix (Google Advance Search, n.d.).

E.1 Guidelines for complying with PPE requirements

Use this checklist to help determine the PPE requirements at your work place. You can use the available tools in the far right column to help you accomplish the step. Check off the boxes in the far left column as you complete each step.

Done	Step	Tools
O	Do a work place walkthrough and look for hazards (including potential hazards) in all employees' workspaces and work place operating procedures.	Checklist #1, Option 1: PPE Hazard Assessment or
O	Consider engineering, administrative, and/or work practice methods to control the hazards first. Identify those existing/potential hazards and tasks that require PPE.	Checklist #2, Option 2: JHA PPE Hazard Assessment
O	Select the appropriate PPE to match the hazards and protect employees.	
O	Communicate PPE selection to each at-risk employee. Provide properly fitting PPE to each employee required to use it.	
O	Train employees on the use of PPE and document it.	PPE Training Certification Form
O	Test employees to make sure they understand the elements of the PPE training.	Sample PPE Training Quiz *(required)*
O	Follow up to evaluate effectiveness of PPE use, training, policies, etc. against the hazards at your work place.	

O Yes O No   All employees have been trained

O Yes O No   Employees are using their PPE properly and following PPE policies and procedures

O Yes O No   Supervisors are enforcing use of required PPE

(If you checked any No boxes, go back through the steps and correct the deficiencies.)

O Yes O No   Have things changed at your work place? (e.g., fewer injuries/ illnesses)

E.2 Hazard assessment for PPE

This tool can help you conduct a hazard assessment to determine if your employees need to use personal protective equipment (PPE) by identifying activities that may create hazards for your employees. The activities are grouped according to what part of the body might need PPE.

This tool can serve as written documentation that you have completed a hazard assessment. Make sure that the blank fields at the beginning of the checklist (indicated by *) are filled out (check Instruction #4).

Instructions:

1. Do a walk through survey of each work area and job/task. Read through the list of work activities in the first column, putting a check next to the activities performed in that work area or job.
2. Read through the list of hazards in the second column, putting a check next to the hazards to which employees may be exposed while performing the work activities or while present in the work area. (e.g., work activity: chopping wood; work-related exposure: flying particles).
3. Decide how you are going to control the hazards. Consider engineering, work place, and/or administrative controls to eliminate or reduce the hazards before resorting to using PPE. If the hazard cannot be eliminated without using PPE, indicate which type(s) of PPE will be required to protect your employee from the hazard.
4. Make sure that you complete the following fields on the form (indicated by *) to certify that a hazard assessment was done:
   a. *Name of your work place
   b. *Address of the work place where you are doing the hazard assessment
   c. *Name of person certifying that a workplace hazard assessment was done
   d. *Date the hazard assessment was done

E.2.1 PPE Hazard Assessment Certification Form

*Name of work place: _____

*Work place address: _____

Work area(s): _____

*Assessment conducted by: _____

*Date of assessment: _____

Job/Task(s): _____

*Required for certifying the hazard assessment.   Use a separate sheet for each job/task or work area

EYES

Work activities, such as:		Work-related exposure to:	Can hazard be eliminated without the use of PPE?
☐ abrasive blasting	☐ sanding	☐ airborne dust	Yes ☐ No ☐
☐ chopping	☐ sawing	☐ flying particles	
☐ cutting	☐ grinding	☐ blood splashes	If no, use:
☐ drilling	☐ hammering	☐ hazardous liquid chemicals	☐ Safety glasses ☐ Side shields
☐ welding		☐ intense light	☐ Safety goggles ☐ Dust-tight
☐ punch press operations		☐ other: _____	☐ Shading/Filter (# ___) goggles
☐ other: _____			☐ Welding shield
			☐ Other: _____

FACE

Work activities, such as:		Work-related exposure to:	Can hazard be eliminated without the use of PPE?
☐ cleaning	☐ foundry work	☐ hazardous liquid chemicals	Yes ☐ No ☐
☐ cooking	☐ welding	☐ extreme heat/cold	
☐ siphoning	☐ mixing	☐ potential irritants: _____	If no, use:
☐ painting	☐ pouring molten	☐ other: _____	☐ Face shield
☐ dip tank operations	metal		☐ Shading/Filter (# ___)
☐ chemical handling			☐ Welding shield
☐ other: _____			☐ Other: _____

HEAD

Work activities, such as:	Work-related exposure to:	Can hazard be eliminated without the use of PPE?
☐ building maintenance	☐ beams/structures	Yes ☐ No ☐
☐ confined space operations	☐ pipes	
☐ construction	☐ exposed electrical wiring or	If no, use:
☐ electrical wiring	components	☐ Protective Helmet
☐ walking/working under catwalks	☐ falling objects	☐ Type A (low voltage)
☐ walking/working under conveyor belts	☐ machine parts	☐ Type B (high voltage)
☐ walking/working under crane loads	☐ other: _____	☐ Type C
☐ utility work		☐ Bump cap (not ANSI-approved)
☐ other: _____		☐ Hair net or soft cap
		☐ Other: _____

HANDS/ARMS

Work activities, such as:

- [ ] baking
- [ ] cooking
- [ ] grinding
- [ ] welding
- [ ] working with glass
- [ ] using computers
- [ ] using knives
- [ ] dental and health care services
- [ ] other: _____
- [ ] material handling
- [ ] sanding
- [ ] sawing
- [ ] hammering
- [ ] Unjamming equipment

Work-related exposure to:

- [ ] blood
- [ ] irritating chemicals
- [ ] tools or materials that could scrape, bruise, or cut
- [ ] extreme heat/cold
- [ ] other: _____

Can hazard be eliminated without the use of PPE?

Yes [ ]   No [ ]

If no, use:
- [ ] Gloves
  - [ ] Chemical resistance
  - [ ] Liquid/leak resistance
  - [ ] Temperature resistance
  - [ ] Abrasion/cut resistance
  - [ ] Slip resistance
- [ ] Protective sleeves
- [ ] Other: _____

FEET/LEGS

Work activities, such as:

- [ ] building maintenance
- [ ] construction
- [ ] demolition
- [ ] food processing
- [ ] foundry work
- [ ] logging
- [ ] plumbing
- [ ] trenching
- [ ] use of highly flammable materials
- [ ] welding
- [ ] material handling
- [ ] other: _____

Work-related exposure to:

- [ ] explosive atmospheres
- [ ] explosives
- [ ] exposed electrical wiring or components
- [ ] heavy equipment
- [ ] slippery surfaces
- [ ] tools
- [ ] dropped tools, material, etc.
- [ ] other: _____

Can hazard be eliminated without the use of PPE?

Yes [ ]   No [ ]

If no, use:
- [ ] Safety shoes or boots
  - [ ] Toe protection
  - [ ] Electrical protection
  - [ ] Puncture resistance
  - [ ] Anti-slip soles
  - [ ] Metatarsal protection
  - [ ] Heat/cold protection
  - [ ] Chemical resistance
- [ ] Leggings or chaps
- [ ] Foot-Leg guards
- [ ] Other: _____

BODY/SKIN

Work activities such as:

- [ ] baking or frying
- [ ] battery charging
- [ ] dip tank operations
- [ ] fiberglass installation
- [ ] irritating chemicals
- [ ] sawing
- [ ] knife or other sharp tools
- [ ] other: _____

Work-related exposure to:

- [ ] chemical splashes
- [ ] extreme heat/cold
- [ ] sharp or rough edges
- [ ] other: _____

Can hazard be eliminated without the use of PPE?

Yes [ ]   No [ ]

If no, use:
- [ ] Vest, Jacket
- [ ] Coveralls, Body suit
- [ ] Raingear
- [ ] Apron
- [ ] Welding leathers
- [ ] Abrasion/cut resistance
- [ ] Other: _____

BODY/WHOLE

Work activities such as:		Work-related exposure to:	Can hazard be eliminated without the use of PPE?
☐ building maintenance		☐ working from heights of 4 feet or more	Yes ☐ No ☐
☐ construction		☐ working near water	If no, use:
☐ utility work		☐ other: _____	☐ Fall Arrest protection/Restraint: Type: _____
☐ order pulling			☐ PFD: Type: _____
☐ warehouse operation			☐ Other: _____
☐ other: _____			*(See Footnote 1)

LUNGS/RESPIRATORY

Work activities such as:		Work-related exposure to:	Can hazard be eliminated without the use of PPE?
☐ cleaning	☐ pouring	☐ irritating dust or particulate	Yes ☐ No ☐
☐ mixing	☐ sawing	☐ irritating or toxic gas/vapor	☐ hearing protection, Type
☐ painting		☐ other: _____	
☐ fiberglass installation			
☐ compressed air or gas operations			
☐ other: _____			*(See Footnote 1)

EARS/HEARING

Work activities such as:		Work-related exposure to:	Can hazard be eliminated without the use of PPE?
☐ generator	☐ grinding	☐ loud noises	Yes ☐ No ☐
☐ ventilation fans	☐ machining	☐ loud work environment	
☐ motors	☐ routers	☐ noisy machines/tools	
☐ sanding	☐ sawing	☐ punch or brake presses	
☐ pneumatic equipment		☐ other: _____	
☐ punch or brake presses			
☐ use of conveyors			
☐ other: _____			*(See Footnote 1)

E.3 Job hazard analysis assessment for PPE

The job hazard analysis (JHA) approach to doing a hazard assessment for PPE is useful in larger businesses with many hazards and/or complex safety issues. It also helps you assign a *Risk priority code* to the hazard to determine the course of actions you need to take to control the hazard (Chapter 8).

Follow the instructions as you conduct your hazard assessment and fill in the hazard assessment form. Customize the form to fit the needs of your work place.

This tool can also serve as written documentation that you have done a hazard assessment to document your hazard assessment for PPE. Make sure that the blank fields at the bottom of the form are filled out.

- Name of your work place
- Address of the work place where you are doing the hazard assessment
- Name of person certifying that a workplace hazard assessment was done
- Date the hazard assessment was done

E.3.1 Job Hazard Analysis Assessment for PPE
E.3.1.1 Instructions

1. Conduct a walkthrough survey of your business: For each job/task step, note the presence of any of the following hazard types (see table below), their sources, and the body parts at risk. Fill out the left side of the hazard assessment form. Gather all the information you can.
   a. Look at all steps of a job and ask the employee if there are any variations in the job that are infrequently done and that you might have missed during your observation.
   b. For purposes of the assessment, assume that no PPE is being worn by the affected employees even though they may actually be wearing what they need to do the job safely.
   c. Note all observed hazards. *This list does not cover all possible hazards that employees may face or for which personal protective equipment may be required.* Noisy environments or those, which may require respirators must be evaluated with appropriate test equipment to quantify the exposure level when overexposure is suspected.

Hazard type	General description of hazard type
Impact	Person can strike an object or be struck by a moving or flying or falling object.
Penetration	Person can strike, be struck by, or fall upon an object or tool that would break the skin.
Crush or pinch	An object(s) or machine may crush or pinch a body or body part.
Harmful dust	Presence of dust that may cause irritation, or breathing or vision difficulty. May also have ignition potential.

Hazard type	General description of hazard type
Chemical	Exposure from spills, splashing, or other contact with chemical substances or harmful dusts that could cause illness, irritation, burns, asphyxiation, breathing or vision difficulty, or other toxic health effects. May also have ignition potential.
Heat	Exposure to radiant heat sources, splashes or spills of hot material, or work in hot environments.
Light (optical) Radiation	Exposure to strong light sources, glare, or intense light exposure, which is a byproduct of a process.
Electrical contact	Exposure to contact with or proximity to live or potentially live electrical objects.
Ergonomic hazards	Repetitive movements, awkward postures, vibration, heavy lifting, etc.
Environmental hazards	Conditions in the work place that could cause discomfort or negative health effects.

2. Analyze the hazard: For each job task with a hazard source identified, use the job hazard analysis matrix table and discuss the hazard with the affected employee and supervisor. Fill out the right side of the hazard assessment form:

   a. Rate the SEVERITY of injury that would *reasonably* be expected to result from exposure to the hazard.

   b. Rate the PROBABILITY of an accident actually happening.

   c. Assign a RISK CODE based upon the intersection of the SEVERITY and PROBABILITY ratings on the matrix.

Job hazard analysis matrix

Severity of injury		Probability of an accident occurring				
Level	Description	A Frequent	B Several times	C Occasional	D Possible	E Extremely improbable
I	Fatal or permanent disability	1	1	1	2	3
II	Severe illness or injury	1	1	2	2	3
III	Minor injury or illness	2	2	2-3	3	3
IV	No injury or illness	3	3	3	3	3

Risk priority

Code	Risk level	Action required
1	High	Work activities must be suspended immediately until hazard can be eliminated or controlled or reduced to a lower level.
2	Medium	Job hazards are unacceptable and must be controlled by engineering, administrative, or personal protective equipment methods as soon as possible.
3	Low	No real or significant hazard exists. Controls are not required but may increase the comfort level of employees.

3. Take action on the assessment: Depending on the assigned Risk level/ Code (or Risk priority), take the corresponding action according to the table above:

   a. If Risk priority is LOW (3) for a task step → requires no further action.

   b. If Risk priority is MEDIUM (2) → select and implement appropriate controls.

   c. If Risk priority is HIGH (1) → immediately stop the task step until appropriate controls can be implemented.

> A high risk priority means that there is a reasonable to high probability that an employee will be killed or permanently disabled doing this task step and/or a high probability that the employee will suffer severe illness or injury!

4. Select PPE:

   a. Try to reduce employee exposure to the hazard by first implementing engineering, work practice, and/or administrative controls. If PPE is supplied, it must be appropriately matched to the hazard to provide effective protection, durability, and proper fit to the worker. Note the control method to be implemented in the far right column.

5. Certify the hazard assessment:

   a. Certify on the hazard assessment form that you have done the hazard assessment and implemented the needed controls.

   b. Incorporate any new PPE requirements that you have developed into your written accident prevention program.

E.3.2 Job Hazard Analysis for Personal Protective Equipment (PPE) Assessment

Job/Task: Location:

Job/Task Step	Hazard Type	Hazard Source	Body Parts At Risk	Severity	Probability	Risk Code	Control Method[1]

(1)Note: Engineering, work practice, and/or administrative hazard controls such as guarding must be used, if feasible, before requiring employees to use personal protective equipment.

Certification of Assessment

*Name of work place: *Address

*Assessment Conducted By: Title: *Date(s) of Assessment

Implementation of Controls Approved By: Title: Date:

E.4 Example personal protective equipment training certification form

Employee's Name: _____   Employee ID No. _____

Job Title/Work area: _____

Employer: _____

Trainer's Name (person completing this form): _____

Date of Training: _____

Types of PPE employee is being trained to use:

_____   _____

_____   _____

_____   _____

The following information and training on the personal protective equipment (PPE) listed above were covered in the training session:

____ The limitations of personal protective equipment: PPE alone cannot protect the employee from on-the-job hazards.

____ What work place hazards the employee faces, the types of personal protective equipment that the employee must use to be protected from these hazards, and how the PPE will protect the employee while doing his/her tasks.

____ When the employee must wear or use the personal protective equipment.

____ How to use the personal protective equipment properly on-the-job, including putting it on, taking it off, and wearing and adjusting it (if applicable) for a comfortable and effective fit.

____ How to properly care for and maintain the personal protective equipment: look for signs of wear, clean and disinfect, and dispose of PPE.

Note to employee: *This form will be made a part of your personal file. Please read and understand its contents before signing.*

(Employee) I understand the training I have received, and I can use PPE properly.

_____   _____
Employee's signature   Date

(Trainer must check off)

____ Employee has shown an understanding of the training.

____ Employee has shown the ability to use the PPE properly.

_____   _____
Trainer's signature   Date

E.5 Example personal protective equipment training quiz, (required)

(This is a sample quiz that you can use to make sure an employee has understood the training and can demonstrate the proper use and care of personal protective equipment. Also quiz an employee who has been retrained due to improper use of the PPE in performing his/her job tasks. You can keep this form in the employee's file with the PPE Certification Form.)

1. What are the limitations of personal protective equipment?
2. List the types of personal protective equipment you must use when doing your work/tasks.
3. What are the hazards in your job for which you must use each type of PPE, and when must you use your personal protective equipment?
4. What are the procedures for the proper use, care, and maintenance of your PPE?
5. What should you look for to determine that your PPE is in good working condition?
6. What do you do when your PPE is no longer usable?
7. (Trainer/Supervisor) Have the employee demonstrate putting on, wearing and adjusting, and taking off each PPE properly. Also have employee demonstrate how to clean and disinfect each PPE.

Has employee demonstrated proper use and care of each PPE?

PPE #1: _____ Yes _____ No _____

PPE #2: _____ Yes _____ No _____

PPE #3: _____ Yes _____ No _____

PPE #4: _____ Yes _____ No _____

The employee has answered all the questions adequately and has demonstrated the ability to properly use and care for the PPE needed to do his/her job.

_____   _____
Trainer's/Supervisor's signature   Date

_____   _____
Employee's signature   Date

E.6 Sample PPE policies

E.6.1 Instructions

In addition, the Consultation Section of the Department of Labor and Industries may be called on for assistance at any time.

THE FOLLOWING PERSONAL PROTECTIVE EQUIP-
MENT (PPE) POLICIES PROVIDE A POSSIBLE FORMAT
THAT CAN BE CUSTOMIZED for YOUR WORK PLACE.

REMEMBER: YOUR SAFETY AND HEALTH PROGRAM
CAN ONLY BE EFFECTIVE IF IT IS PUT INTO PRACTICE!

E.7 Personal protective equipment policies

(Customize by adding the name of your business)

E.7.1 Introduction

The purpose of the Personal Protective Equipment Policies is to protect the
employees of (Name of your business) from exposure to work place hazards
and the risk of injury through the use of personal protective equipment
(PPE). PPE is not a substitute for more effective control methods and its use
will be considered only when other means of protection against hazards are
not adequate or feasible. It will be used in conjunction with other controls
unless no other means of hazard control exist.

Personal protective equipment will be provided, used, and maintained
when it has been determined that its use is required to ensure the safety
and health of our employees and that such use will lessen the likelihood of
occupational injury and/or illness.

This section addresses general PPE requirements, including eye and
face, head, foot and leg, hand and arm, body (torso) protection, and protection from drowning. Separate programs exist for respiratory protection and
hearing protection as the need for participation in these programs is established through industrial hygiene monitoring. (List other programs or policies requiring PPE, such as hearing protection, respiratory protection, fall
protection, etc., that you may have at your work place) are also addressed in
(State the section or location in your Accident Prevention Program where
they are found).

The (Name of your business) Personal protective equipment policies
includes:

- Responsibilities of supervisors and employees
- Hazard assessment and PPE selection
- Employee training
- Cleaning and Maintenance of PPE

E.7.2 Responsibilities

*(Customize this page by modifying or adding any additional responsibilities and
deleting those that may not apply to your company.)*

*Safety Person (or designated person responsible for your work place safety and
health program.)*

*Note: Depending on your business and the number of employees you have, you
may simply have a "designated safety coordinator" (who may be a supervisor/lead
worker) or a larger organized safety and health unit. Customize this section to fit
the needs of your p.*

(Safety Coordinator or designated person) is responsible for the development, implementation, and administration of (Name of your business)'s PPE policies. This involves

1. Conducting workplace hazard assessments to determine the presence of hazards, which necessitate the use of PPE.
2. Selecting and purchasing PPE.
3. Reviewing, updating, and conducting PPE hazard assessments whenever
   a. a job changes,
   b. new equipment is used,
   c. there has been an accident,
   d. a supervisor or employee requests it,
   e. or at least every year.
4. Maintaining records on hazard assessments.
5. Maintaining records on PPE assignments and training.
6. Providing training, guidance, and assistance to supervisors and employees on the proper use, care, and cleaning of approved PPE.
7. Periodically re-evaluating the suitability of previously selected PPE.
8. Reviewing, updating, and evaluating the overall effectiveness of PPE use, training, and policies.

E.7.3 Supervisors (leads, etc., and/or designated persons)

Supervisors (leads, etc., and/or designated persons) have the primary responsibility for implementing and enforcing PPE use and policies in their work area. This involves

9. Providing appropriate PPE and making it available to employees.
10. Ensuring that employees are trained on the proper use, care, and cleaning of PPE.
11. Ensuring that PPE training certification and evaluation forms are signed and given to (Safety Person or designated person responsible for your work place safety and health program).
12. Ensuring that employees properly use and maintain their PPE, and follow (Name of your business) PPE policies and rules.
13. Notifying (Name of your business) management and the Safety Person when new hazards are introduced or when processes are added or changed.
14. Ensuring that defective or damaged PPE is immediately disposed of and replaced.

E.7.4 Employees

The PPE user is responsible for following the requirements of the PPE policies. This involves

15. Properly wearing PPE as required.
16. Attending required training sessions.
17. Properly caring for, cleaning, maintaining, and inspecting PPE as required.
18. Following (Name of your business) PPE policies and rules.
19. Informing the supervisor of the need to repair or replace PPE.

Employees who repeatedly disregard and do not follow PPE policies and rules will be (Write in the actions management will take concerning this matter.)

(Customize this page by modifying or adding any additional responsibilities and deleting those that may not apply to your company.)

E.7.5 Procedures

E.7.5.1 Hazard Assessment for PPE

(Safety Person or designated person), in conjunction with supervisors, will conduct a walk-through survey of each work area to identify sources of work hazards. Each survey will be documented using the Hazard Assessment Certification Form, which identifies the work area surveyed, the person conducting the survey, findings of potential hazards, and date of the survey. (Safety Person or designated person) will keep the forms in the (Specify exact location, e.g., your company's business files).

(Safety person or designated person) will conduct, review, and update the hazard assessment for PPE whenever

- a job changes,
- new equipment or process is installed,
- there has been an accident,
- whenever a supervisor or employee requests it,
- or at least every year.

Any new PPE requirements that are developed will be added into (Name of your business)'s written accident prevention program.

E.7.5.2 Selection of PPE

Once the hazards of a workplace have been identified, (Safety Person or designated person) will determine if the hazards can first be eliminated or reduced by methods other than PPE, that is, methods that do not rely on employee behavior, such as engineering controls (Appendix B).

If such methods are not adequate or feasible, then (Safety Person or designated person) will determine the suitability of the PPE presently available; and as necessary, will select new or additional equipment, which ensures a level of protection greater than the minimum required to protect our employees from the hazards (Appendix C). Care will be taken to recognize the possibility of multiple and simultaneous exposure to a variety of hazards. Adequate protection against the highest level of each of the hazards will be recommended for purchase.

All personal protective clothing and equipment will be of safe design and construction for the work to be performed and will be maintained in a sanitary and reliable condition. Only those items of protective clothing and equipment that meet NIOSH or ANSI (American National Standards Institute) standards will be procured or accepted for use. Newly purchased

PPE must conform to the updated ANSI standards, which have been incorporated into the PPE regulations, as follows:
- Eye and Face Protection ANSI Z87.1-1989
- Head Protection ANSI Z89.1-1986
- Foot Protection ANSI Z41.1-1991
- Hand Protection (There are no ANSI standards for gloves, however, selection must be based on the performance characteristics of the glove in relation to the tasks to be performed.)

Affected employees whose jobs require the use of PPE will be informed of the PPE selection and will be provided PPE by (Name of your business) at no charge. Careful consideration will be given to the comfort and proper fit of PPE in order to ensure that the right size is selected and that it will be used.

E.7.5.3 Training

Any worker required to wear PPE will receive training in the proper use and care of PPE before being allowed to perform work requiring the use of PPE. Periodic retraining will be offered to PPE users as needed. The training will include, but not necessarily be limited to, the following subjects:
- When PPE is necessary to be worn
- What PPE is necessary
- How to properly don, doff, adjust, and wear PPE
- The limitations of the PPE
- The proper care, maintenance, useful life, and disposal of the PPE

After the training, the employees will demonstrate that they understand how to use PPE properly, or they will be retrained.

Training of each employee will be documented using the Personal Protective Equipment Training Documentation Form *(or whatever form your company uses)* and kept on file. The document certifies that the employee has received and understood the required training on the specific PPE he/she will be using.

The PPE Training Quiz will be used to evaluate employees' understanding and will be kept in the employee training records.

E.7.5.3.1 Retraining

The need for retraining will be indicated when:
- an employee's work habits or knowledge indicates a lack of the necessary understanding, motivation, and skills required to use the PPE (i.e., uses PPE improperly),
- new equipment is installed,
- changes in the work place make previous training out-of-date,
- changes in the types of PPE to be used make previous training out-of-date.

E.7.5.4 Cleaning and Maintenance of PPE

It is important that all PPE be kept clean and properly maintained. Cleaning is particularly important for eye and face protection where dirty or fogged lenses could impair vision. Employees must inspect, clean, and maintain their PPE according to the manufacturers' instructions before and after each use. *(Attach a copy of the manufacturers' cleaning and care instructions for all PPE provided to your employees).* Supervisors are responsible for ensuring that users properly maintain their PPE in good condition.

Personal protective equipment must not be shared between employees until it has been properly cleaned and sanitized. PPE will be distributed for individual use whenever possible.

Defective or damaged PPE will not be used and will be immediately discarded and replaced.

Note: *Defective equipment can be worse than no PPE at all. Employees would avoid a hazardous situation if they knew they were not protected; but they would get closer to the hazard if they erroneously believed they were protected, and therefore would be at greater risk.*

It is also important to ensure that contaminated PPE, which cannot be decontaminated is disposed of in a manner that protects employees from exposure to hazards.

E.7.5.5 Safety Disciplinary Policy

(Customize by adding your company name here) believes that a safety and health Accident Prevention Program is unenforceable without some type of disciplinary policy. Our company believes that in order to maintain a safe and healthful workplace, the employees must be cognizant and aware of all company, State, and Federal safety and health regulations as they apply to the specific job duties required. The following disciplinary policy is in effect and will be applied to all safety and health violations.

The following steps will be followed unless the seriousness of the violation would dictate going directly to Step 2 or Step 3.

1. A first time violation will be discussed orally between company supervision and the employee. This will be done as soon as possible.
2. A second time offense will be followed up in written form and a copy of this written documentation will be entered into the employee's personnel folder.
3. A third time violation will result in time off or possible termination, depending on the seriousness of the violation.

(Customize this page by adding any additional disciplinary actions and deleting those that may not apply to your company.)

Appendix F Example of Safety Rules – Codes of Safe Practice

Work shall be well planned and supervised to prevent injuries when working with equipment and handling heavy materials. Employees will be trained in properly material handling.

Employees shall not handle or tamper with any energy sources (electrical, hydraulics, thermal, mechanical, etc.) in a manner not within the scope of their duties, unless they have received instructions from their supervisor/employer.

All injuries shall be reported promptly to the supervisor so that arrangements can be made for medical and/or first-aid treatment. First aid materials are located in _____, emergency, fire, ambulance, rescue squad, and doctor's telephone numbers are located on _____, and fire extinguishers are located at _____.

F.1 Suggested safety rules
- Do not throw material, tools, or other objects from heights (whether structures or buildings) until proper precautions are taken to protect others from the falling objects.
- Wash your hands thoroughly after handling hazardous substances.
- Flammable liquids shall not be used for cleaning purposes.
- Arrange work so that you are able to face ladder and use both hands while climbing.

F.2 Use of tools and equipment
- Keep hammers in good condition to avoid flying nails and bruised fingers.
- Files shall be equipped with handles; never use a file as a punch or pry.
- Do not use a screwdriver as a chisel.
- Do not lift or lower portable electric tools by the power cords; use a rope.
- Do not leave the cords of these tools where cars or trucks will run over them.

F.3 Machinery and vehicles
- Do not attempt to operate machinery or equipment without special permission, unless it is one of your regular duties.
- Loose or frayed clothing, dangling ties, finger rings, and similar items must not be worn around moving machinery or other places where they can get caught.
- Machinery shall not be repaired or adjusted while in operation.

(Small Business Safety and Health Management Series OSHA 2209-02R 2005)

Appendix G Example Safety Review of New/Relocated Equipment Major Modification Sign-Off Form

G.1 Do not operate equipment until this tag is completed

CPR #	Project title
Type of equipment	Catalog #
MFG Serial #	Plant/facility location
Comments: (as applicable)	

G.1.1 Installation Completed

This equipment has been properly installed and the proper guarding and safety equipment has been put in place. Have discussed installation with Division.

Project manager

	Signature	Date

Comments

This equipment has been properly installed and the proper guarding and safety equipment has been put in place.

Maintenance manager

	Signature	Date

Comments

I have reviewed this equipment from a safety standpoint. This equipment is accepted.

Operation manager

	Signature	Date

Comments

I have reviewed this equipment from a safety standpoint. This equipment is accepted.

Production supervisor

	Signature	Date

Comments

I have reviewed this equipment from a safety standpoint. This equipment is accepted.

Safety coordinator/manager

| | Signature | Date |

Comments

Appendix H Other Analytical Tools for Consideration

A number of other analytical tools such, as "what if," "checklist," hazard and operability study (HAZOP), failure mode and effect analysis (FMEA), or "fault-tree" analysis can be used to determine possible process breakdowns. You then can design prevention/controls for the likely causes of these unwanted events.

H.1 Process hazard analysis

A process can be defined as any series of actions or operations that convert raw material into a product. A process terminates in a finished product ready for consumption or in a product that is the raw material for subsequent processes. The process hazard analysis is used to assess the types of hazards found within a process.

OSHA's process safety management (PSM) of highly hazardous chemicals defines process as any activity involving a highly hazardous chemical, including any use, storage, manufacturing, handling, or on-site movement of such chemicals, or a combination of these activities. The objective of this standard is to protect employees by preventing or minimizing the consequences of chemical incidents involving highly hazardous chemicals.

The PSM is relevant and useful to the full range of workplaces, not only those subject to the standard's requirements.

The PHA is a detailed study of the actions and operations to identify to the degree possible hazards that may develop. Every element of the process must be studied. Each action of every piece of equipment, each substance present, and every action taken by an employee must be assumed initially to pose a hazard to employees. PHA is applied to show that each element either has no appreciable hazard, that a hazard(s) that is controlled in every foreseeable circumstance, or has an uncontrolled hazard (Preventing Chemical Accidents, Introduction to Process Hazard Analysis, First Edition, n.d.; Process Safety Management OSHA 3132, 2000).

H.2 "What-if" analysis

The What-If analysis begins by identifying points within a process where a loss-producing situation could develop. A series of What-If questions traces "what else" might happen, and assesses all feasible or possible outcomes or unintended consequences. Additional prevention and controls for possible unplanned and/or undesirable events are developed and implemented.

For more complex processes, the "What If" study is best organized through the use of customized "checklists." Aspects of the process a re assigned to analysis team members with the greatest experience or skill in areas of concern. As a What-If study could include but not be limited to audits of equipment operator practices and job knowledge, the suitability of equipment and materials of construction, the chemistry of the process and its control systems, and the operating and preventive maintenance records (Task Analysis Tools Used Throughout Development, Human Error Analysis, n.d.).

H.3 What-if/checklist review team

The What-If review team is selected from a wide range of disciplines, such as production/operations, maintenance, engineering/technical, safety, etc. Each team member is provided with basic information about the operation to be studied. This information includes data on known hazards from tools, equipment, and materials, the process technology being used, current protocols, procedures, standard operating procedures, loss producing incidents including injuries, health effects, physical damage, and previous hazard reviews.

A physical initial tour of the operation is conducted to methodically survey the operation from receipt of raw materials to final delivery of the finished product to the customer's site. At each step, the team generates a list of "what-if" questions regarding the hazards, potential scope of risk and overall safety of the operation. When the review team has completed the initial list of questions about what it has observed, a customized checklist is developed to stimulate additional questions that must be addressed.

The review team develops a hazard assessment report that addresses each question and provides recommendations that should be implemented, specifying the any additional actions or studies needed (Job Hazard Analysis 3071, 2002).

H.4 Hazard and operability study (HAZOP)

Hazard and operability study (HAZOP) is a method for systematically comparing each element of a process system against its potential for "critical parameters deviation" from the intended design conditions that could create hazards and operability problems. An HAZOP analysis team studies the process piping and instrument diagrams and/or plant model then analyzes the effects of potential deviations from design conditions in process flow, temperature, pressure, and time. Keywords, such as "more of," "less of," "part of," are used in describing each potential deviation (Job Hazard Analysis 3071, 2002).

H.5 Failure mode and effect analysis (FMEA)

The FMEA is a methodical study of operational component failures that begins with a review of system flowcharts and diagrams. Examples of components that might potential fail are instrument transmitters, controllers, valves, pumps, etc. – all process related process components. These items are listed on a data tabulation sheet and individually analyzed for the following:

- Potential mode of failure (i.e., open, closed, on, off, leaks).
- Consequence of the failure; effect on other components and effects on whole system. Hazard class (i.e., high, moderate, low).
- Probability of failure.
- Detection methods.
- Compensating provision/remarks.

Potential multiple concurrent failures are included in the analysis. The last step in the analysis an assessment of the data for each component or multiple component failure and develop a series of recommendations appropriate to risk management (Job Hazard Analysis 3071, 2002).

H.6 Fault tree analysis (FTA)

The FTA begins with the definition of an undesirable outcome and pulls together all of the components necessary for that occurrence.

A fault tree analysis can be either a qualitative or a quantitative model of the undesirable outcomes, such as a toxic gas release or explosion, which could result from a specific initiating event. It begins with a graphic representation (using logic symbols) of all possible sequences of events that could result in an incident. The resulting diagram looks like a tree with many branches. The diagram lists the sequential events (failures) for different independent paths to the top or undesired event. Probabilities (using failure rate data) are assigned to each event and then to calculate the probability of occurrence of the undesired event.

The technique is particularly useful in evaluating the effect of alternative actions on reducing the probability of occurrence of the undesired event (Job Hazard Analysis 3071, 2002).

H.7 Phase or activity hazard analysis

Phase hazard analysis is a useful tool for construction and other industries that involve a rapidly changing work environment, different contractors, and widely different operations. A phase is defined as an operation involving a type of work that presents hazards not experienced in previous operations, or an operation where a new subcontractor or work crew is to perform work. In this type of hazard analysis, before beginning each major phase of work, the contractor or site manager should assess the hazards in the new phase. Appropriate supplies and support are coordinated as well as preparation for hazards expected through a plan to eliminate or control them (EM 385-1-1 Safety and Health Requirements Manual, 2014).

To find these evolving hazards for elimination or control, the same techniques that are used in routine hazard analysis, change analysis, process analysis, and job analysis. The major additional challenge is to identify those hazards that develop when combinations of activities occur in close proximity as employees for several contractors with differing expertise may be intermingled. A coordinated plan must be implemented to ensure all exposed groups or parties how to protect themselves from the hazards associated with the activities of nearby colleagues as well as the hazards presented by combinations of the overlapping work zones (EM 385-1-1 Safety and Health Requirements Manual, 2014).

The Corp of Engineer uses an activity hazard analysis that must be developed before each activity. According to EM 385-1-,1 before beginning each activity involving a type of work presenting hazard not experienced in previous project operations or where a new work crew or subcontractor is to perform the work, activity hazard analyses shall be performed by the contractors performing the work activity (EM 385-1-1 Safety and Health Requirements Manual, 2014).

CHAPTER EIGHT

Defining Associated Risk

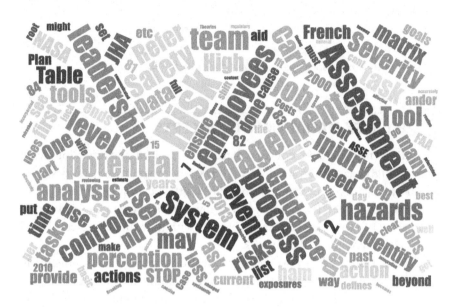

"Dice have no memory; they change all of the time."

— *CSI TV*

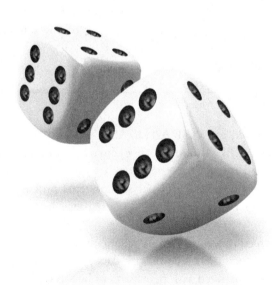

Job Hazard Analysis. http://dx.doi.org/10.1016/B978-0-12-803441-5.00008-8

Chapter Objectives

At the end of this chapter, you should be able to:

- Discuss a logical format that outlines hazards associated with specific job steps and related tasks.
- Define risk management and its principles.
- Discuss various risk models used to review organizations.
- Discuss the use of a risk matrix.
- Identify the importance of incorporating risk into the JHA process.

8.1 RISK MANAGEMENT CONCEPTS

Risk management concepts have been around and used for many years in high hazard industries. However, safety programs are still designed around regulatory compliance using only postloss data with limited use of basic risk principles. Risk management involves the systematic application of an array of tools used to identify hazards within organizations combined with an assessment of inherent risk.

An open line of two-way communications is essential to effectively spread information through the organization about its scope of risk. For this to be effective, the intent of the risk management process should be clearly defined and communicated accurately and objectively to the leadership team and employees. Risk management elements should be incorporated into each component of the organization for a safety system to be effective and for an understanding of the current level any potential risk.

8.2 RISK

Risk as defined in ANSI/AIHA/ASSE Z10 is "an estimate of the combination of the likelihood of an occurrence of a hazardous event or exposure(s), and the severity of injury or illness that may be caused by the event or exposures. Risk analysis concepts provide a method of establishing and prioritizing events" (The American Society of Safety Engineers, 2012).

A shift in perception is needed in an organization to ensure that there is a need to make decisions based on risk data and not strictly on loss data. If this perception is changed, risk management becomes the foundation for the safety system and the organization has a better potential for minimizing loss-producing events (US Air Force, 2011).

8.3 JHA INTEGRATION WITH RISK MANAGEMENT CONCEPTS

JHA provides a method for improving risk analysis when used to identify existing and potential hazards and the consequences of exposure to hazards. Job content is identified by reviewing the combination of required actions, job environment, tools, equipment, and materials used, and affected employees.

8.4 FIRST STEPS

The first step in the JHA process is to develop a clear and concise picture of the components of the job, its interrelated steps, and the specific tasks needed to complete those steps (Federal Aviation Administration (FAA), 2000). As part of developing a JHA process consideration should be given to identifying whether the job is routine or non-routine. Nonroutine jobs require additional refresher training as time between activities may reduce the knowledge of the controls needed. Many maintenance and construction jobs are high risk and require special considerations for timing of training, guidelines, and controls that should be implemented.

Direct employee involvement in establishing the interactions required is essential to determine how the job is completed. Their insights are needed if effective controls and overall job performance improvements are to be developed (Chapter 10).

8.5 GENERAL RISK MANAGEMENT THEORIES AND MODELS

8.5.1 National Aeronautics and Space Administration (NASA)

General risk management criteria and models have been developed that provide a graphical presentation of risk complexity. One model (Continuous Risk Management (CRM)) used by NASA was implemented thorough a methodical risk management approach required of all NASA programs and projects (Figure 8.1). Unfortunately, while NASA has a rigorous process, it has suffered major catastrophes with the loss of two space shuttles

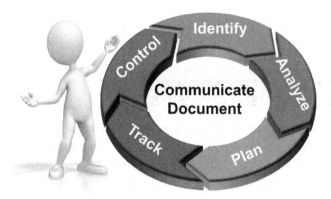

Figure 8.1 *Overview of the National Aeronautics and Space Administration (NASA) Continuous Risk Management Process.*

and in its early history, the loss of an Apollo crew in a capsule fire. Space flight is one of extreme high risk and while the engineering may clearly define the loss potential the organization's safety culture and its leadership style has overridden the best efforts of its safety system (NASA, n.d.; List of spaceflight-related accidents and incidents, n.d.; US DOE, 2005). While the tools and intent may be present, too often tragic events have occurred as the understanding of the scope of risk was not made clear or not accepted by the leadership team. This history emphasizes why we have stressed the need for increased communication and political skills in the development of the JHA process and any safety system.

8.5.2 French and Bell's Organizational Development Model

A concept that we have found useful was adapted from an organizational model developed by French and Bell. The model's components consist of Goals, Structure, Human-Social, Technology, Task, and Environment (French & Bell, 1984). The following provides a description on how this concept can provide a framework for better JHA structure.

- "Job" (steps and tasks) for "Goals:" "What is the objective of the Job? What is the job to be accomplished?
- "People" (employees, other exposed individuals): Who will be completing the job and what other employees or individuals may be exposed to it.
- "Tools/Equipment/Materials:" What is the combination and types of tools, equipment/technology and materials necessary to complete the job? Each item may have inherent hazards and associated risk present at various stages of a job's steps and tasks.

- "Environment:" What is the nature of the work environment and its general condition? Consideration is given to anything that defines where the job is being performed – night/day, lighting, housekeeping, temperature, air quality, etc.
- "Policy/Procedures:" What are the current administrative policies, standard operating procedures, guidelines, and rules that govern the job?

The French and Bell organizational development model allows for a structured approach that can assess the interactions that produce a successful "goal," i.e., the completion of a task. The amount of overlap or interaction between the individual components can be defined. The job can be viewed as dynamic with each part identified, and reviewed for modification, gradual change and how it has evolved (US Air Force, 2011; MITRE's Systems Engineering Process Office, n.d.).

The question for every job, especially those with a high hazard severity potential is: "What should be done by the leadership team to create a set of conditions that reduces to the highest degree possible the potential for a loss-producing event?" To answer this question, looking beyond the JHA process is needed with an assessment of the many influences impacting how the process is implemented.

8.5.3 Federal Aviation (FAA) Model

The FAA provides an eight process for conducting a risk assessment: (Federal Aviation Administration (FAA), 2008a)

1. Define the objective: The first step is to define the objectives of the system and ask the question: What are we trying to accomplish?
2. Define and describe the system: Describe how the system elements interact: Human, tools/equipment/materials, environment, and policies and procedures.
3. Hazard identification: Identify hazards and consequences of exposure. Hazards are identified by analyzing the tasks grouped by function. During the identification of each task, the risk analysis assesses the potential consequences of exposure to the hazards. The classic problem solving format "Who, What, Where, When, Why, and How (How much? How Many?") Is used to define the root cause. This method is called the "5W2H" method that is used in Six Sigma techniques to help to identify a root cause.
4. Risk analysis. Analyze hazards and identify the risks. Assessment is the application of quantitative and qualitative measures to determine

the level of risk associated with specific hazards. This process uses the estimated probability and potential severity of an incident (MITRE's Systems Engineering Process Office, n.d.). The risk analysis reviews hazards to determine what can happen. The inability to quantify and/or the lack of historical data on a particular hazard does not exclude the hazard from the need for analysis.

5. Risk assessment: Group steps/tasks and prioritize risks. Risk assessment combines the impact of risks and compares them against defined acceptable level criteria. These criteria can include the consolidation of risks into categories that can be jointly mitigated combined and used in decision making.

6. Decision-making: Developing action plans. Once a list of tasks has been prioritized, the list is reviewed to determine how to address each risk, beginning with the highest priority. The leadership team develops an action plan to apply control methods that have been selected. In addition, the leadership team provides the resources and individuals needed to put these measures in place. The "Hierarchy of controls" is used during this phase as outlined in Figure 7.3.

7. Validation and control: Evaluate result of actions for further planning needs. Evaluate the effectiveness of the action planning process. This evaluation will include identification of data to be collected and then the review of data. "Residual" risk (any remaining risks) can be acceptable, unacceptable, or remain unknown. If acceptable, documentation is required to show the rationale for accepting the risk. If it is unacceptable, an action plan is established for additional controls. If listed as unknown, then the process continues the data collection.

8. Modify system/process, as applicable: If the identified risk changes or action plans do not produce the intended effect, a determination should be made as to why. Was the wrong hazard addressed? Was the hazard missed? Does the system/process need to be modified? Reevaluate the process beginning at hazard identification (Federal Aviation Administration (FAA), 2000). After controls are in place, the new process should be periodically reevaluated to ensure effectiveness. The risk management process continues throughout the life cycle of the system, mission or activity (MITRE's Systems Engineering Process Office, n.d.).

Refer to Figure 8.2 used by The Federal Aviation Administration (FAA).

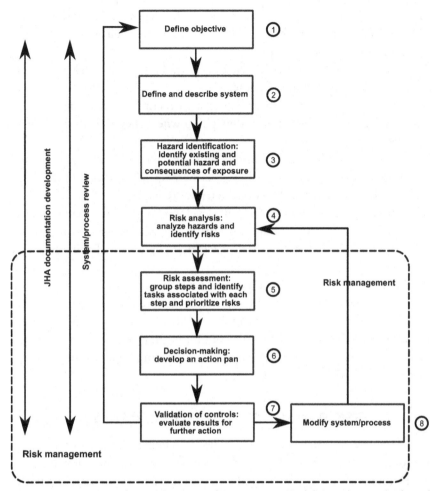

Figure 8.2 *Overview of an Eight Step Risk Assessment Model. Based on and adapted from System Safety Process Steps. Federal Aviation Administration (FAA) Safety Risk Management Order, 8040.4.*

 ## 8.6 THE AMERICAN SOCIETY OF SAFETY ENGINEERS (ASSE) RISK ASSESSMENT INSTITUTE

The ASSE Risk Assessment Institute provides a seven-step process for conducting a risk assessment: (American Society of Safety Engineers, n.d.)

1. Gather data: An organization should complete an in-depth inventory of all hazards and related risks.

2. Set scope and limits of the assessment: The depth and extend of a risk assessment can range from a high level overview of all aspects of an organization to individual jobs.
3. Charter and develop a risk reduction team: This step parallels the development of a JHA team (Chapter 4).
4. Conduct the risk assessment: The actual identification of hazards and risks begins by pinpointing and mapping where they exist in the various processes used.
5. Document results: During this documentation process, a format is established of who, what, where, how, and why for all information that is to be stored or "curated" for future retrieval (Chapter 15).
6. Follow-up on actions taken: The development of documentation, resources, and their organization is critical in ensuring that a comprehensive follow-up on what controls have been implemented and whether it is effective.
7. Sustain and continuously improve the risk reduction process.

The models discussed are examples that outline the basic elements required in a risk assessment and can be modified to meet the special needs of an organization. As a process for continuous improvement, they provide validation of decisions, desired results, and determination of the need for further action (Figure 8.3).

8.7 RISK MANAGEMENT RESPONSIBILITIES

Effective risk management specifies and defines the levels of responsibility and authority of leadership team and may include the following:

- Defining unacceptable risk and ensuring that a full understanding of the potential negative impact of risk has been assessed.
- Assessing risks, developing risk reduction alternatives, and defining residual risk concerns and issues.
- Identifying unnecessary or ineffective risk controls for further analysis.
- Selecting risk reduction options from recommendations.
- Accepting or rejecting risk based on the benefit to be derived.
- Training and educating employees on the selected risk management tools and techniques (Chapter 12).
- Ensuring that risks are taken only at the appropriate organizational level, and as needed, elevating risk decisions to a higher leadership level. This shift implies that the next level of leadership has a full understanding of associated risk and its control.

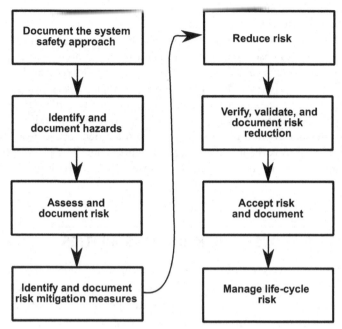

Figure 8.3 *Overview of Establishing Task Priorities. Based on and adapted from Department of Defense Standard Practice (2012).*

- Integrating risk assessment methods into the business planning process to ensure that time and money are budgeted for implementation of necessary controls (Carter and Simon, 2001; MITRE's Systems Engineering Process Office, n.d.; The American Society of Safety Engineers, 2012).

8.8 LEADERSHIP'S RISK RESPONSIBILITIES

Leadership's responsibilities include:
- Consistently using risk assessment and management concepts for identifying potential loss-producing events.
- Ensuring that employees follow appropriate risk control procedures and protocols as defined by the risk assessment and JHAs.
- Elevating risk concerns and issues beyond their control or authority to more senior leadership for resolution (MITRE's Systems Engineering Process Office, n.d.).

Lesson Learned #1

During an incident investigation session with supervisors, the initial incident investigation had a recommendation for retraining an injured employee on a particular standard operating procedure. A job hazard analysis was completed to fully assess the job and what the employee was trying to accomplish and the procedure referenced and under discussion was requested as part of the analysis. It turned out that the standard was non-existent! This lead to further discussion of the need to do the proper research on references used. It took the job hazard analysis to point out the gap and prevent an employee from being disciplined for violating a fictional SOP!

8.9 EMPLOYEE'S RISK RESPONSIBILITIES

Employee's responsibilities and specific roles include:
- Understanding the reasons for risk controls and ensuring they are followed.
- Maintaining a constant awareness of the potential severity associated with specific procedures, task, or operations.
- Immediately communicating to their direct leadership team when either risk reduction measures do not work, are unrealistic, and reporting ineffective high-risk procedures or controls (MITRE's Systems Engineering Process Office, n.d.).
- Working with coworkers to ensure that all appropriate protocols and procedures are followed as well as assisting each other in maintaining effective controls.
- Not taking any unnecessary risk.

8.10 RISK ACCEPTANCE

"Risk management is a logical process that weighs the potential cost of losses against the possible benefits of various levels of control ranging from no control implemented to instituting. But we must learn to balance the possible negative consequences of risk against the potential benefits" (US Air Force, 2011).

A decision making process should show the logic and assessment of how and why that risk was considered acceptable and how the level of risk did not unduly set in motion possible harm to any individual or group, environment, third party, etc. The decision to accept a risk should not be made on strictly "return on investment" criteria. It should consider the impact on the community, consumers, environment, legal duties, and many other "costs" considerations.

Case Study #1

The Ford Motor Company made a risk decision with its Pinto design using a cost benefit analysis that showed the savings to Ford would exceed any potential lawsuits. The company paid dearly for that decision. It failed to comprehend the potential impact on the brand and how the public would react to a callous decision concerning a life threatening design (The Top Automotive Engineering Failures: The Ford Pinto Fuel Tanks, 2011).

Case Study #2

Takata Corporation made a risk decision by not recalling exploding airbags for a lengthy period of time because a particular car model was not initially included in an original recall (Clifford and Blackwell, 2015).

To reduce the "perception that if no losses have occurred then no "risk" is present," the leadership team should ask a series of questions about each job function:

- How often does the exposure to a specific hazard(s) occur?
- What is the frequency that the job should be done or completed?
- What is the probability that a loss-producing event might occur during any of the job's steps and tasks? Has general industry information been researched and provided insights on what might happen?
- What could be the consequences of exposure given the combination of people, activity, tools, equipment, materials, and the environment?
- What is the potential cost of a loss-producing event considering all negative consequences versus the benefit of completing the job?
- Do the total benefits outweigh the total cost? (US Air Force, 2011) Costs is all "cost" as mentioned, beyond just the financial considerations.

8.11 WHY ARE UNNECESSARY RISKS TAKEN?

Unnecessary risks are voluntarily taken when the alleged benefits at some level outweigh the implied consequence. In addition, a lack of experience, ignorance of the possible consequences and possibly a general attitude that "it can't happen", "its fate, it would happen anyway", or "I'm better than others and can't be hurt" gets factored into the decision.

Further, when an individual deals with any type of hazard-related condition, a built-in human trait is to judge their environment based on past experiences. We observe a situation; scan our memory for a similar situation experienced in the past, and then act, based what we remember without thinking of the consequences (Roughton & Crutchfield, 2013).

"People's views on risks and their value judgments are not static, but change according to circumstances."

– (Mullai, 2006)

Lesson Learned #1

A colleague told the story of an employee cleaning a printer roller by wrapping a rag around his hand and holding it against moving rollers. The employee's response was, "I've done this for many years and never been caught!!" Several weeks later, he was finally caught and had a serious hand injury. He thought himself above the risk as his experience implied.

When one of the authors begin his career in the printing industry, there was a saying, "A good printer always has a missing finger!" The industry considers this acceptable!

Once a hazardous activity is completed one time and nothing happens, if the activity was though beneficial, it will be repeated without considering the risk.

To put this in perspective, the following story stresses how behaviors can continue over time:

A man's wife would cook ham often and when she cooked the ham, he noticed that she always cut both ends off the ham. One day he asked his wife: "Why do you cut the ends off." She replied, "Because my mother always did it." He asks, "Can we call your mother and ask her why she cuts the ends off." Her mother's response was "Because my mother always did it."

This was very interesting, so he wanted to pursue this a little more. So the grandmother was asked, "We would like to know why you cut off the end of the ham before you put it in the pan?" Grandmother stated "Because, in my day, the pans were too small and the ham would not fit into my pan so I had to cut the ends off to make it fit."

This influence of the grandmother moved through several generations without question! Only after several generations was the key question asked – Why?

Sometimes we accept that something looks right and we do it ourselves without asking questions. We keep doing the same activity until we experience a loss-producing event.

Using the ham story example, we see things we do not understand, but continue doing the same thing over and over again without asking questions. One way to resolve habitual behaviors similar to the above situation is by developing and maintaining a "questioning attitude" while performing any job (US DOE, 2009a). This "questioning attitude" helps to encourage an individual to "Stop" when they are unsure about a particular condition by asking "Why am I doing this?" Refer to Table 8.1 for a method for developing a questioning attitude.

"The important thing is not to stop questioning; curiosity has its own reason for existing."

– Albert Einstein

Based on and adapted using (US DOE, 2009b).

8.12 HAZARD RECOGNITION TOOLS, BUILDING THE FOUNDATION FOR RISK PERCEPTION

A risk evaluation tool, the risk matrix, has been used to develop an understanding of operational risk for a number of years. The US military has adopted the concept to address risk in its daily operations and activities and recommends that individual as well as operational risk are identified by the leadership team (Department of the Navy Office of the Chief of Naval Operations, 2010).

This risk matrix is based on and adapted for demonstration purposes from the Department of Defense (DOD) Standard Practice (Air Force Safety Agency, 2000; Federal Aviation Administration (FAA), 2008b) (Figure 8.4).

Risk assessment tools used in industry approach the risk matrix concept as a management tool and not one that directly involves the employee. However, use of a personal risk assessment tool can be an effective way to

Table 8.1 Developing a questioning attitude

- Stop, Look, and Listen. Proactively search for work situations that flag uncertainty (see When to Use the Tool).
- Ask Questions. Gather relevant information.
- Proceed if sure. Continue the activity if the uncertainty has been resolved with facts, otherwise, do not proceed in the face of uncertainty!
- Stop When Unsure. If inconsistencies, confusion, uncertainties, or doubts still exist, do the following.

Risk assessment matrix				
Severity Probability	Catastrophic	Critical	Marginal	Negligible
Frequent	High	High	Serious	Medium
Probable	High	High	Serious	Medium
Occasional	High	Serious	Medium	Low
Remote	Serious	Medium	Medium	Low
Improbable	Medium	Medium	Medium	Low
Eliminated	Eliminated			

Figure 8.4 *Example Risk Assessment Matrix. Based on and adapted for demonstration purposes Department of Defense Standard Practice (2012).*

address risk at the "grass roots level" and for determining appropriate immediate actions.

> *"When undertaking a risk assessment, the consequence or 'how bad' the risk being assessed is must be measured. In this context, consequence is defined as: the outcome or the potential outcome of an event. Clearly, there may be more than one consequence of a single event"* (The National Patient Safety Agency, 2008).

Use of a standardized personal risk assessment tool builds a bridge between the differences and variations in individual risk perception. A combination of the employee and leadership team discussing potential risk is the best approach to address risk perception. A personal risk assessment tool and a discussion process enhances the employees' knowledge in identifying, recognizing, evaluating, and controlling of associated risk.

8.13 THE RISK GUIDANCE CARD, A POTENTIAL SOLUTION

The risk guidance card can be used to address ongoing employee perceptions or concerns about job hazards. The risk guidance card can be used with a work team and/or employees as part of a prejob assessment. The card provides a "Go/No Go" decision method as the employee(s) performs assigned tasks (Roughton & Crutchfield, 2008, 2013). The risk guidance card is used until the perception is mutually consistent between the concerned employee(s) and leadership team.

A risk assessment matrix is placed on the risk card to allow evaluation of the estimates of what is the perceived potential event severity and the frequency of exposure to a hazard. A brief list of guidelines and questions are placed on the card to guide the assessment and discussions.

> "A risk assessment matrix is a useful tool to identify the level of risk and the levels of management approval required for any Risk Management Plan. There are various forms of this matrix, but they all have a common objective to define the potential consequences or severity of the hazard versus the probability or likelihood of the hazard" (Safety Management System Toolkit, 2007).

The intent of the risk guidance card is to allow employees to assess levels of perceived risk, and if believed by the employee to be unacceptable, begin a dialogue with the appropriate leadership level on whether to accept or reject the risk and what controls are to be implemented. This provides a way to reduce the probability that a high risk is accepted without prior discussion with leadership team members.

Refer to Table 8.2 for an example to define probability and severity.

8.14 USING THE RISK GUIDANCE CARD

To use the risk guidance card, the employees ask the following questions:
- Given what I see and believe about the current situation or condition, what are the consequences of exposure and whether something can go wrong?
- What are the odds or probability that something harmful or damaging can happen? Will that incident be marginal, critical, or severe?
- What in this task can cause injury or damage?
- What should be done about this situation or condition?

The objective is get the exposed employee(s) to define the potential harm explicitly in terms of the adverse consequence(s) from the hazard and its level of risk. Brief, simple definitions are used to define probability and severity ratings to begin the overall discussion (Tables 8.3 and 8.4) (Improving Health, Improving Services (Risk Form Assessment), 2012; Department of the Army, 2008; US Air Force, 2011; Roughton & Crutchfield, 2013; Roughton, 1995).

Table 8.2 Identifying probability and severity

Probability		Severity	
Unlikely.	Rare chance of occurrence, some possibility injury exist	Marginal.	Minor injury, no first aid
Likely.	An event or an injury as happened in the past	Critical.	Minor injury, potential first aid
Very likely.	Harm is certain – An obvious condition	Severe.	High change of an injury or permanent disability

The objective is to Identify conditions(s) and/or behavior(s) before performing task.

STOP – THINK – AND ASK Questions

When they do not understand the hazard!!use a questioning attitude to determine the likelihood of an injury

What is the frequency of this task?	Seldom. Less than 1 time per shift/day	Occasionally. At least daily, no more than 3 times per shift/day	Frequently. More than 3 times per shift/day

Remember – As the frequency of an event increases so does the probability for an injury

Questions to ask for before conducting any task

What is involved in this task that can hurt me or my coworkers?
How can/we keep from getting hurt while performing this task?
If I get hurt how serious could it be?
How likely is it to happen?
What should be done about it?

Source: Roughton & Crutchfield (2013); Roughton (1995).

Table 8.3 Probability rating

Unlikely	Rare occurrence, the possibility of an injury or damage exist
Likely	Reasonable – a strong possibility exist for a loss-producing event
Very likely	High possibility of a loss producing event

Source: Roughton & Crutchfield (2013); Roughton (1995)

Table 8.4 Severity rating

Marginal	Minor injury, first aid
Critical	Injury requiring medical attention or damage repair
Severe	High chance of a serious injury involving or permanent disability or major damage

For example, when an employee uses the risk guidance card and their perception of the hazard is identified as a Risk Rating of 1, 2, or 3 (RED), then the task is stopped and the leadership team is contacted immediately.

This perceived Risk Rating of 1, 2, or 3 is discussed in detail with a member of the leadership during which the employee(s) will share their concerns. The key rule is that the leadership team member cannot override the concerns of the employee without first providing a solution or clearly demonstrating how the hazard and its associated risk are or can be controlled. Both the leadership team member and employee(s) should mutually agree with the analysis before the task can be continued.

If no agreement can be reached between that level of leadership and the employee(s) then the concerns will be discussed with the next level of leadership. This discussion will include the employee, the employee's direct leader and the next level of leadership, etc. until there is an agreement between all parties. This process continues until everyone is in mutual agreement as to the level of risk and potential outcomes.

An objective of the Risk Guidance Tool is to develop a situational awareness of the potential for a loss-producing event. For a visual representation of the risk assessment, the Risk Guidance Tool uses a color code. An example of the use of color is found in the US Navy's Operational Risk Management (ORM) Fundamentals:
- Green indicates errors may occur, but errors will be caught by the individual.
- Yellow indicates the potential for consequential errors have increased.
- Red indicates errors may occur that cannot be caught and, therefore, become consequential to the task or mission. (Department of the Navy Office of the Chief of Naval Operations, 2010)

Given the need for an organization to meet specific production or goals, the pressure to maintain a schedule of activity will consciously or unconsciously pressure employees to see risk as acceptable even when conditions or the situation indicates otherwise (see Figure 8.5). For an example of the Risk Guidance Card (Figure 8.6).

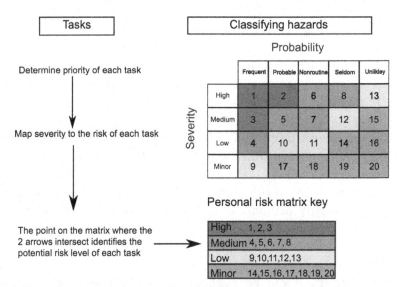

Figure 8.5 *Personal Risk Assessment Hazard Classification Tool, A Risk Guidance Card to help Assess Risk of Assignments. Based on and adapted from Risk Assessment Matrix, Department of Defense Standard Practice.*

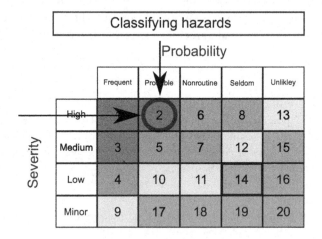

Figure 8.6 *Annotated Personal Risk Assessment Hazard Classification Tool, A Risk Guidance Card to Help Assess Risk of Assignments. Based on and adapted from Risk Assessment Matrix, Department of Defense Standard Practice Safety System System Safety, MIL-STD-882E (2012).*

SUMMARY

The concept of risk should be clearly defined and should be included as a major element in the job hazard analysis (JHA) process. Using only loss-related data that is solely based on injuries, incident rates and/or damage does not provide a full understanding of the potential for loss-producing events.

Risk management concepts have been around and used for many years in high hazard industries. However, many safety programs are still designed around regulatory compliance using post loss criteria and only limited use basic risk management principles.

An open line of two-way communication between all levels of the organization is essential to effectively spread information through the organizational about its scope of risk.

The JHA provides a method for improving the risk analysis when used to identify existing and potential hazards and the consequences of exposure to hazards. Job content is identified by reviewing the combination of required actions, job environment, tools, equipment, and materials used, and affected employees and other personnel.

The understanding of risk assessment concepts is essential to the accepting of risk. One of the primary objectives of the JHA is to locate and identify the risk inherent in the completion of a job, its steps and tasks. Several models provide suggested the steps to follow in the review of risk.

The acceptance of risk without an understanding of the consequences of exposure and/or loss-producing events that can result in a litigious climate of lawsuit frenzy can be discovery in even a cursory review of the loss history of documented events.

Risk assessment tools used in industry approach the risk matrix concept as a management tool and not one that directly involves the employee. However, use of a personal risk assessment tool can be an effective way to address risk at the "grass roots level" and for determining appropriate immediate actions.

The Risk Guidance Card, in the form of a small card, can be used to address ongoing employee perceptions or concerns about job hazards. The risk guidance card can be used with a work team and/or employees as part of a "prejob assessment." The card provides a "Go/No Go" decision method as they perform assigned tasks.

A successful safety system is one in which risks are continuously identified and analyzed for relative importance and impact. Risks are mitigated, controlled and tracked by effectively using tools and resources such as the JHA, observation, inspections, employee participation, quality control methods such as Six Sigma, etc.

CHAPTER REVIEW QUESTIONS

1. What is essential between all levels of an organization?
2. Define Risk?
3. What does the JHA provide?
4. Describe NASA's Continuous Risk Management Process.
5. How does the French and Bell model apply to the JHA process?
6. What are various reason we take risk?
7. Can a financial ROI be used in risk assessment? What else should be used?
8. What are the leadership and employee responsibilities?
9. Why can a risk card be a useful tool for risk assessment?
10. How is the risk assessment card used?

BIBLIOGRAPHY

Air Force Safety Agency. (2000). *Air force system safety handbook.* Kirtland AFB NM 87117-5670, Public Domain, Modified for Use.
American Society of Safety Engineers. (n.d.). Risk Assessment Institute. Retrieved from http://bit.ly/1GYTij1
Carter, G.R. & Simon S. (2001). *Construction safety risk–improving the level of hazard identification.* In ESREL 2001 European Safety Reliability International Conference, Torino, Italy.
Clifford, A., & Blackwell, R.B. (2015). *Massive Takata airbag recall: Everything you need to know, including full list of affected vehicles.* Car and driver. Retrieved from http://bit.ly/1D8eFdR
Department of Defense Standard Practice. (2012). *System safety,* MIL-STD-882E. Public Domain.
Department of the Army. (2008). *Army system safety management guide.* Pamphlet 385-16, Public Domain. Retrieved from http://bit.ly/11f0gib
Department of the Navy Office of The Chief of Naval Operations. (2010). *Operational risk management (ORM) fundamentals.* Pubic Domain. Retrieved from http://bit.ly/VuvB8D
Federal Aviation Administration (FAA). (2000). *Principles of system safety,* Chapter 3. Public Domain, Adpated for use. Retrieved from http://1.usa.gov/YiEZvJ
Federal Aviation Administration (FAA). (2008a). *Safety management system, Manual–Version 2.1,* Public Domain. Retrieved from http://1.usa.gov/WSds8S
Federal Aviation Administration (FAA). (2008b). *System safety handbook,* Chapter 15, Public Domain, Based on and Adapted for Use. Retrieved from http://1.usa.gov/1FDhENy
French, W., & Bell, C. (1984). *Organizational development: Behavioral science interventions for organizational movement.* Englewood Cliffs, NJ: Prentice-Hall.
Improving Health, Improving Services (Risk Form Assessment). (2012). Lincoln, LN4 2HN: NHS Lincolnshire.: NHS Lincolnshire, Cross O'Cliff, Bracebridge Heath, Public Domain. Retrieved from http://bit.ly/XOLXZo

List of spaceflight-related accidents and incidents. (n.d.). Wikipedia. Retrieved from http:// en.wikipedia.org/wiki/List_of_spaceflight-related_accidents_and_incidents

MITRE's Systems Engineering Process Office. (n.d.). *Risk management toolkit*, Public Domain.

Mullai, A. (2006). *Risk management system: Risk assessment frameworks and techniques*. Turku, Finland: DaGoB Project Office, Turku School of Economics.

NASA Headquarters. (n.d.). *NASA risk management handbook*. Washington, D.C. 20546: National Aeronautics and Space Administration. Retrieved from http://1.usa.gov/1xc8l7l

Roughton, J. (1995). *Job hazard analysis: An essential safety tool*. J. J. Keller's OSHA Safety Training Newsletter, (pp. 131–134).

Roughton, J., & Crutchfield, N. (2008). *Job hazard analysis: A guide for voluntary compliance and beyond. chemical, petrochemical & process*. MA: Elsevier/Butterworth-Heinemann, Retrieved from http://amzn.to/VrSAq5.

Roughton, J., & Crutchfield, N. (2013). In B. Heinemann (Ed.), *Safety culture: An innovative leadership approach*. MA: Butterworth Heinemann, Retrieved from http://amzn. to/1qoD4oN.

Safety Management System Toolkit. (2007). Developed by the Joint Helicopter Safety Implementation Team of the International Helicopter Safety Team, *The international helicopter safety symposium*, Montréal, Québec, Canada. Retrieved from http://bit.ly/YaSCOg

The American Society of Safety Engineers. (2012). *Occupational health & safety management systems*. ANSI/AIHA/ASSE Z10. Retrieved from http://bit.ly/1MsT6MG

The National Patient Safety Agency. (2008). *A risk matrix for risk managers*. 4-8 Maple Street, London. Retrieved from http://bit.ly/12hoCH4

The Top Automotive Engineering Failures: The Ford Pinto Fuel Tanks. (2011, May). Popular Mechanics. Retrieved from http://bit.ly/1C2zEDh

United States Air Force. (2011). *Mishap prevention program*. Instruction 91-202. Retrieved from http://1.usa.gov/XMhhrU

US DOE. (2009a). *Concepts and principles, human performance improvement handbook* (Vol. 1). US Department of Energy. Retrieved from http://bit.ly/1DfdJVU

US DOE, 2009b. *Human performance tools for individuals, work teams, and management, human performance improvement handbook* (Vol. 2). US Department of Energy. Retrieved from http://bit.ly/14kc6Lj

US DOE. (2005). *Columbia space shuttle accident and Davis-Besse reactor pressure-vessel head corrosion event.* (2005). US Department of Energy Action Plan Lessons Learned, Public Domain. Retrieved from http://1.usa.gov/YOWYft

CHAPTER NINE

Planning for the Job Hazard Analysis

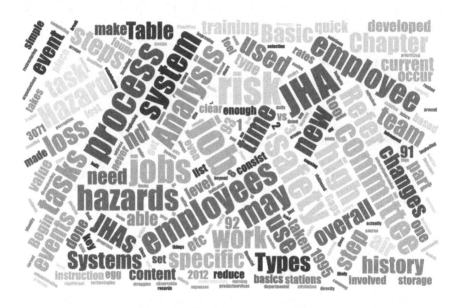

"We do not want production and a safety program, or production and safety, or production with safety. But, rather, we want safe production."

—*Dan Petersen*

Chapter Objectives

At the end of the chapter, you should be able to:

- Discuss the importance and benefits of the JHA.
- Discuss how the JHA committee is selected?
- Define the basics for selecting jobs for analysis
- Discuss how jobs are to be analyzed, selected, and prioritized?
- Define a process for developing a job inventory and its importance

Job Hazard Analysis. http://dx.doi.org/10.1016/B978-0-12-803441-5.00009-X

9.1 BENEFITS OF DEVELOPING JHA'S

In Chapter 1, "Why focus on the job hazard analysis," developing a JHA process was discussed as having benefits that go beyond just regulatory compliance. The JHA process can bridge the gap between basic regulatory compliance and a safety system that provides a comprehensive risk-based structure.

Benefits of a JHA
- Detects and reduces the potential for loss-producing events.
- Provides job orientation/training instruction content on how to safely perform the steps and tasks. It provides a quick refresher instruction for infrequent and nonroutine jobs.
- The job requirements are made clear and concise for employees and the leadership team.
- Assist in identifying methods to improve quality, aid in improving job efficiency, and reduce operational costs.
- Employees are involved the overall job improvement efforts.

9.2 BEGINNING THE PROCESS

Safety systems consist of a number of elements that address the content for controls of specific observable hazards in an organization. The use of generic safety materials can jumpstart a system by establishing a basic administrative format for immediate use. The need for generic materials will always remain as organizations evolve and change over time. A simple change in a location's leadership or even individuals can result in a safety system imploding and disappearing.

These generic or "Plug-n-Play" programs are normally built around regulatory compliance. The regulatory criteria give the perception that the risk are controlled. As a result, the safety system is not part of the overall operational process and is considered an "add-on" that is not integrated into overall organizational structure. Safety system elements are then not considered essential to the overall success of the organization.

What does all this have to do with completing a JHA? If JHA is not considered a part of how jobs are designed then employee selection, training, safety system budgets, and other needs can be wasted. Startup operations tend to suffer from high injury rates and major loss-producing situations as the organization struggles to stabilize how things get done.

> **Lesson Learned #1**
>
> A company was implementing an ergonomic program for workstations. A multiyear injury history had indicated that the current design was creating an unacceptable level of injuries. The ergonomic review found a need for new chairs, adjustable workstations, and other capital expenses. However, the financial budget process was on a 3-year cycle and even if the desired changes were approved, they would not be implemented for 3 years. The job were never actually designed for the newer technologies and accompanying new hazards.

9.3 THE "FEEL" OF THE WORKPLACE

The "feel" of the workplace can be lost unless systems are in place that constantly monitor ongoing change(s), for example, employee and leadership turnover, organizational restructuring, new technology, field product/services change, etc. A structured process aids in ensuring that the leadership team understands the benefits of developing and using JHAs and how they can create value to the organization. Since the safety professional is the interface between the leadership team and other support groups, it is up to the safety professional to communicate to the leadership team and employees how the safety systems and the JHA are integrated.

9.4 CONDUCTING THE JHA

Conducting the JHA begins by ensuring that the committee selected understands the term "Job." In this discussion, it is used to both identify a job as a title that includes many activities and as a specific individual activity. Refer to Chapter 2 where we defined the term "job" in detail. The following phases are required to begin a JHA process:

- Develop an inventory of jobs: This inventory brings together as much information as possible about what is being done in the course of everyday activities. Resources would include existing job descriptions, training records, and insights from discussions with employees and industry information. The interviews with departmental leadership is essential as departments may have developed their own job descriptions depending on how decentralized the organization may be. This information provides a high level overview of what is expected of employees.

- Develop a list of known hazardous jobs: The inventory is reviewed for content and the nature of each job. Jobs with hazards that present high risks are ranked based on which are most likely to occur and with the most severe consequences of a loss-producing event. These jobs are the first priority for further analysis.
- Involve employees in developing the prioritized list for JHA development: Employee participation in the process minimizes possible oversights of specific hazards unseen by those who do not do the job daily. Including employees increases the quality analysis of job components. The key is for all employees to "buy in" to the future solutions and share the ownership in the JHA process and safety system.
- Review loss history: Loss-producing events are "warning signs" or indicators that the existing preventative measures or current controls (if any) may not be adequate to reduce losses. The documents and history of injuries (OSHA logs, claims reports, incident investigations), damages to equipment or facilities (work orders, repair reports) may be spread across multiple departments and require additional time and approval to access. Multiyear histories can be used if no significant changes have been made in operations and analyzed by department and job type.
- Conduct a preliminary job review: A structured format is used to break the job into its required steps and tasks as well as all the items necessary to get the job done. When preparing to develop a JHA, the employee is directly observed performing the job and each step and task listed in sequence. Each step has possible multiple tasks that should be reviewed. Describe each required action with only enough information necessary and not too detailed. If the same job is performed by other employees, several reviews may be completed to verify a consistent approach is in use.

Hazards and associated risk within each step are discussed with employees as to what they know about the current work environment. This information is compared against the loss history of the job to assess where in each job the highest probability of loss exists. Chapter 10 will cover this review at length.

- Establish a plan to remove or control hazards identified as soon as possible: During the initial development of the job inventory, uncontrolled hazards may be identified. These hazards need immediate attention and corrective actions should be taken as soon as possible as they have a high probability of generating a loss-producing event and cannot wait for a full JHA development.

- Finally, review the information collected with the leadership team and employees to ensure that the committee has not overlooked important elements.

9.5 JHA IMPLEMENTATION OBSTACLES

A JHA process takes time and effort in order to effectively define, document, and develop new or modified controls. Although JHA is an effective tool, it should be considered part of a continuous improvement process, a "living document" that will change from time-to-time as new opportunities for improvements are discovered. This potential for improvement will outweigh any drawbacks (Job Hazard Analysis, 3071, 2002).

As an organization may have a very large number of jobs to review, a budget for time, and resources is essential. Each analysis takes considerable time and attention and a schedule is needed to work through entire job inventory. Leadership commitment and support is necessary to make the JHA process possible. Resources and coordination in additional to time and budget include access to equipment, materials, and tools in use.

A plan and criteria for approaching affected employee is needed for observation and evaluation of the job, steps, and tasks. Special consideration is needed for areas sensitive to leadership/employee relationships. Open communication and effective positive two-way communication is essential to resolve any issues or concerns that may develop (Conducting a Job Hazard Analysis (JHA), n.d.; Roughton, 1995).

9.6 THE IMPORTANCE OF EMPLOYEES TO THE JHA PROCESS

As discussed in Chapter 7, employee participation is one of the key considerations for any successful safety system and the JHA process. Employees may become more receptive to change when they are engaged and the opportunity to be involved in decisions that impact on their work and completion of tasks (Roughton, 1995).

9.7 SELECTING THE JHA ADMINISTRATOR

A designated person should be selected to coordinate the overall JHA process and act as the clearinghouse for documents used in analyzing jobs. The person selected should have a combination of the following traits:

- Be able to communicate verbally, in writing, and in presentations to all levels of the organization.
- Be able to communicate the value and benefits of the JHA process.
- Respected by peers as knowledgeable about operations and have an understanding of the various processes and methods used by the organization.
- Be able to apply risk assessment and problem-solving techniques to uncover hidden hazards and associated risk.
- Understand the nature and relationship of hazards and associated risk with loss producing events.
- Understand the basics of project management and keep the project organized and moving toward its main objectives.

(Roughton & Florczak, 1999)

This individual should have the authority to make recommendations that may occur during implementation. The JHA administrator uses a variety of methods and procedures:

- Provide input and advice to the various committees developing JHAs.
- Assist with evaluating the completeness and effectiveness of the JHAs.
- Assist in using the JHAs in loss-producing event investigations.
- Assist in the periodic evaluation of JHAs to ensure that they are current with the operational process and technology.
- Assist in reviewing the JHAs with employees to ensure an understanding of what is expected of them and if they have any concerns with new procedures or actions required.

(Managing Worker Safety and Health, n.d.)

9.8 SELECTING THE JHA COMMITTEE

A cross-functional committee should be used to conduct job risk assessments, reviewing loss history, job related documents, interviews, and overall data collection. The committee directs the JHA process through the following:

- Use a charter to clearly define how they will operate and manage the JHA process (Chapter 4).
- Hold regular meetings and provide written documentation of meeting minutes to the JHA process administrator.
- Encourage employee participation by communicating the value and use of JHAs.
- Analyze job data on steps and tasks, identified hazards, and associated risk assessments, and recommended controls.
- Review employee suggestions and concerns and bring these to the attention of the JHA process administrator.
- Ensure that insights provided by employees are accepted in a positive manner and timely feedback is provided.
- Communicate immediately to the leadership team when high severity hazards and associated risks are identified and appropriate controls should be implemented.

(Roughton & Crutchfield, 2008)

If the organization does not use committees, the culture may not support the abnormality of a standalone committee. Determine how assignments and responsibilities are delegated and how projects are managed before embarking on a committee approach.

9.9 THE JHA COMMITTEE CHARTER

A charter is used to guide the JHA committee and clearly define how it will operate. The charter should include:

- A clear statement that describes the job and safety improvement opportunities for the organization.
- The mission and objectives of the committee and why it was established.
- Describes the procedures to be followed by the committee.
- The scope of the JHA process and the limits on the committee.
- The timeframe of the charter and committee membership.
- The date and time the committee will begin activity.
- The ownership of the JHAs completed.
- The communications methods and documentation of the process.
 (Conducting a Job Hazard Analysis (JHA), n.d.; Roughton, 1995)

Unless already provided as part of the overall organizational training, the committee should be educated on the basics on how to work as a committee, responsibilities of committee membership, how to hold meetings, and how to present and communicate findings.

9.10 JHA AS A PROBLEM SOLVING TOOL

JHA can be used as a problem-solving tool that can define the root cause of problems associated with a job. A job can be viewed as a series of causes and effects of elements that work together to complete an action. Each element brings inherent hazards that have a level of risk (probability and severity). Refer to risk assessment in Chapter 8, "Defining Associated Risk" and Figure 9.1.

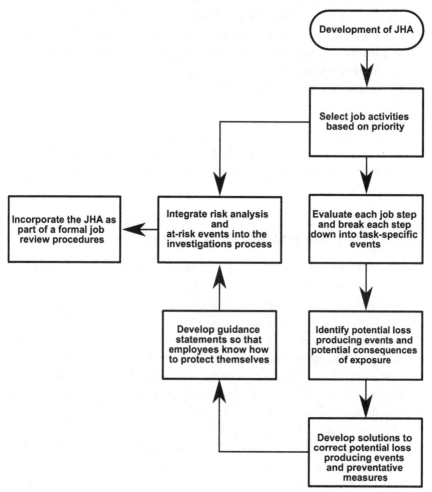

Figure 9.1 *Basic Job Hazard Analysis Model, Roughton & Crutchfield (2008).*

> The Corps of Engineers uses a task hazard analysis (THA) on construction sites. The THA is developed prior to performing any new task. No task will proceed until a THA has been conducted and all affected site employees are trained (US Army Corps of Engineers, 2014).

To ensure that the committee has a common knowledge of the terms that use in the JHA process, refer to Table 9.1 for an overview of basic JHA terms and types of risk..

Overview of Basic Types of Risk.

Table 9.1 Overview of basic JHA terms types of risk

Term	Discussion
Job	A job can be defined as any activity (mental or physical or both) that has been assigned to an employee as a responsibility. ("Managing Worker Safety and Health," n.d.) A Job can be further defined as a sequence of steps with specific tasks that are designed to accomplish a desired goal.
Steps	Steps are specific elements in a job. A step can be defined as a segment necessary to advance one of a series of actions, processes, or measures taken to achieve a goal. A job is completed by following a sequence of steps.
Task	A task can be defined as an activity required to complete a step. Multiple tasks may be required within each step. Tasks are detailed actions taken to complete a step.
Hazard	"A hazard is a condition, set of circumstances, or inherent property that can cause injury, illness" ("Occupational Health & Safety Management Systems," 2012) (Appendix I) (Managing Worker Safety and Health, n.d.). Hazards increase the probability that injury or harm will occur.
Exposure	An exposure is when anyone (employees, objects, etc.) enters a "danger zone" by virtue of the proximity to the hazard (Roughton & Florczak, 1999; Roughton & Crutchfield, 2013).
Consequences of exposure	Consequences are defined as "something that logically or naturally follows from an action or condition. The effect, result, or outcome of something occurring earlier" (Consequence, n.d.).
At-risk events	At-risk events are activities that place employees or individuals into exposure to a hazard and is associated risk.

Table 9.2 Overview of Basic Types of Risk

Term	Discussion
Risk	"An estimate of the combination of the likeli- hood of an occurrence of a hazardous event or exposure(s), and the severity of injury or ill- ness that may be caused the event of exposures" ("Occupational Health & Safety Management Systems," 2012). Risk also includes potential property damage (Chapter 8).
Identified risk	The type of "risk, which has been determined through various analysis techniques" (Air Force System Agency, 2000).
Unidentified risk	This is "risk that has not been determined. It is real, It is important, but not measurable. Some risks are never known" (Air Force System Agency, 2000).
Unacceptable risk	"Risk which cannot be tolerated by the managing activity. It is a subset of identified risk which is either eliminated or controlled" (Air Force System Agency, 2000).
Acceptable risk	"Identified risk which is allowed to persist without further engineering or management action. It is accepted by the managing activity,…it is the user who is exposed to this risk" (Air Force System Agency, 2000).
Residual risk	The risk remaining after response or mitigation (existing measures and incremental strategies). Residual risk must be less than the initial risk analysis (Air Force System Agency, 2000) (Figure 9.2).

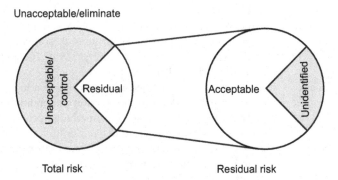

Figure 9.2 *Types of Risk–Total Risk Versus Residual Risk. Based on and adapted using the Air Force System Agency (2000).*

9.11 SELECTING THE JOBS FOR ANALYSIS

To evaluate specific jobs effectively, both knowledge and experience of the work process, an understanding of how to conduct the JHA, and how to best implement controls and/or preventative measures are important (Managing Worker Safety and Health, n.d.).

When selecting jobs for analysis, combinations of actual physical hazards, the actions of the employee, and/or gaps in the safety system are considered, discussed in more detail in Figure 13.3.

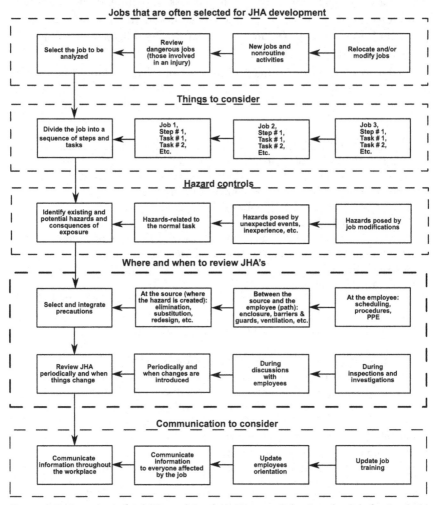

Figure 9.3 *Overview of Job Hazard Analysis Process, Selecting the Job for Analysis.*
Based on and adapted using Job Safety Analysis, Worksafe; Roughton and Crutchfield (2008)

Begin by reviewing jobs that have high-potential risk severity and the highest rates of disabling injuries or damage based on initial job inventory assessment. These jobs can provide the potential for immediate improvement. Corrective actions may be able to showcase savings in workers' compensation claims, improved job efficiency as hazards are avoided or reduced. Jobs that are new or have had specific tasks, changes in a process and/or procedure should be the next priority. Jobs with multiple complex steps and tasks are good candidates for analysis as their process complexity leads to potential procedural issues.

Jobs that are automated should be considered and can offer real surprises. They have the appearance of controlled risk and limited in loss potential. However, they may have hidden risk should the automation fail or procedures for maintenance and operation not be followed (Roughton & Crutchfield, 2013) (Figure 9.3).

Refer to Table 9.3 for some typical types of jobs that should be considered high priority.

Table 9.3 Typical jobs types to be considered as high priority

- High frequency of injuries, illnesses, or damage.
- High degree of risk as found in industry history or from risk assessment.
- High duration of task, time requirements to complete.
- High physical forces on the employee and or equipment.
- Posture required of the person i.e., Ergonomics.
- Point of operation requiring employee vs. machine interface or exposure.
- High pressure, mechanical, pneumatic, fluid, etc.
- Excessive vibration.
- Environmental exposures.
- Non-routine tasks involving high risk where experience can be limited by time.
- High turnover or rotation of employees, new employees with limited experience.
- Near misses or close-calls, at-risk events, or loss-producing events.
- Recent process or operational changes or relocation of equipment, new equipment or process, new tools, materials, or work environment.
- New job and/or tasks with little or no injury statistical data.
- Jobs that require a high degree of risk and requirement special training and knowledge skills and/or decision making.
- Job complex enough to require written instructions.
- Review jobs requiring industrial hygiene, ergonomic or environmental special surveys or monitoring.

Adapted and modified from Conducting a Job Hazard Analysis (JHA) (n.d.); US DOE (2009).

9.12 NONROUTINE TASKS

Interviews should ask about special nonroutine activities that should be undertaken to keep production or services on schedule, for example, spill cleanup, equipment jams, storage rack entry requiring working at a height, miscellaneous use of aerosol products, anything that is not specifically within the primary production process flow (Job Hazard Analysis, 3071, 2002).

Procedures to keep nonroutine jobs visible to the leadership team and in the JHA process are critical as these jobs may entail high-risk maintenance tasks and/or high-energy source exposures. In general, a priority on maintenance related jobs can be essential.

For all nonroutine jobs, a special safety briefing prior to starting the task should be implemented. The procedures should include determining if new hazards have developed due to changes in the job and additional controls are necessary before continuing.

Lesson Learned #2

In one severe, high-loss property loss, a welder undertook a quick nonroutine repair at an egg laying plant. This type of operation consists of large egg-laying houses that are highly combustible (chickens, feed, wastes) and highly automated. A hot work permit was required. The welder considered the job simple and to save time chose to quickly make the repair without following the procedures. The welding torch heated the opposite side of the metal being welded and combustible materials ignited. The fire was intensified by the ventilation system used to keep air movement in the laying house. The result was the loss of the entire egg laying house, its equipment, and thousands of chickens.

Lesson Learned #3

An employee noticed a pallet of material that needed to be straighten on the upper tier of a storage rack. Being a good employee, he saw a need and went to set it right. He climbed into the rack and began moving the pallet. He lost his balance and fell twenty feet to the warehouse floor, survived the fall but was seriously injured. In the search for non-routine jobs to analyze, ask about situations that need a quick response.

> ## SUMMARY

One goal for the job hazard analysis (JHA) process is to become self-sustaining and effective. The goal first begins by establishing a JHA committee that can provide experience, expertise, and assistance in developing the process. A properly structured committee working on the JHA process increases the effectiveness of the safety system.

The JHA process can bridge the gap between basic regulatory compliance and a safety system that provides a comprehensive risk-based structure.

The JHA process begins by shifting the mental perception about hazard controls and safety-related programs. The nature of controls and programs is that they imply that each program is essentially stand-alone.

The "feel" of the workplace can be lost unless systems are in place that constantly monitor ongoing change(s) such as employee and leadership turnover, organizational changes, new technology, field product/services change, etc. A structured process aids in ensuring that the leadership team understands the benefits of developing and using JHAs and how they can create value to the organization.

Conducting the JHA begins by ensuring that the committee selected understands the term "Job." In this discussion, it is used to both identify a job as a title that includes many activities and as a specific individual activity.

A JHA process takes time and effort in order to effectively define, document and develop new or modified controls. Although the JHA is an effective tool, it should be considered part of a continuous improvement process, a "living document" that will change from time-to-time as new opportunities for improvements are discovered.

A designated qualified person should be selected to manage the overall process and act as the clearinghouse for materials used in developing and analyzing JHAs.

A cross-functional committee should be used to conduct job risk assessments, reviewing loss history, job related documents, interviews and overall data collection.

A charter is suggested to guide the JHA committee and clearly define how it will operate.

If a central safety committee is used, a committee member could be designated to guide and administer the JHA process. This person would use the cross-functional teams with diversity and expertise useful for development of the JHA portfolio. The teams could be permanent in standing or "Ad Hoc" formed for special short-term projects.

The JHA can be used as a problem-solving tool that can define the root cause of problems associated with a job. A job can be viewed as a series of causes and effects of various elements that work together to complete an action or service.

Begin by reviewing jobs that have high potential risk severity and the highest rates of disabling injuries or damage based on initial job inventory assessment. These jobs can provide the potential for immediate improvement.

Nonroutine jobs can be difficult to identify or even locate as they may not be found in any formal job or tasks list. If no formal list of nonroutine jobs is available for use in identifying nonroutine JHAs, the approach is to use experienced employees and leaders to develop a list through discussions and continued job site observations.

CHAPTER REVIEW QUESTIONS

1. What does the JHA bridge between?
2. Do generic safety programs serve a purpose?
3. How can the "feel" of the workplace be lost?
4. What are the phases to follow when beginning a JHA process?
5. What are the obstacles to a JHA process?
6. Why is it important to get employees involved in the JHA process?
7. What are the qualities for a JHA administrator?
8. How is a JHA committee selected and guided?
9. How are jobs selected for analysis?
10. Discuss the issues with determining and locating nonroutine jobs?

BIBLIOGRAPHY

Air Force Safety Agency. (2000). *Air force system safety handbook*. Kirtland AFB NM 87117-5670, Public Domain, Modified for Use.
Conducting a Job Hazard Analysis (JHA). (n.d.). Oregon Occupational Safety and Health Division (Oregon OSHA), Public Domain, Permission to Reprint, Modify, and/or Adapt as necessary. Retrieved from http://bit.ly/WXGJhK
Consequence. (n.d.). Dictionary.com. Retrieved from http://bit.ly/1HqekVC
Job Hazard Analysis, 3071. (2002). *Occupational safety and health administration (OSHA)*. Occupational Safety and Health Administration (OSHA), Public Domain, Modified and/or Adapt as necessary. Retrieved from http://1.usa.gov/11zbazr
Managing Worker Safety and Health. (n.d.). Missouri Occupational Safety and Health Administration (OSHA), Office of Cooperative Programs, Public Domain, Adapted for Use. Retrieved from http://on.mo.gov/15C4FyS

Occupational Health & Safety Management Systems. (2012). The American Society of Safety Engineers, ANSI/AIHA/ASSE Z10. Retrieved from http://bit.ly/1MsT6MG

Roughton, J. (1995). *How to develop a written job hazard analysis. National environmental training association conference presentation.* Orlando, Florida: Professional Development Course (PDC).

Roughton, J., & Crutchfield, N. (2008). *Job hazard analysis: A guide for voluntary compliance
and beyond. chemical, petrochemical & process.* MA: Elsevier/Butterworth-Heinemann, Retrieved from http://amzn.to/VrSAq5.

Roughton, J., & Crutchfield, N. (2013). In B. Heinemann (Ed.), *Safety culture: An innovative
leadership approach.* Butterworth Heinemann, Retrieved from http://amzn.to/1qoD4oN.

Roughton, J., & Florczak, C. (1999). *Job safety analysis: A better method.* Chicago, IL: Safety and
Health, National Safety Council, pp. 72–75.

US Army Corps of Engineers. (2014). EM 385-1-1, *Safety and health requirements manual.*
Public Domain. Retrieved from http://1.usa.gov/1Fu8Yfo

US DOE. (2009). *Concepts and principles, human performance improvement handbook* (Vol. 1). US
Department of Energy. Retrieved from http://bit.ly/1DfdJVU

Appendix I Description of Common Hazards

Hazards	Hazard descriptions
Acceleration/ deacceleration	When something speeds up or slows down too quickly
Biological	Airborne and bloodborne viruses, animals, insects, vegetation
Chemical (corrosive)	A chemical that, when it comes into contact with skin, metal, or other materials, damages the materials. Acids and bases are examples of corrosives.
Chemical (flammable)	A chemical that, when exposed to a heat ignition source, results in combustion. Typically, the lower a chemical's flash point and boiling point, the more flammable the chemical. Check MSDS for flammability information.
Chemical (toxic)	A chemical that exposes a person by absorption through the skin, inhalation, or through the blood stream that causes illness, disease, or more severe consequences. The amount of chemical exposure is critical in determining hazardous effects. Check Material Safety Data Sheets (MSDS).
Chemical Reactions (potential explosion)	Chemical reactions can be violent; can cause explosions, dispersion of materials and emission of heat.

Hazards	Hazard descriptions
Electrical (fire)	Use of electrical power that results in electrical overheating or arcing to the point of combustion or ignition of flammables, or electrical component damage.
Electrical (loss of power)	Safety-critical equipment failure as a result of loss of power.
Electrical (shock/short circuit)	Contact with exposed conductors or a device that is incorrectly or inadvertently grounded, such as when a metal ladder comes into contact with power lines. As little as 60Hz alternating current (common house current) is very dangerous because it can stop the heart
Electrical (static/ ESD)	The moving or rubbing of wool, nylon, other synthetic fibers, and even flowing liquids can generate static electricity. This creates an excess or deficiency of electrons on the surface of material that discharges (spark) to the ground resulting in the ignition of flammables or damage to electronics or the body's nervous system.
Electrical (contact)	Inadequate insulation, broken electrical lines or equipment, lightning strike, static discharge etc.
Ergonomics (human error)	A system design, procedure, or equipment that is error-provocative, i.e., a switch turns something on when pushed up.
Ergonomics (strain)	Damage of tissue due to overexertion (strains and sprains) or repetitive motion.
Ergonomics, Eight risk factors	High frequency: There are a lot of repetitions of the same movement in a task.
	High duration: The employee must repeat the same movement over an extended period of time.
	High force: The employee must exert force to complete the task. This may include lifting, pushing, pulling, reaching, etc.
	Posture: Stress from overextending body parts, or improper body position is part of the task.
	Point of operation: The location of the employee or tool in relation to the material or product, increases the stress impact of other risk factors
	Mechanical pressure: Hand-held tools have hard, sharp edges or short handles.
	Vibration: Impact tools, power tools, bench-mounted buffers and grinders produce excessive vibration.
	Environmental exposure: The employee works in or temperature extreme environments.

(Continued)

Hazards	Hazard descriptions
Excavation (collapse)	Soil collapses in a trench or excavation as a result of improper or inadequate shoring. Soil type is critical in determining the likelihood of a hazard
Explosives (chemical reaction)	Explosions result in large amounts of gas, heat, noise, light, and over-pressure
Explosion (over pressurization)	Sudden and violent release of a large amount of gas/ energy due to a significant pressure difference such as rupture in a boiler or compressed gas cylinder
Fall (slip, trip)	Conditions that result in falls (impacts) from height or traditional walking surfaces (such as slippery floors, poor housekeeping, uneven walking surfaces, exposed ledges, etc.)
Fire/Heat	Temperatures that can cause burns to the skin or damage to other organs. Fires require a heat source, fuel, and oxygen
Flammability/ Fire	For combustion to take place, the fuel and oxidizer must be present in gaseous form
Mechanical	Pinch points, sharp points and edges, weight, rotating parts, stability, ejected parts and materials, impact. Skin, muscle, or body part exposed to crushing, caught-between, cutting, tearing, shearing items, or equipment.
Mechanical failure	Typically occurs when devices exceed designed capacity or are inadequately maintained.
Mechanical/ Vibration (chaffing/ failure)	Vibration that can cause damage to nerve endings, or material fatigue, i.e., examples, abraded slings and ropes, weakened hoses and belts
Noise	Noise levels (>85 dBA 8 h TWA) that result in hearing damage or inability to communicate critical information
Pressure	Increased pressure in hydraulic and pneumatic systems
Radiation	Nonionizing (burns), Ionizing (destroys tissue)
Radiation (ionizing)	Alpha, Beta, Gamma, neutral particles, and X-rays that cause injury (tissue damage) by ionization of cellular components
Radiation (nonionizing)	Ultraviolet, visible light, infrared, and microwaves that cause injury to tissue by thermal or photochemical means.

Hazards	Hazard descriptions
Struck against	Injury to a body part as a result of coming into contact of a surface in which action was initiated by the person. For example, a screwdriver slips
Struck by (mass, acceleration)	Accelerated mass that strikes the body causing injury or death. For example, falling objects and projectiles.
Temperature extreme (heat/cold)	Temperatures that result in heat stress, exhaustion, or metabolic slow down such as hypothermia.
Violence in the workplace	Any violent act that occurs in the workplace and creates a hostile work environment that affects employees' physical or psychological well being
Visibility	Lack of lighting or obstructed vision that results in an error or other hazard.
Weather phenomena (snow/rain/wind/ice)	Naturally occurring events

(Conducting a Job Hazard Analysis (JHA), n.d.; Job Hazard Analysis, 3071, 2002)

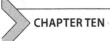
Breaking the Job Down into Individual Components

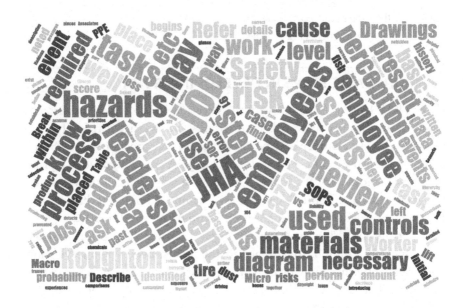

"Seek first to understand, then to be understood."

—*Stephen Covey*

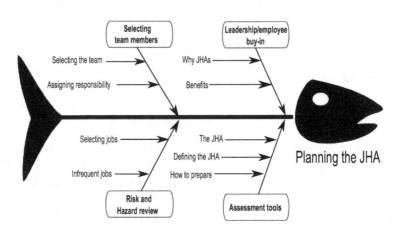

Planning the JHA

Job Hazard Analysis. http://dx.doi.org/10.1016/B978-0-12-803441-5.00010-6

Chapter Objectives

At the end of the chapter, you should be able to:

- Define the basic steps in JHA development.
- Discuss how perceptions about hazards can be defined.
- Identify methods on how to break the job down into steps and tasks.
- Define steps and tasks within a job.
- Define the methods used in breaking a job down.
- Describe the contents of a JHA tool kit.

10.1 BASIC STEPS IN DEVELOPING A JHA

The JHA process begins with the selection of jobs ranked by priority based on loss history and/or known hazards and associated risk. The end product is the development of a written standard operating procedure (SOP) as well as safety procedures and protocols. The JHA is not intended to replace work instructions or SOPs, as these provide the formal in-depth details of a job. JHA remains the core document for detailing exposures to hazards and developing preventative measures (Job Hazard Analysis, 3071, 2002).

After the initial job inventory has been completed and priorities have been established for jobs to be analyzed, the process begins by interviewing employees and other individuals who are familiar with the specific job under review. The interviews should cover as many individuals as possible who may have knowledge of the job elements and how it is being completed.

The perception of the leadership team and employees about the level of risk acceptance should be determined. Table 10.1 provides a summary of a leadership team's hazard perception versus employee hazard perception.

To have an effective safety process that detects and corrects hazards, the organization needs to ensure that it stays in the upper left quadrant of the matrix where knowledge is open with no-hidden issues, information about hazards is communicated, and the appropriate preventative measures and controls are taken (Figure 10.1).

10.2 INDIVIDUAL JOB COMPONENTS

The job should be considered as a whole system that accounts for all the actions and elements necessary for its performance. A job is more than a sequence of steps or activities (Keller & Associates, 2000). Visualize the job as a funnel that, as steps and tasks are completed, filters out the hazards and associated risks (Figure 10.2).

Table 10.1 Leadership team hazard perception versus employee hazard perception

Leadership team perception	Employee perception	
	Know about hazard	**Do not know about the hazard**
Know about hazard	In an ideal situation, both the leadership team and the employees know about hazard(s). A process should determine if controls are in place and effective.	The leadership team recognizes the hazard(s) but employees who perform the task do not recognize the hazard. A communication gap with potential liability issues if not corrected.
Do not know about the hazard	Employees know the hazard(s) of the task and the leadership team does not recognize the hazard(s). Poor communication between the leadership team and the employee.	Neither the leadership team nor employees know the hazard(s) of the task. Only dumb luck has prevented a loss-producing event. Worse Case Scenario.

At the top of this funnel, a large amount of detailed information enters and should be analyzed. As the job is filtered (analyzed), it is broken into manageable "steps". These steps are analyzed for finer elements or specific tasks identified as necessary to complete each step (Roughton & Crutchfield, 2008). The JHA process sequence is as follows:

- Select the appropriate job for analysis.
- Break the job down into individual steps, i.e., the sequence of actions required to complete the job).
- Break each step down further by determining the tasks required within each step.
- Identify all tools, equipment or technology, materials (including chemicals) required by each task to complete each step. Be complete and not leave anything out or assume not important.
- Describe the nature of the work environment – temperatures, air quality, any dust, vapors, fumes, time of day/night, general housekeeping, where the job takes place, etc. – all aspects of the environment.
- Identify and review the current administrative procedures and all written documents used by the job.
- Identify employees and/or other individuals who might be present when the job is done and who are exposed to its activities.
- Define the existing and/or potential hazards and the consequences of exposure to the hazard(s) for each step and task.

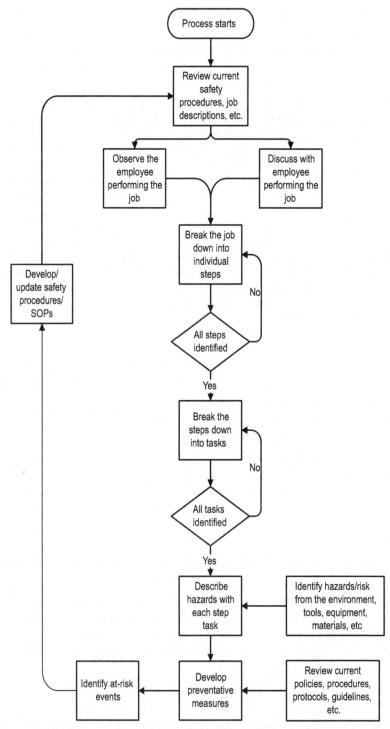

Figure 10.1 *Basic Illustration and Overview of the Job Hazard Analysis Process. Based on and adapted using Conducting a Job Hazard Analysis (JHA) (n.d.); Roughton and Crutchfield (2008).*

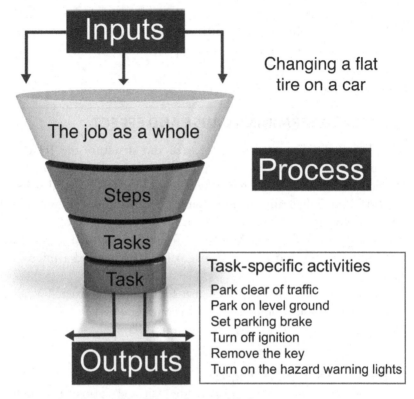

Figure 10.2 *The Job Funnel for filtering Steps and Tasks.*

- Document any past at-risk event(s) or history of loss-producing event(s.) What actions and behaviors are present? What are the factors that may be driving a specific behavior? (Conducting a Job Hazard Analysis (JHA), n.d.; Managing Worker Safety and Health, n.d.).
- Assess and calculate a risk score associated with each step based on the activities, tools, equipment, materials, environment, etc. Use the risk matrix to determine the probability and severity of the risk, as discussed in Chapter 8.
- Identify preventative measures/controls that can be used to eliminate and/or minimize each identified hazard. Use the "Hierarchy of Controls" and Haddon's concepts as discussed in Chapter 7.
- Assess for "residual risk" by revising the risk score. One important point is to ensure that the residual risk is less than the initial risk. If no

substantial decrease in risk is noted, review and determine if additional controls should be implemented.

- The final stage of a JHA is to develop an SOP that integrates controls into guidelines and procedures.

10.3 DETERMINING CAUSE AND EFFECT

The technique used to categorize and structure the JHA is the "cause and effect" diagram, which provides a visual picture of the job, its steps, and tasks. This diagram developed by Ishikawa is also known as a "Fishbone" diagram (Fishbone, n.d.). The fishbone allows the JHA developer to list all of the elements of the job as well all of the tasks as they relate to specific steps. Additional fish bones are used to collect the data outlined above at both the macro level (steps) and a micro view (tasks).

Refer to Figures 10.3 and 10.4 that have been constructed as an example of the combination of elements to consider when changing a car tire (Roughton & Crutchfield, 2008; Roughton, 1995).

The Cause and Effect Diagram

The fishbone diagram consists of a box (the "fish head") placed on the right hand side of the diagram. A brief description of the job is placed in the box. A horizontal "backbone" is drawn from this box to the left. "Ribs" that represent the selected causes are placed along the backbone. The ribs listed are steps, tools/equipment/materials, environment, procedures, rules, protocols, and people (Fishbone, n.d.).

10.4 USING A CHECKLIST

The fishbone diagram allows the JHA developer to review at a glance each part of the job and assess how the pieces fit together. The JHA may find that the various elements of the job do not match, i.e., physical hazards may not match the proper preventative measures. The tasks design may not consider the current environment or where the job is performed. Different people may be doing the job and not received the needed level of training.

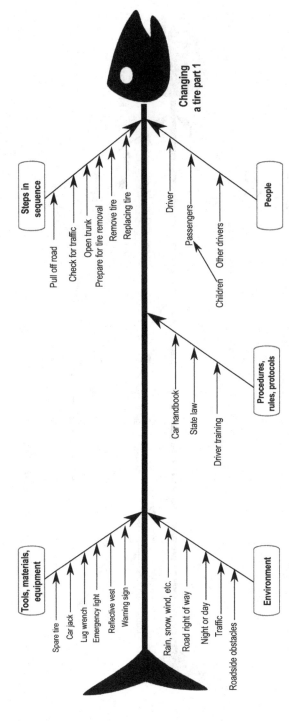

Figure 10.3 *Macro Level–High Level View of the Cause and Effect of Changing a Tire.*

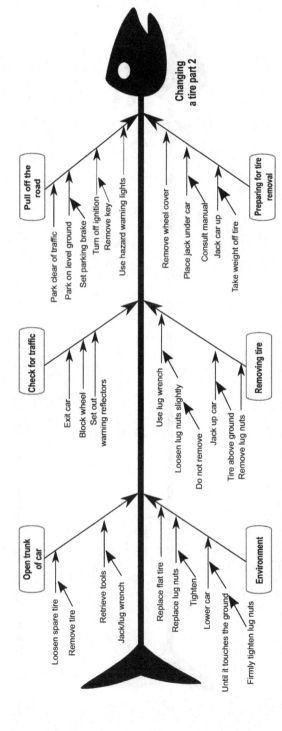

Figure 10.4 *Micro Level–Low Level View of the Cause and Effect of Changing a Tire.*

A checklist can be used to gather answers to questions that the JHA developer may want to further review (Gawande, 2009; Hazard Assessment Checklist, n.d.).

> For example, if the job requires lifting of 50 pound bags of a material, are the assigned employees' able to lift that amount or has an ergonomic issue been built into the job? If a chemical is present, are the procedures in place for its control and up to date? Under equipment, is the correct PPE in use? If electrical equipment is in use, does anything in the environment increase the electrical risk, i.e., water in area?

Refer to Appendix J for a "Sample Facility Checklist" and other helpful resources that can be used as a guide.

10.5 GATHERING INFORMATION FOR BREAKING DOWN THE JOB

Two methods, the discussion method and the observation method, can be used in combination to develop customized checklists that assess if hazards and risks are controlled within a job. These are used to clarify and verify information found in job descriptions, current SOPs, operational guidelines, and other documents received in the job inventory stage.

10.5.1 Discussion method

The JHA developer and designated employees discuss the required steps and tasks listing known hazards, past loss-producing events, and in general how the job should be accomplished. The discussion method collects the range of employee experience with the various job activities, providing comparisons of experiences and what is currently considered an acceptable risk (Managing Worker Safety and Health, n.d.; Roughton & Crutchfield, 2013).

These discussions should attempt to determine what precursors exist that can invoke human error as well as any design flaws that may be present (US DOE, 2009) (Chapter 2).

The interviews should determine if time and/or other pressures are creating unnecessary stress that are distracting employees and creating the perception that shortcuts are necessary to complete a job within required time frames. These shortcuts may have become the expected normal way to do a job and are error invoking. The job may be require improvised workarounds that are necessary to overcome poor design and bad task layout.

> **Case Study #1**
>
> An employee got his hand caught in a machine's in-running nip point while trying to make a minor machine adjustment. When the injury was investigated, the incident review team could not identify any condition that created a hazard nor why the employee would stick his hand knowingly into the moving piece of equipment. The safety rule was that all equipment should be shut down and locked out before any type of maintenance or adjustments.
>
> Witnesses to the event stated, "What do you (leadership) do when a piece of equipment stops? You always ask the question "Why is the equipment down?" and will constantly ask the same question over and over until the equipment is up and running again. We do not need that type of pressure. So we (employees) have decided that if a minor adjustment is to be made, we will not shut the equipment down but take a chance and make the adjustment while it is running."
>
> This case study highlights how leadership, by stressing that the employees keep equipment running, created an unintended consequence that drove the employee behavior to take short cuts. The employees' perception was that since few injuries had occurred, the risk of being caught in a piece of equipment was perceived as less than the consequences of dealing with leadership's constant pressure on production.
>
> The better approach would have been to first ask: "Anyone injured? Is everyone okay?" and then "What do we need to do now? How soon can maintenance get here to find out what is wrong?"

10.5.2 Observation method

The observation method involves being at the job location or work area and seeing how the job is being performed. While observing the job, ongoing discussions with employees are used to assess their perception of existing or potential hazards and their understanding of the risk and potential consequences (Roughton, 1996). This technique provides the opportunity to ask questions after each job step and tasks in "real time" and allows a firsthand view of the job.

After observations are completed and data is collected and recorded, involved employees should be included in reviewing the data analysis to ensure that all basic job elements have been listed in the right sequence (Roughton, 1996).

The observation method involves watching experienced employees perform the job step-by-step and task-by-task. The major advantages a combination of job observation, group discussion, and data verification includes:

- Tapping into the knowledge of experienced the leadership team and employees who are directly involved in the job.
- Not relying on just SOPs, which may be out of date or employee recall from memory of how the job is performed.
- Reducing the probability that existing and potential hazards and their risk consequences are not overlooked or missed.
- Direct recognition of existing hazard(s) and starting the development of possible preventative measures and/or controls for each defined step and its tasks.
- Encouraging the leadership team and employees to take "ownership" of the process and the JHA.
- Developing the leadership team and employees skills in coaching and/or training of inexperienced individuals in JHA requirements for safe job completion (Managing Worker Safety and Health, n.d.).
- Developing risk management protocols to assess future risk and the potential severity of an injury or loss-producing event (Managing Worker Safety and Health, n.d.).
- Identifying other potential at-risk events or behaviors that may be present and previously not known.

10.6 DEVELOPING A TOOL KIT FOR THE JHA PROCESS?

A suggested JHA toolkit should include basic tools and materials to capture all elements of the job under review. These might include electronic equipment, graph paper, tape measure, flashlight, or other aids to document and measure what is occurring.

10.7 ELECTRONIC EQUIPMENT

Digital cameras, tablets, and smart phones provide a quick and economic way to capture the information about a job under review. Photos and videos can be used in discussions with employees so that they can point out areas of concern as well as documenting the job activities for future use. Tablet and smart phone apps are available for capturing, then editing videos and photos, insert comments, and images. Technology continues to evolve and improve making the JHA easier to complete and far more comprehensive in detail.

Video is essential in evaluating body position, stress points, repetitiveness, movements, etc., as well as use of tools, equipment, and materials. As tasks are performed the video can provide slow motion and stop action to can provide additional insights for evaluation.

> Subtle and different elements that may not have directly been observed become apparent. Employees may not be aware of certain movements and actions they make that have become the habitual normal yet harmful behavior. Reviewing the videos and photos in a group setting involving employees and leadership can be especially useful as a training and awareness communication tool.
>
> The video can be used to ensure that everyone sees and understands what issues are present needing a solution.

10.8 OTHER APPLICATIONS

A combination of spreadsheets, word documentation, and graphics software is essential to developing a quality JHA work product. The ability to hyperlink documents, pictures, notes, and all other information improves the ease of development and use. Most organizations use products from Microsoft© or Apple© that provide a full family of tools for presentation, documents, and spreadsheets.

> Caution note: Areas that could require legal review.
>
> Before taking videos and photos, permission should be coordinated with the leadership team due to proprietary processes, equipment, and operations. In addition, obtaining individual employee permission for inclusion in videos and pictures should be in place.
>
> Finally, review the area for clearly blatant safety violations such as missing machine guards, poor housekeeping, electrical issues, lack of PPE, etc. When reviewing pictures and videos, what is happening in the background might be of critical importance requiring immediate action.

10.8.1 Drawings and Sketches

Video and photos should be accompanied with drawings or sketches that explain the full job under review. A drawing or sketch of the work area provides the details on the placement of materials, tools and equipment as well as the general patterns of employee movements, tools and materials in use, and flow of the process. Drawings provide a way to show the various photo and video angles that can provide the best perspectives. A simple drawing of the work process and workstation might be all that is needed to begin the evaluation of the workflow. The drawing can be shared with employees who can provide an indication of what are the dominant features of the work environment (Job Safety Analysis, n.d.).

The drawings, sketches, and diagrams can show where overlapping jobs and/or tasks have created a greater potential for a loss-producing event. Drawings and sketches can be linked to the JHA document either scanned or drawn using digital software.

10.9 CRITERIA FOR JOB OBSERVATIONS

Jobs should be observed being performed under normal conditions, movements, use of tools, equipment, etc. and the primary environmental conditions (noise, lighting, dust, etc.) that may be present. If the job is performed on multiple shifts, the JHA should be conducted on those shifts as well, as jobs may vary from shift to shift. Only the tools, materials and equipment routinely or regularly used should be observed (Roughton, 1996).

If discussions imply that variations in tools, equipment and/or materials are occurring, further inquiry as to why this is allowed or thought necessary. If allowed, then a new JHA is developed using the modified conditions.

The discussions with employees should ask if any nonroutine job steps or tasks have on occasion been completed or the job completed under adverse or extreme environmental or production conditions. These nonroutine situations will require further review and consideration for special controls or administrative policies. The extreme environmental conditions or production conditions are studied and a new JHA developed if these are expected in the future.

10.10 REALITY CHECK

If the discussed outline is followed, the value of the process should be clear to the leadership team.

Questions for a JHA quality review
- What resources (tools, equipment, materials, supplies, etc.) are required to do the job?
- What basic step starts and what step completes the job? Establish an agreed upon beginning and ending of the job. Ten to fifteen steps are considered the maximum number of steps that should be analyzed. More than 15 steps may imply that the job is too complex.
- Determine the action sequence of what occurs, step-by-step including the tasks as listed under each step. Departures from the normal procedures should be noted as these can potentially cause a loss-producing event and may be an indication of operational process problems that need immediate attention.
- Describe each step in sequence. Begin each step with an easy to understand action word, i.e., remove, lift, or pry, etc. (Roughton, 1996; Roughton & Crutchfield, 2008).

SUMMARY

The JHA process begins by selecting designated jobs, ranked in order by priority, and ends with standard operating procedures (SOP) and enhanced hazard controls and associated risk reduction.

The perception of the leadership team and employees about the level of risk acceptance should be determined. The objective is changing the level of risk acceptance by assessing the hazards and making the actual risk visible.

The job should be considered as a whole system that accounts for all the actions and elements necessary for its performance. A job is more than a sequence of steps or activities. Visualize the job as a funnel that, as steps and tasks are completed, filters out the hazards, and associated risks.

The technique used to categorize and structure the JHA is the "cause and effect" diagram, which provides a visual picture of the job, its steps and tasks. This diagram developed by Ishikawa or is also known as a "Fishbone" diagram.

Two methods, discussion method and observation method, can be used in combination to develop customized checklists that assess if hazards and risks are controlled within a job. These are used to clarify and verify information found in job descriptions, current SOPs, operational guidelines, and other documents received in the job inventory stage.

A suggested JHA toolkit should include basic tools and materials to capture all elements of the job under review. These might include electronic equipment, graph paper, tape measure, flashlight, or other aids to document and measure what is occurring.

If the process outlined is followed, the value of the process should be clear to the leadership team who hopefully has been supportive of the JHA. If concerns still remain, review the process and adjust its implementation to resolve any concerns and/or issues as presented.

CHAPTER REVIEW QUESTIONS

1. How does the JHA process begin?
2. Discuss the Perception Matrix and how it might be used.
3. Why should a job be considered as a whole system?
4. Discuss why the JHA might be viewed as filter?
5. What is the benefit of using a Fishbone Diagram?
6. What is the difference between a Step and a Task?
7. What are two methods for gathering job information?
8. What tools should be used during JHA development?
9. What is a JHA Quality Review and why is it important?

BIBLIOGRAPHY

Conducting a Job Hazard Analysis (JHA). (n.d.). Oregon Occupational Safety and Health Division (Oregon OSHA), Public Domain, Permission to Reprint, Modify, and/or Adapt as necessary. Retrieved from http://bit.ly/WXGJhK

Fishbone. (n.d.). iSixSigma. Retrieved from http://bit.ly/14v46Gn

Gawande, A. (2009). *The checklist manifesto: How to get things right.* New York: Henry Holt and Company.

Hazard Assessment Checklist. (n.d.). Cal-OSHA Occupational Safety and Health Administration. Retrieved from http://bit.ly/1CBAZC2 – pdf version.

Job Hazard Analysis, 3071. (2002). *Occupational safety and health administration (OSHA).* Occupational Safety and Health Administration (OSHA), Public Domain, Modified and/or Adapt as necessary. Retrieved from http://1.usa.gov/11zbazr

Job Safety Analysis. (n.d.). WorkSafe. Retrieved from http://bit.ly/1CQguB4

Keller, J.J., & Associates. (2000). *The compass: Management practice specialty news, why you've been handed responsibility for safety* (pp. 1,4).

Managing Worker Safety and Health. (n.d.). Missouri Occupational Safety and Health Administration (OSHA), Office of Cooperative Programs, Public Domain, Adapted for Use. Retrieved from http://on.mo.gov/15C4FyS

Roughton, J. (1995). *How to develop a written job hazard analysis. National environmental training association conference presentation.* Orlando, Florida: Professional Development Course (PDC).

Roughton, J. (1996). *Job hazard analysis: A critical part of your job as supervisor is evaluating and controlling workplace hazards.* Canada: Occupational Health and Safety, pp. 41–44.

Roughton, J., & Crutchfield, N. (2008). *Job hazard analysis: A guide for voluntary compliance and beyond. chemical, petrochemical & process.* MA: Elsevier/Butterworth-Heinemann, Retrieved from http://amzn.to/VrSAq5.

Roughton, J., & Crutchfield, N. (2013). In B. Heinemann (Ed.), *Safety culture: An innovative leadership approach.* MA: Butterworth Heinemann, Retrieved from http://amzn.to/1qoD4oN.

Safety and Health Program Assessment Worksheet. (2007). Oregon Occupational Safety and
    Health Division (Oregon OSHA), Public Domain, Permission to Reprint, Modify, and/
    or Adapt as necessary. Retrieved from http://bit.ly/XLNphg
Self-Inspection Checklist. (n.d.). Michigan Occupational Safety and Health Administration
    (MIOSHA), Public Domain, Based on and Adapted for Use. Retrieved from http://
    www.michigan.gov/documents/cis_wsh_cet0156_107628_7.doc.
US DOE. (2009). *Concepts and principles, human performance improvement handbook* (Vol. 1)
    (pp. 41–44). US Department of Energy. Retrieved from http://bit.ly/1DfdJVU

Appendix J Sample Facility Checklist

Yes	No	NA	Checklist Item
			Are the materials on the walking surface or floor that could cause a tripping hazard?
			Is lighting required? Is it lighting adequate?
			Are electrical, chemical, thermal, mechanical or kinetic, biological, acoustic (noise), or radiation hazards associated with the task? Are any of these hazards likely to develop? Are dusts, fumes, mists, or vapors in the air?
			Do environmental hazards such as: chemicals, radiation, welding rays, heat, or excessive noise, result from the performance of the task?
			Are dusts, fumes, mists, or vapors in the air?
			Can contact be made with hot, toxic, infectious, or caustic substances? Could the employee be exposed to radiation sources?
			Are tools, machines, and equipment in need of repair?
			Does excessive noise exists that could affect communication? Is there likelihood that the noise can cause hearing loss?
			Are job procedures in place? Are these procedures understood by all employees and followed and/or modified as applicable?
			Are emergency procedures defined for the job? Are employees trained in emergency procedures?
			Are employees who operate vehicles and equipment authorized and properly trained?
			Are industrial trucks or motorized vehicles properly equipped with brakes? Are there overhead guards, backup signals, horns, steering gear, seat belts, etc.? Are they properly maintained?

Yes	No	NA	Checklist Item

Are employees wearing the appropriate PPE? How was it specified and selected? Was a PPE assessment conducted? Refer to Appendix F and G for an example of PPE assessment.

Have any employees complained of headaches, breathing problems, dizziness, strong odors, or other indicators of health related issues?

Are there confined or enclosed spaces? Have they been tested for oxygen deficient atmospheres, toxic vapors, or flammable materials? Is ventilation adequate? Who has the reports and when were they completed? Have they been reviewed recently?

Are workstations and tools designed to account for ergonomically related movement or issues, bending, twisting, stretching, motions etc.? Is the employee required to make movements that are rapid, stressful, a stretch, bend, etc. Is the employee required to make movements that could lead to or cause hand or foot injuries, strain from lifting, and the hazards of repetitive motions? Can employees strain themselves by pushing, pulling, lifting, bending, or twisting? Can they overextend or strain themselves while doing a task. Is the flow of work properly organized? Is the employee at any time in an off-balance position?

Are body positions, machinery, pits or holes, and/or hazardous operations adequately guarded? Are fixed objects in the area whose location and design may cause injury, from sharp edges, location, or shape?

Are lockout procedures used for machinery deactivation during maintenance and/or unjamming equipment?

Is the employee positioned at a machine in a way that is potentially dangerous?

Can reaching over moving machinery parts or materials cause an injury to the employee? Is the danger of striking against, being struck by, or contacting a harmful object present? Could employees be injured if they are forcefully struck by an object or contact a harmful material?

Yes	No	NA	Checklist Item
			Can employees be caught in, on, by, or between objects? Can they be injured if their body, their clothing or equipment is caught on an object that is either stationary or moving?
			Can employee be pinched, crushed, or caught between either a moving object and a stationary object, or two moving objects?
			Is equipment difficult to operate and have the potential to be used incorrectly?
			Is there a potential for a slip, trip, or fall? Can employees fall from the same level or a different level?
			Can suspended or residual energy cause harm to employee?
			Can weather conditions, i.e., ice, snow, water, etc. affect employee safety? Is the employee exposed to extreme heat or cold?
			What other hazards not discussed may be present? Have the potential causes of injuries been traced to their source (root cause)?

Adapted and combined (Job Hazard Analysis, 3071, 2002; Job Safety Analysis, n.d.).

Other Helpful Resources:

Cal-OSHA Hazard Assessment Checklist (Hazard Assessment Checklist, n.d.)

Oregon OSHA Safety and Health Program Assessment Worksheet (Safety and Health Program Assessment Worksheet, 2007)

Michigan Occupational Safety and Health Administration (MIOSHA) Self-Inspection Checklist (Self-Inspection Checklist, n.d.)

CHAPTER ELEVEN

Putting the Puzzle Pieces Together

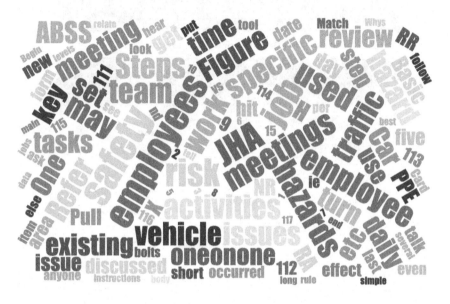

"Feel inspired and inspire others. Do you know your Why? The purpose, cause, or belief that inspires you to do what you do?"

—*Simon Sinek*

Job Hazard Analysis. http://dx.doi.org/10.1016/B978-0-12-803441-5.00011-8

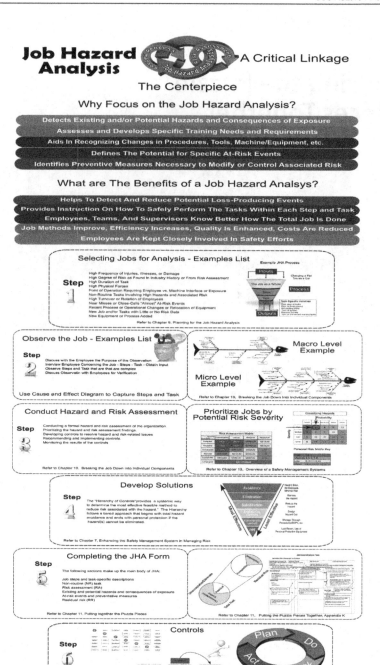

Chapter Objectives

At the end of the chapter, you should be able to:

* Identify the key considerations for conducting a JHA.
* Complete a JHA form using the methods provided in this chapter.
* Assess and integrate risk analysis into the JHA.
* Identify the importance of considering residual risk in the JHA.
* Identify the basics for listing controls and preventive measures.
* Discuss the importance of reviewing the JHA with employees.

11.1 TELLING THE JHA STORY

When conducting a JHA, the process attempts to tell the story of what is happening in the job. The "Five Why's" plus "H" questions (Who, What, Where, When, Why, and How) are used to categorize information to begin telling the story. The story becomes a clear and concise picture when used with accompanying data and feedback from employees.

Depending on the complexity of the JHA (the story), the JHA developer might ask questions in several different ways. Refer to Tables 11.1–11.6 for a basic description of The Five "Why's" and "H" for consideration.

Table 11.1 Asking the WHO question

WHO
* Is involved?
* Is affected by the JHA?
* Is the best person to develop the JHA?
* Is missing in the review of the JHA?
* Has more information about the hazards in the related tasks?
* Else should I talk to about developing the JHA?

Table 11.2 Asking the WHAT question

WHAT
* Is the end result of the JHA (What is the point of the story?)
* Does the JHA developer need to understand?
* New insights and perceptions were experienced by the JHA developer or employees?
* Are the tools, material, and equipment used?
* Are the environmental conditions?

Table 11.3 Asking the WHERE question

WHERE
- Is the job completed?
- Is the information needed to develop the JHA?
- Is this JHA going to be used?
- Are the policies, procedures, etc. for this job?

Table 11.4 Asking the WHEN question

WHEN
- Is the job done? Which shift, time of day, continuously, etc.?
- Are employees trained for the job?
- Is preventive maintenance scheduled?
- Have injuries or damage occurred with this job?
- Was the job last reviewed?

Table 11.5 Asking the WHY question

WHY
- Does this job need to be analyzed?
- Are employees not following procedure?
- Have the risk not been recognized earlier?
- Are documents not kept current?

Very few people and organizations can clearly articulate WHY they do what they do. Why is a purpose, a cause or a belief? It provides a clear answer to Why we get out of bed in the morning, Why our company even exists and why that should matter to anyone else.

– (Sinek, 2009)

Table 11.6 Asking the HOW question

HOW
- Clear is the JHA information presented?
- Will things be different after the JHA has been developed?
- Long will this JHA be effective?
- Will the JHA be communicated to the employees?
- Will control be implemented?

Based on and adapted from Strubler (n.d.)

Refer to Appendix K for "Examples Information on How to Tell the JHA Story":
- Sample instructions on how to change a tire on a car
- Sample JHA prehazard assessment worksheet

- JHA on changing a tire
- Annotated JHA on changing a tire
- Comparison JHA on changing a tire, traditional versus new version job hazard analysis

11.2 COMPLETING THE JHA FORM

A comprehensive JHA form is the document that provides the complete description of all aspects of the job – Where it takes place; What is required; Who does it, When it is done, and How it is completed.

The following sections are step-by-step examples on how to complete the JHA from information gathered.

11.3 THE HEADER

The header is designed to provide anyone reviewing the JHA with basic information about the nature of the job.

The follow elements make up the header:
- Job description
- Department
- Date developed
- Page numbering
- Performed by
- Employee signature
- PPE required

11.4 JOB DESCRIPTION

The job description is a very basic statement about what activity will be accomplished. It describes the job in as few words as possible, i.e., changing a tire, lawn mower operation, casing a die, etc. This description is written in terms familiar with employees performing the job.

For maximum benefit, the job description and breakout of steps and tasks should be written to match the reading levels of the majority of the workplace (typically an 8th grade reading level). The use of pictures as previously discussed in Chapter 10 enhances and aids in communicating the steps and task as identified. The key is to keep the content as simple as possible by avoiding technical jargon and using bullets to convey actions.

11.5 DEPARTMENT

This section identifies the department or area where the job is performed.

11.6 DATE DEVELOPED

The date that the JHA was completed – This date is used to document the initial review and changes when a review and/or update of the JHA is completed. The old JHA should be kept for reference to ensure that all new changes can be tracked.

11.7 PAGE NUMBERING

Page numbers are used to ensure that the JHA is complete.

11.8 PERFORMED BY

This section documents the name of the individual(s) or committee members who developed the JHA. Documents should always be associated with an individual(s). When a change is made, the contributing person(s) is listed and the form shown as revised.

11.9 PERSONAL PROTECTIVE EQUIPMENT (PPE) REQUIRED

PPE is the last section to complete after all of the hazards of each task are defined and after alternative controls have been implemented. Refer to Chapter 7, Appendix E for "Personal Protective Equipment (PPE)" Assessment forms, etc. that be used to identify all related PPE.

11.10 BODY OF JHA

This section captures the data collected from the cause and effect diagram and visual observations of the job steps and tasks. This section provides detailed instructions to the employees on hazards associated with specific task and provides a comment for each task on specific actions or control to be implemented.

The following sections make up the main body of JHA:

- Job steps and task-specific descriptions
- Nonroutine (NR) task
- Risk assessment (RA)
- Existing and potential hazards and consequences of exposure
- At-risk events and preventative measures
- Residual risk (RR)

11.11 JOB STEPS AND TASK-SPECIFIC DESCRIPTION

This section details the job in a logical sequence by reviewing job steps and then defining the specific tasks that relate to a specific step.

The use of the cause and effect diagram allows the committee to brainstorm the sequence of events and then make observations to verify their logic. Documenting the sequence of steps is the way of determining each necessary element of the job as it is performed. This is the most critical parts of conducting a JHA.

Tracking the sequence of steps is important because if the steps are out of sequence, the relationship between the steps and the existing and potential hazards and consequences of exposures, at-risk events, and the preventative measure(s) cannot be properly documented. The cause and effect diagrams will have provided a detailed view of the required steps and their related tasks that will be used to complete this section.

We have observed leadership teams and employees struggling to identify the sequence of steps in a job even though they have supervised or personally done the job for years. They clearly know how the job is completed but over time, the sequence of steps have become habits completed without thought.

Gradual changes, shortcuts, and modifications may have been developed by individuals doing the job. The JHA provides the map to keep desired actions within specific boundaries. In addition, if a job requires specific decision making (if X happens, do Y – "Rule Based") or requires a specific knowledge or expertise (knowledge based), the criteria can be included in the documentation (US DOE, 2009a).

The following JHA example provides guidance in looking at each step to determine if specific elements can be combined. For example, the following are key steps and require a number of tasks for successfully changing a flat tire:

- Pull car off the road
- Check for traffic

Job steps and task-specific description	NR	RA	Existing and potential hazards and/or consequences of exposure	At-risk events and preventive measures	RR
Pull car off the road					
• Park clear of traffic					
• Park on level ground					
• Set parking brake					
• Turn off ignition					
• Remove the key					
• Turn on the hazard warning lights					
Check for traffic					
• Exit car					
• Block wheel					
• Set flares/reflectors					

Figure 11.1 *Job Steps and Task-Specific Description.*

- Open trunk
- Preparing for tire removal
- Removing tire
- Replacing tire, etc.

Each key step is identified, and then the sequence of tasks specific to that step is listed. These tasks are listed below each appropriate step.

An important point to remember is that if a job has fewer than 3 steps then a JHA may not be needed. If it has more than 10–15 steps then more than one JHA may be required. The objective is to keep the job flow clear and concise and not to make the JHA overly complicated or it will not be used (Conducting a Job Hazard Analysis (JHA), n.d.) (Refer to Figure 11.1 for details on how to apply "Job Steps and Task-Specific Description").

11.12 NONROUTINE JOBS

Nonroutine elements may be critical task to an operation and are identified by placing an "X" in the column listed as "NR". When breaking the steps down into its individual tasks, look for steps or tasks not performed on a routine basis. These tasks may be done infrequently because they are used only at rule-based decision points and completed only if a process rule tells the employee to take action under certain conditions.

Job steps and task-specific description	NR	RA	Existing and potential hazards and/or consequences of exposure	At-risk events and preventive measures	RR
Pull car off the road					
• Park clear of traffic	X				
• Park on level ground					
• Set parking brake					
• Turn off ignition					
• Remove the key					
• Turn on the hazard warning lights					
Check for traffic					
• Exit car					
• Block wheel					
• Set flares/reflectors					

Figure 11.2 *Documenting Nonroutine Task.*

For example, starting a piece of equipment, performing preventative maintenance, doing piece work where specific equipment is used on a random basis, etc. are actions that may only be required under certain conditions. Necessary controls may have been forgotten in the interim.

The job steps and tasks–specific description will remove the need to review the entire JHA when only a few of the tasks are being performed. The leadership team, employee, or anyone about to perform the job can quickly scan the JHA for the nonroutine tasks noted as an X and review the specific hazards associated with the task before starting work.

If a job has nonroutine actions, before any step or task is begun, a formal review and refresher discussion about the required controls and safety procedures should be conducted.

When defining each step or task, ask the following questions: "Is this a nonroutine step?" "How does it affect other tasks?" (Figure 11.2)

11.13 RISK ASSESSMENT

After developing required steps and tasks, the level of risk is determined and placed under the "RA" section. As in the nonroutine column, an RA column makes it easier to be reviewed by employees and the leadership team.

The risk level is based on the risk analysis as presented in Chapter 8, Defining Associated Risk, in Figures 8.5 and 8.6 to help assess risk of assignments (Figure 11.3).

Job steps and task-specific description	NR	RA	Existing and potential hazards and/or consequences of exposure	At-risk events and preventive measures	RR
Pull car off the road					
• Park clear of traffic	X	H			
• Park on level ground					
• Set parking brake					
• Turn off ignition					
• Remove the key					
• Turn on the hazard warning lights					
Check for traffic					
• Exit car		H			
• Block wheel					
• Set flares/reflectors					

Figure 11.3 *Documenting Initial Risk Assessment for the Task.*

Tasks with high risk are given a higher priority and may require immediate actions. A step may, on the other hand, include tasks with only marginal risk and have limited safety requirements. If a job step is shown to have catastrophic potential, the job is immediately shut down until the risk is brought to an acceptable level with immediate controls implemented.

11.14 EXISTING AND POTENTIAL HAZARDS AND CONSEQUENCES OF EXPOSURE

The assumption is made that no controls in place. This column answers the question: "What are the possible negative physical consequences of exposure to a specific hazard?"

The JHA developer should "Think outside of the box," and consider as many combinations of consequences to hazardous exposures as possible. The use of the cause and effect diagram with the five elements provides the ability to visualize how combinations create risk based on the hazards present.

For example, if an employee puts a hand into running equipment, what is the probability of that hand being caught by the machine? What could be the severity of the event? The more an employee is exposed to an at-risk event, the greater the chance that the hand will be caught. The frequency of exposure to the hazard increases the probability of getting caught in the piece of equipment with serious severity.

'The existing and potential hazards and consequences of exposure are identified for each listed task. The steps and tasks are reviewed alongside the tools, equipment, and materials used (what are their hazards?) and the work environment. Refer to Figure 11.4 for an example on how to apply "Existing And Potential Hazards And Consequences Of Exposure Documentation."

Job steps and task-specific description	NR	RA	Existing and potential hazards and/or consequences of exposure	At-risk events and preventive measures	RR
Pull car off the road					
			Traffic – speed and conditions		
• Park clear of traffic	X	H	Getting hit by an oncoming vehicle		
• Park on level ground					
• Set parking brake			Environment - weather, ground surface,		
• Turn off ignition			conditions		
• Remove the key					
• Turn on the hazard warning lights			Vehicle condition		
Check for traffic					
			Traffic speed		
• Exit car		H			
• Block wheel			Getting hit by an oncoming vehicle		
• Set flares/reflectors					

Figure 11.4 *Existing and Potential Hazards and Consequences of Exposure Documentation.*

11.15 AT-RISK EVENTS AND PREVENTATIVE MEASURES

The at-risk event and preventative measures listed, act as a guidance statement to convey safe methods. At-risk events and preventative measures are now matched against existing and potential hazards and the consequences of exposure. Refer to Figure 11.5 for an example on describing "At-Risk Events Documentation."

Job steps and task-specific description	NR	RA	Existing and potential hazards and/or consequences of exposure	At-risk events and preventive measures	RR
Pull car off the road					
			Traffic – speed and conditions	Operate vehicle safety	
• Park clear of traffic	X	H	Getting hit by an oncoming vehicle		
• Park on level ground					
• Set parking brake			Environment - weather, ground surface,		
• Turn off ignition			conditions		
• Remove the key					
• Turn on the hazard warning lights			Vehicle condition		
Check for traffic					
			Traffic speed	Exit/entry from car	
• Exit car		H			
• Block wheel			Getting hit by an oncoming vehicle		
• Set flares/reflectors					

Figure 11.5 *At-Risk Events Documentation.*

11.16 PREVENTATIVE MEASURES

The "Hierarchy of Controls" and "Haddon's Energy Countermeasures" as provided in Chapter 7, are used to select controls. This column provides guidance on how employee(s) performing the job will know what methods and actions to follow to protect themselves.

The use of general statements such as "watch out", "be careful", "use caution" or "be safe," "think about," or "be mindful of" should not be used. Specific statements are used to clearly describe the actions to be taken and how the steps/tasks are to be safely performed.

Specific statements, which describe both actions to be taken and how they are to be performed are preferable. The preventative measures listed in the right hand column should match each hazard that has been identified (Figure 11.6).

Job steps and task-specific description	NR	RA	Existing and potential hazards and/or consequences of exposure consideration	At-risk events and preventive measures	RR
Pull car off the road				Operating vehicle safety	
• Park clear of traffic	X	H	Traffic – speed and conditions	• Ensure that brake is set so that	
• Park on level ground			Getting hit by an oncoming vehicle	vehicle will not move.	
• Set parking brake				• Make sure that vehicle is parked	
• Turn off ignition			Environment - weather, ground	off of the roadway so that it is	
• Remove the key			surface, conditions	clear of traffic.	
• Turn on the hazard warning lights				• Ensure that vehicle is parked on	
			Vehicle condition	a level surface to prevent it from	
				moving when it is jacked up	
				• Vehicle maintenance	
Check for traffic				Exit/entry from car	
			Traffic speed		
• Exit car		H		• Have clear view of on-coming	
• Block wheel			Getting hit by an oncoming vehicle	traffic when existing vehicle	
• Set flares/reflectors				• Park out of road and right of way	

Figure 11.6 *Preventative Measures and Guidance Statements Documentation.*

11.17 RESIDUAL RISK

The last stage of the JHA is to conduct a final risk assessment that determines what level of risk remains. The "residual risks" of each task are identified in this column. The residual risk should always be less hazardous than the initial risk. If the residual risk is the same, nothing has been accomplished to (Figure 9.2). Refer to Figure 11.7 for a documenting the residual risks of the task documentation.

Job steps and task-specific description	NR	RA	Existing and potential hazards and/or consequences of exposure	At-risk events and preventive measures	RR
Pull car off the road				Operating vehicle safety	

• Park clear of traffic
• Park on level ground
• Set parking brake
• Turn off ignition
• Remove the key
• Turn on the hazard warning lights
	X	H	Traffic – speed and conditions
			getting hit by an oncoming vehicle
			
			Environment - weather, ground
			surface, conditions
			
			Vehicle condition
				• Ensure that brake is set so that
				  vehicle will not move.
				• Make sure that vehicle is
				  parked off of the roadway so
				  that it is clear of traffic.
				• Ensure that vehicle is parked
				  on a level surface to prevent it
				  from moving when it is jacked
				  up
				• Vehicle maintenance
					M

Check for traffic • Exit car • Block wheel • Set flares/reflectors		H	Traffic speed Getting hit by an oncoming vehicle	Exit/entry from car • Have clear view of on-coming traffic when existing vehicle	H

Figure 11.7 *Types of Risk–Total Risk Versus Residual Risk Documentation.*

11.18 FINAL REVIEW AND APPROVALS

Approvals are required when the JHA is completed to ensure the analysis has been reviewed and accepted by the JHA developer(s), the leadership team and the JHA committee. The completed JHA is reviewed by employees for content, clarity, and completeness (Roughton & Crutchfield, 2008). Sections that are vague, missing information, or confusing to the employees should be revisited and rewritten (Roughton & Crutchfield, 2008).

11.19 ANOTHER AREA FOR CONSIDERATION
11.19.1 Activity-Based Safety System

The activity-based safety system (ABSS) in an approach that leverages direct communication by establishing basic activities that are consistently completed at specific times and places. Specifics activities are performed, tracked, and reviewed to provide ongoing real-time safety-related performance measurements. The ABSS extends the influence of the safety system throughout the organization. It is designed to enhance safety awareness and in turn strengthen the safety culture. ABSS establishes communication links that are used to rapidly transmit concerns and issues between levels of the organization. This increases the probability that hazards and risk-related issues are addressed without delay (Figure 11.8).

To begin the ABSS process, review existing safety system related activities and decide on which activities are adding value to the system. Once all existing safety activities are identified, the decision can be made to remove, modify, and/or replace the nonvalued activities.

The key intent of ABSS is to complement specific safety-related efforts that may be already in place. All safety activities should be integrated with existing safety system elements to formalize the communication process throughout the organization.

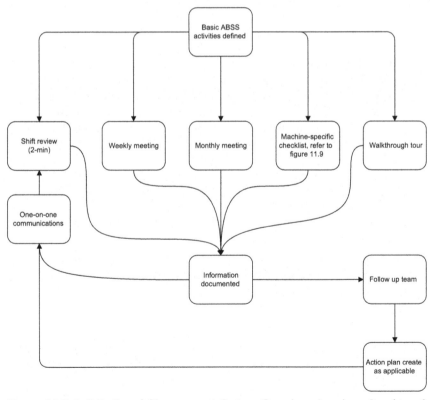

Figure 11.8 *Activity-Based Management System Overview. Based on Roughton & Crutchfield, 2013.*

11.19.2 Advantage of Using ABSS

The advantage is that it uses the experience of the leadership team to build safety-related issues information for discussion with employees. When fully implemented, each member of the leadership team should be able to develop area-specific topics to which employees can relate.

11.19.3 How ABSS Works

Meetings and other various methods are used to convey a safety message. To save time, organizations use canned predetermined topics that are used at safety meetings. While these types of topics may be beneficial, this canned approach restricts the leadership team from using their own creativity and expertise. A standardized script does not always take into account the nature of the work activity and is a "one size fits all" approach.

> "Training must match the application
>   Training packages that include a written script, and sometimes a video, and are designed to solve safety problems are plentiful. In many cases, the trainer only conveys what is provided, reading a prepared script that may or may not apply to the specific working conditions. As a result, trainees recognize the information is not relevant and imparting the information becomes more difficult than it needs to be" (Safety culture in Nuclear Installations, 2002).

ABSS consist of the following basic elements:
- Employee meetings (Daily preshift reviews, weekly meetings, monthly meeting).
- One-on-one discussions with employees.
- Area walkthrough tours (housekeeping, hunting for hazards, etc.).
- Machine/equipment-specific checklist.
- Follow-up team.
- Performance metrics.

It is a communication system that discusses and identifies immediate hazards and associated risk of area-specific safety issues that can be discussed on a daily basis (Chapter 8).

11.20 SAFETY MEETINGS

All employees should have an understanding of the requirements and importance of safety-related issues in their organization. For an organization to be successful in sustaining a safety system, all levels of the organization should conduct safety-related meetings.

Meetings can range from a free form format to agenda driven and are used for maintaining general safety awareness directly with each work group, present specific topics for discussion, and provide safety-specific information and required regulatory compliance training.

11.21 DAILY PRESHIFT REVIEW

The daily preshift review is a short, simple meeting that is held with each work group by their direct leader. This meeting is short and to the point, long enough to ensure that all those involved receive the required safety-related topic of the day.

It is important that this meeting be held preshift or prework assignment held every day. These meeting should become a daily habit, held at the same time, and in the same area without fail. It sets the stage for activities and communications before the shift begins.

These preshift meeting becomes more important during a crisis or when you are under production pressures. It may help in overcoming a desire to take chances in the attempt to get back to a normal situation or maintain production without considering the risk.

"A magnifying effect occurs as each of the employees in turn influence and communicates through their own personal network. As employees talk to each other in break rooms, at lunch, friends off the job, etc. the message continues to travel throughout the organization" (Roughton & Crutchfield, 2013).

11.22 MULTISHIFT OPERATION

It is important that the transfer of safety and hazard-related information and knowledge between shifts is conducted. Prior to the preshift review, the leadership team from the previous shift should ensure that safety or operational issues during the previous shift are communicated to the on-coming shift.

11.23 WEEKLY MEETINGS

Regular weekly meetings should be conducted at a specific time and place. This meeting is more formal than the preshift reviews and sets the tone for the week's safety agenda and brings closure to the past week's efforts.

A weekly safety meeting would last about thirty minutes or until all of the safety-related discussions have been addressed and completed. It may require more time to discuss safety-related topics, new issues, injuries in other areas or facilities with similar exposures, or other changes in the organization (Roughton & Crutchfield, 2013).

The weekly meeting is used to recap and summarize any open discussions from the daily preshift meeting to ensure that no obstacles or miscommunications continue to exist.

11.24 MONTHLY MEETINGS

The monthly meeting is for an in-depth training and/or refresher on organizational policies, procedures, protocols, guidelines, etc. This meeting is more formal than the weekly meetings and may be 1 h in length or until all of the safety-related training has been completed.

The monthly meeting brings together larger groups and provides a way of sharing diverse set of ideas and could include outside speakers, members of the leadership team to provide an overview of the organization performance, etc.

11.25 ONE-ON-ONE DISCUSSIONS WITH EMPLOYEES

The one-on-one discussion or direct face-to-face conversation provides real-time feedback between the leader and employee. Many employees will not speak up in meetings due to shyness, fear, mistrust, or other reasoning. By using a direct approach, employees can discuss openly with the leader the information from safety meetings and any other concerns that they would not bring up in front of their peers.

"Face-to-Face Discussion

Opportunities for employees to have face-to-face discussion support other communication activities and enable them to make a more personal contribution.

Tours and formal consultation meetings are options but others include:

- Planned meetings (or team briefings) at which information can be cascaded. These can include targeting particular groups of workers for safety critical tasks;
- Health and safety issues on the agenda at all routine management meetings (possibly as the first item); monthly or weekly "tool-box" talks or "tailgate" meetings at which supervisors can discuss health and safety issues with their teams, remind them of critical risks and precautions and supplement the organization's training effort.

These also provide opportunities for employees to make their own suggestions (perhaps by "brainstorming") about improving health and safety arrangements.

(Successful Health and Safety Management, hsg65, 1997)

These one-on-one discussions are centered on safety concerns. They should be conducted in the employee's work environment where the employee feels more comfortable, not in the supervisor's office.

11.26 SAFETY WALKTHROUGH TOUR

Safety inspections, observations, and walkthroughs are a core feature of safety systems. The safety walkthrough is an essential component of ABSS and is conducted as a joint effort by a diverse team that can consist of supervision, management, senior leadership, and employees as applicable.

The objective is to have a group that brings a variety of perceptions, backgrounds, expertise, and different points of view into the work environment. The participation of a member of the leadership team is to provide awareness and to provide a presence to all employees that this effort is considered important and a value to the organization.

This walkthrough is typically no more than one hour in length and is not to be treated as a formal inspection. It is an awareness and general observation tool that allows the group to interact with employees to identify specific concern about hazards.

At the conclusion of a walkthrough, safety-related issues identified should require have risk assessment and corrective action plan implemented.

11.27 MACHINE/EQUIPMENT-SPECIFIC CHECKLIST

The next component of ABSS is a machine/equipment-specific checklist. This checklist is used to focus on specific, identified safety-related issues for each piece of machinery and/or equipment in the organization. It is developed and updated by employees and the leadership team (Figure 11.9) (Appendix L).

The checklist is not intended to be a maintenance checklist, as it is to be a quick reference to ensure that the primary hazards are reviewed and controlled. Once the checklist format and content is completed and agreed

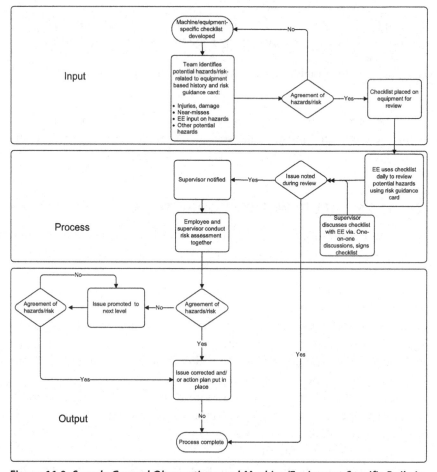

Figure 11.9 *Sample General Observations and Machine/Equipment-Specific Daily Inspection Checklist Development.* Based on Roughton & Crutchfield, 2013.

upon, it is physically placed on the equipment so that it can be reviewed on a daily basis by the operator and used in the one-on-one discussion with the leader. The checklist is not static and is considered a living document as additional information is received.

To effectively use this checklist, employees of each shift will review the machine or equipment before production begins, rate each checklist item with the risk guidance card, and record the risk rating and if the machine/equipment is in acceptable or unacceptable condition (Chapter 8).

This checklist can be used as part of the one-on-one discussions with employees where the leader and employee will discuss elements on the list and validate that the review is acceptable to both the employee and the leader. If the employee who reviews the checklist finds that an item is unacceptable, based on the assigned risk code using the risk guidance card, the leadership is contacted and a review is conducted together at the machine or equipment.

In reviewing the checklist as described earlier, and if there is a safety issue identified, an agreement must be reached between the employee and the leader as to the nature, type of the hazard, and the potential risk before the equipment can be put back in operation.

Refer to Chapter 8 for a detail discussion on the risk guidance card. If no agreement is reached, the next level of the leadership team is contacted and a second discussion begins. The intent of having these discussions is to reduce the potential and probability that employees will continue to operate machinery or equipment that is not functioning as intended, believing that they have no alternative but to use the machinery or equipment in an unsafe condition.

11.28 FOLLOW-UP TEAM

A follow-up team is important in that it ensures that all safety-related work order request are addressed and completed in a timely manner. This team should consist of a maintenance technician, several employees, and a leader depending on the number of work orders that are under review (Chapter 8).

The follow-up team provides an unbiased review of each safety-related work order created, scheduled, and completed within a designated time period or that remains outstanding. The team is charged with reviewing all safety-related work order, using the risk guidance card to establish a priority for corrective action or moving the request to the next level of decision makers (Chapter 8).

The team is designed to break down any barriers that may exist between involved parties. To close this potential gap, the team uses a peer-to peer approach to ensure that the safety-related hazard and associated risk is assessed.

The intent is to involve the employee, ensure that the work order is valid, that the hazard and associated risk is valid and needs to be corrected. When the work order is completed, a member of the follow-up team discusses the issue/conditions with the employee who requested a hazardous issue be corrected. If the employee agrees with the fix then the work order is signed off and closed. The follow-up team can present the status of safety-related work orders at weekly/monthly meetings. The status is posted both electronically and hardcopy for all employees to review.

11.29 ABSS ROLES AND RESPONSIBILITIES

The following is a basic overview of roles and responsibilities for each level of the leadership team.

11.29.1 Supervisor/Lead Person

The supervisor/lead person's role is the key in presenting a common and consistent message to their area of responsibility. The supervisor documents the various activities of the ABSS process in a safety activity report (Appendix N).

Supervisors should participate each week in the following safety activities:
- Develop and present daily shift reviews.
- Conduct daily one-on-one discussions with employees.
- Review machine/equipment-specific safety checklist.
- Coordinate with the follow-up team to correct safety-related issues.
- Participate in monthly walkthroughs

11.29.2 Middle Management

Middle management should participate in safety-related activities as determined by the leadership team. This involvement reinforces the safety culture and promotes overall commitment to the safety system. They should participate each month in the following safety activities:
- Attend at least one daily shift review.
- Contact at least five employees to conduct a one-on-one discussion with employees.
- Reviewing machine/equipment-specific safety checklist with operators
- Safety walkthrough tours

11.29.3 Senior Management

Senior management should participate in or conduct safety walkthroughs at a minimum of one time per quarter. All areas of physical responsibility should be reviewed annually. They should participate quarterly in the following safety activities:

- Attend at least one daily shift reviews.
- Contact at least five employees to conduct a one-on-one discussion with employees.
- Reviewing machine/equipment-specific safety checklist with operators
- Safety walkthrough tours

Senior management should have an open door policy, conduct a round table meeting with selected employees semi-annually, unannounced visits to selected areas semi-annually to meet one-on-one with employees are random.

11.29.4 Safety Professional

Safety professionals are expected to participate each week in the following safety activities:

- Assist supervision in developing daily shift reviews.
- Conduct at random, five one-on-one discussions with employees.
- Conduct at random, five reviews of machine/equipment-specific safety checklists.
- Coordinate with the follow-up team to correct safety-related issues.
- Assist leadership in safety walkthrough tours

The safety professional provides support by through safety-related materials, suggestions, and guidance. The safety profession does not conduct meetings (Figure 11.10).

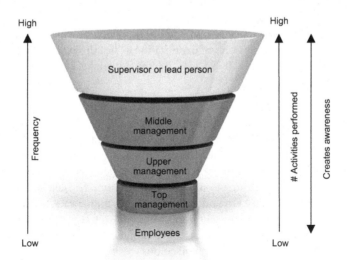

Figure 11.10 *Frequency of Activities Performed by Level.* Based on Roughton & Crutchfield, 2013.

11.30 MEASURING THE SUCCESS OF ABSS

Safety performance metrics and safety system elements are of no benefit unless they are clearly and routinely communicated throughout the organization.

"The majority of measures should be leading indicators that focus on proactive activities on the part of all employees—measures that track what people are doing daily to prevent accidents. With such measures in place, immediate and certain consequences can be engineered in to ensure those activities occur"(Agnew & Daniels, 2011).

"It is often said that only those things that get measured, get done; and that, since only certain things can be measured, it is hardly a surprise when managers or organizations are assessed on short term criteria."
(Safety culture in Nuclear Installations, 2002)

"Performance indicators or metrics are parameters measured to reflect the critical success factors of an organization. The purpose of these measures is to provide facility personnel with a way of knowing whether planned activities are occurring as originally intended as well as warning of developing problems.

There are two types of indicators:

Lagging – Measures of results or outcomes which represent where you are and what you have accomplished, but do not necessarily predict future accomplishments, and

Leading – Measures of system conditions, which provide a forecast of future performance; measures of organizational "health," which can predict results and achievements" (US DOE, 2009b) (Appendix L).

Basic Tips for ABSS
- Be a good listener and make time for employees. Regular, one-on-one meetings with each employee are important. This is not to be a formal human resources process of personnel review. The goal is to reach out to those employees who best know the workplace and its ongoing potential for change.
- Give employees full attention with no distractions, i.e., take the time to discuss safety, quality, etc. and nothing else. No phone calls, texting, etc.
- Keep the message consistent about the value of the safety system. If mixed messages have been sent concerning safety-related issues, a one-on-one can correct the communication.
- Give regular positive feedback.
  (Roughton & Crutchfield, 2010)

SUMMARY

A successful job hazard analysis (JHA) will involve collecting job data, developing the job steps and task, creating cause and effect diagram(s), the hazard assessment, and using a risk matrix to identify probability and severity.

Use of the JHA provides a structure and method to ensure that activities (jobs and their required steps and tasks) are consistently performed with proper controls in place to reduce the potential consequences of hazardous exposure.

When conducting a JHA, the process attempts to paint a picture of what is happening and the story about the potential and existing hazards. A clear, concise picture with accompanying data provides feedback to the employees on what controls are essential to protect themselves.

The "5 Why's" plus "H" questions (Who, What, Where, When, Why, and How) are used to categorized information and better ensure no gaps in the information.

Checklists should be used to ensure that all of the important elements of the JHA are completed and concise.

A comprehensive JHA form is the document that provides the complete description of all aspects of the job. Where it takes place; What is required to do it; Who does it, When it is being done, and How it is to be completed – all with the intent of linking activity to the level of associated risk.

Tracking the sequence of steps is important because if the steps are out of sequence, the relationship between the steps and the existing and potential hazard and consequences of exposures, at-risk events, and the preventative measure(s) cannot be properly documented.

The last stage of the JHA is to conduct a final risk assessment that determines what level of risk remains.

Approvals are be required when the JHA is completed to ensure the analysis has been reviewed and accepted by the JHA developer(s) and the leadership team. The JHA is submitted to a member of the leadership team for approval at completion.

The activity-based safety system (ABSS) in an approach that leverages direct communication by establishing basic activities that are consistently completed at specific times and places. The ABSS extends the influence of the safety system throughout the organization. ABSS establishes communication links that are used to rapidly transmit concerns and issues between levels of the organization. This increases the probability that hazards and risk-related issues are addressed without delay.

CHAPTER REVIEW QUESTIONS

1. Discuss the use of the cause and effect diagram.
2. What are the 5 W plus H questions?
3. What is the job description?
4. Describe the job steps and task-specific description section of the JHA.
5. Define nonroutine task.
6. Describe the existing and potential hazards and consequences of exposure section of the JHA.
7. Describe the at-risk events and preventative measures section of the JHA.
8. What is residual risk?
9. Describe the ABSS system.

BIBLIOGRAPHY

Agnew, J., & Daniels, A. (2011). *Developing high-impact leading indicators for safety*. Performance Management Magazine. Retrieved from http://bit.ly/WTK66g
Conducting a Job Hazard Analysis (JHA). (n.d.). Oregon Occupational Safety and Health Division (Oregon OSHA), Public Domain, Permission to Reprint, Modify, and/or Adapt as necessary. Retrieved from http://bit.ly/WXGJhK
Job Safety Analysis, OSH Answers Fact Sheets, Reprinted with Permission. (n.d.). Canadian Centre for Occupational Health & Safety (CCOHS). Retrieved from http://bit. ly/1xuqMVl
Oregon OSHA Website, Job Hazard Analysis 103 Workshop, http://www.cbs.state.or.us/external/osha/educate/training/pages/materials.html
Roughton, J., & Crutchfield, N. (2008). *Job hazard analysis: A guide for voluntary compliance and beyond. Chemical, petrochemical & process*. MA: Elsevier/Butterworth-Heinemann, Retrieved from http://amzn.to/VrSAq5.
Roughton, J., & Crutchfield, N. (2010). *Safety culture – six basic safety program elements*. Ezine Articles. Retrieved from http://bit.ly/Z5oolV
Roughton, J., & Crutchfield, N. (2013). In B. Heinemann (Ed.), *Safety culture: An innovative leadership approach*. MA: Butterworth Heinemann, Retrieved from http://amzn. to/1qoD4oN.
Safety culture in Nuclear Installations. (2002). International Atomic Energy Agency (IAEA), Guidance for use in the enhancement of safety culture, IAEA-TECDOC-1329. Retrieved from http://bit.ly/V1KsKt
Sinek, S. (2009). *Start with why: How great leaders inspire everyone to take action*. New York: Penguin, Retrieved from http://bit.ly/1Lfs2zr.
Strubler, D. (n.d.). The difference that continual improvement makes, Principle 4, The Five "W's" and Once"H. Retrieved from http://bit.ly/1M3HZtk
Successful Health and Safety Management, hsg65. (1997). Health and Safety Executive, Crown Publishing, Permission to Reprint. Retrieved from http://bit.ly/YKDzRk
US DOE. (2009). *Concepts and principles, human performance improvement handbook* (Vol. 1). US Department of Energy. Retrieved from http://bit.ly/1DfdJVU
US DOE. (2009b). *Human performance tools for individuals, work teams, and management, human performance improvement handbook* (Vol. 2). US Department of Energy. Retrieved from http://1.usa.gov/11Ex7vE

FURTHER READING

Job Hazard Analysis, 3071(2002). *Occupational Safety and Health Administration (OSHA)*, Public Domain, Modified and/or Adapt as necessary. Retrieved from http://bit.ly/1ZI1Q7y

Appendix K Examples Information on How to Tell the JHA Story

Sample Instructions on How to Change a Tire on a Car
  Sample JHA PreHazard Assessment Worksheet
  JHA on Changing a Tire
  Annotated JHA on Changing a Tire
  Comparison JHA on Changing a Tire, Traditional Versus New Version
  Job Hazard Analysis, Canadian Centre for Occupational Health & Safety (CCOHS)

K.1 Sample instructions on how to change a tire of a car

- Pull off to the side of the road out of traffic. Make sure the car is parked off the road and clear of traffic.
- Park on level ground.
- Set the parking brake. Apply the parking brake and place the transmission in park if it is an automatic. If the car has a standard transmission, place the shift in first gear or reverse.
- Turn off the ignition and remove the key.
- Turn on the hazard warning lights.
- Check for traffic and exit the car. Watch out for on coming traffic as you exit the car.
- Find something to block the front wheels if changing a back tire or block the back wheels if changing the front tire, (to keep the car from rolling.)
- Set safety flares or reflectors five car lengths front and back.
- Open the truck and remove the tire.
- Pull out spare tire.
- Retrieve other tools out of the trunk, such as jack, lug wrench.
- Remove wheel covers.
- Properly place jack under the car. Consult your owners' manual and find where the jack needs to be positioned.
- Jack the car up part of the way so that tire is still touching the ground. Raise the car just enough to take the weight off the tire.
- Using the lug wrench, loosen the lug nuts slightly but do not remove.
- Jack up the car so the tire is above ground.
- Remove the lug nuts from the bolts.
- Remove the flat tire.
- Replace the flat tire with the spare.
- Replace the lug nuts on the bolts and tighten, but not too tight, just enough to hold the tire in place while you lower the car.
- Lower the car until it touches the ground, and then firmly tightens all of the lug nuts.
- Gather everything and put in trunk.
- As soon as possible, have the flat tire repaired and reinstalled.

K.2 Sample JHA prehazard assessment worksheet

JHA control #	Brief job description – cause and effect diagram		PPE Requirements: Required for entire facility		Page ___ of ___

Task description			Existing and potential hazards and/or consequences of exposure	At-risk events	Preventive measures, awareness statement
	RA	NR			RR
	H	X			M
Pull the car off of the road and sure that you			Traffic, speed and conditions	Operating vehicle safety	• Ensure that brake is set so that vehicle will not move.
• Park clear of traffic			Getting hit by an oncoming vehicle		• Make sure that vehicle is parked off of the roadway so that it is clear of traffic.
• Park on level ground			Environment - weather, ground surface, conditions		• Ensure that vehicle is parked on a level surface to prevent it from moving when it is jacked up
• Set parking brake			Vehicle condition		
• Turn off ignition					
• Remove the key					
• Turn on the hazard warning lights					
	RA	NR			RR
					Note how each task may impact the next task
					Ensure that task-specific PPE is listed in this section of the JHA
	RA	NR			RR
Supervisor:				Date:	
Analysis conducted by:				Date:	
Other reviewer(s) (Include employees):				Date:	

Adapted and modified Oregon OSHA (n.d.); US Department of Labor (n.d.)

K.3 JHA - Example of changing a tire

Brief description: Changing a tire   Department: Highway   Date: April, 2014   Last revision:

Performed by: J. Roughton/Nathan Crutchfiled   Employee: Joe tire   Supervisor: Jim production

Personal protective equipment: None required   Note: Recommended PPE will be listed under each specific task based PPE Assessment

Job steps and task-specific description	NR	RA	Existing and potential hazards and/or consequences of exposure	Potential at-risk events and preventive measures	RR
Pull car off the road • Park clear of traffic • Park on level ground • Set parking brake • Turn off ignition • Remove the key • Turn on the hazard warning lights	X	H	Traffic – speed and conditions Getting hit by an oncoming vehicle Environment – weather, ground surface, conditions Vehicle condition	Operating vehicle safety • Ensure that brake is set so that vehicle will not move. • Make sure that vehicle is parked off of the roadway so that it is clear of traffic. • Ensure that vehicle is parked on a level surface to prevent it from moving when it is jacked up	M
Check for traffic • Exit the car • Block the wheel • Set flares/reflectors on the road	X	H	Traffic speed Getting hit by an oncoming vehicle	Exit/entry from car • Pay attention to on-coming traffic when existing vehicle	M

K.3 JHA - Example of changing a tire *(cont.)*

Job steps and task-specific description	NR	RA	Existing and potential hazards and/or consequences of exposure	Potential at-risk events and preventive measures	RR
Open trunk • Loosen spare tire • Remove tire • Retrieve jack and lug wrench		M	Strain/sprain from removing tire and tools from trunk	Eyes on task • Keep eyes on task when removing tire Tools and equipment • Keep back as straight possible when removing tire and tools from trunk Lifting and lowering • Use proper lifting techniques when lifting tire from trunk	L
Preparing for tire removal • Remove wheel covers • Place jack under car • Jack car up • Take weight off tire		M	Strain/sprain from removing wheel covers Struck against vehicle when placing jack under car Struck by vehicle when placing jack up car Terrain/ground surface and condition, shift of jack	Tools and equipment • Select the correct tool for removing wheel covers Eyes on task • Keep eyes on task when removing wheel covers • Keep eyes on task when placing jack under car • Keep eye on task and highway when jacking up car	L
Removing tire • Use lug wrench • Loosen lug nuts slightly • Jack up the car • Remove lug nuts		H	Strain/sprain from using lug wrench Struck against vehicle when loosen lug nuts Struck by vehicle when jack car up	Tools and equipment • Select the correct tool for removing lug nuts • Ensure that jack is positioned under car before continuing Eyes on task • Keep eyes on task when using lug wrench • Keep eyes on task when loosing lug nuts • Keep eye on task and highway when jacking up car	L

Replacing tire	H	Eyes on task	L
• Replace flat tire	Strain/sprain from using lug wrench	• Keep eyes on task when using lug wrench	
• Replace lug nuts	Struck against vehicle when replacing lug nuts	• Keep eyes on task when replacing lug nuts	
• Lower the car	Struck by vehicle when lowering car	• Keep eye on task and highway when lowering car	
	Terrain/ground surface and condition, shift off of jack	Tools and equipment	
		• Select the correct tool for replace lug nuts	
		• Ensure that jack is positioned on solid surface in required set-point of car before continuing	

Note: NR, nonroutine task, Place a check mark for these types of task; RA, risk analysis; RR, residual risk (After JHA Development)

Specific statements, which describe the actions, what actions will be taken, and how the steps/tasks are to be safely performed is must be clearly described:

• Are the at-risk events and preventive measure specifically designed around what the person is to actually do?
• Is the objective or the awareness statement well defined?
• Are action words used describing how to prevent an employee from an injury?
• Are preventive measures practical?
• Is there a common sense approach, given the nature of the tasks performed?
• Do employees have control over at-risk events and preventative measures?
• Can employees control their actions or does it take management commitment and leadership to provide the tools and resources necessary to perform the job safely?

K.4 Example annotated JHA for changing a tire

Brief description: changing a tire	Department: highway	Date April 14, 2014	Last revised: November 1, 2015
Performed By: J. Roughton/Nathan Crutchfiled	Employee signature: Joe tire	Supervisor signature: Jim production	
Personal protective equipment: none required		Note: Recommended PPE will be listed under each specific task based PPE Assessment	

Note: NR = Non-Routine Task – Place a check mark for these types of task. RA=Risk Analysis, RR=Residual Risk (After JHA Development)

Job Steps and Task-Specific Description	NR	RA	Existing and Potential hazards and/or Consequences of exposure consideration	Potential at-risk events and preventive measures	RR
Pull car off the road		H	Employee participation and buy-in via signing the JHA to verify agreement of hazard. Supervisor review and sign off with employee is document in this section.	The PPE Section has two specific uses:	M
• Park clear of traffic				Operator	
• This section is used to break down the job steps into the individual Tasks.				1. **Facility-wide specific PPE:** PPE listed in this section is required for the entire facility, based on the consequences of exposure and the PPE assessment.	
• Remove the key					
• Turn on the hazard warning lights				2. **Task-Specific PPE:** Specific PPE will be identified by each task in this section. This section will ensure that the user understands task-specific PPE as identified in the PPE assessment and how it related to the at-risk event and Preventative Measures associated with the hazard.	
Check for traffic		H	Getting hit by an oncoming vehicle	Exit/	T
• Exit car	X				
• Block wheel					
• Set flares/reflectors	X				
Op...		M	This section highlights existing and potential hazards and consequences of exposure that may result from the specific hazards.	**Eyes on task**	M
• For non-routine task (not completed frequently) an "X" placed in this section.				• Keep eyes on task	
• Drivers do not routinely exit vehicles on right of way.			Str...	**Tools and equipment**	
				• Keep back as straight possible when removing tire and tools from trunk	
This section is where the initial risk assessment is noted. Refer to chapter 8 for details				At-Risk events are integrated into each task to highlight specific behavior(s) associated with the hazard.	
				Defails the preventative measures that are to be used to ensure that the tasks/steps is performed safely.	
				Note: At-risk events can be developed by a team	
				This section is where the residual risk assessment is noted. Refer to Chapter 9 for details	

K.5 Comparison JHA on changing a tire, traditional versus current research

K.5.1 Traditional Version

Sequence of events	Potential accidents or hazards	Preventive measures
Park vehicle	• Vehicle too close to passing traffic • Vehicle on uneven, soft ground • Vehicle may roll	• Drive to area well clear of traffic. Turn on emergency flashers • Choose a firm, level area • Apply the parking brake; leave transmission in gear or in PARK; place blocks in front and back of the wheel diagonally opposite to the flat

K.5.2 New Version

Job: Changing a tire   Department: Highway   Date April, 2014–2015

Performed by: J. Roughton/Nathan Crutchfield   Employee signature: Joe tire   Supervisor signature: Jim production

Personal protective equipment: None requiredw   Note: Recommended PPE will be listed under each specific task based PPE assessment

Job steps and task-specific description	NR	RA	Existing and potential hazards and/or consequences of exposure consideration	Potential at-risk events and preventive Measures	RR
Pull car off the road • Park clear of traffic • Park on level ground • Set parking brake • Turn off ignition • Remove the key • Turn on the hazard warning lights		H	Getting hit by an oncoming vehicle	Operating vehicle safety • Ensure that brake is set so that vehicle will not move. • Make sure that vehicle is parked off of the roadway so that it is clear of traffic. • Ensure that vehicle is parked on a level surface to prevent it from moving when it is jacked up	M

Note: NR, nonroutine task, Place a check mark for these types of task; RA, risk analysis; RR, residual risk (After JHA Development)

K.6 Job hazard analysis, Canadian Centre for Occupational Health & Safety (CCOHS)

One way to increase the knowledge of hazards in the workplace is to conduct a job hazard analysis on individual tasks. A job hazard analysis (JHA) is a procedure which helps integrate accepted safety and health principles and practices into a particular operation. In a JHA, each basic step of the job is examined to identify potential hazards and to determine the safest way to do the job. Other terms used to describe this procedure are job safety analysis (JSA) and job hazard breakdown.

Some individuals prefer to expand the analysis into all aspects of the job, not just safety. This approach known as total job analysis, job analysis or task analysis is based on the idea that safety is an integral part of every job and not a separate entity. In this document, only health and safety aspects will be considered.

The terms "job" and "task" are commonly used interchangeably to mean a specific work assignment, such as "operating a grinder," "using a pressurized water extinguisher," or "Changing a flat tire." JHAs are not suitable for jobs defined too broadly, for example, "Overhauling an engine"; or too narrowly, for example, "positioning car jack."

K.6.1 What are the Benefits of Doing a Job Hazard Analysis?

The method used in this example is to observe a worker actually perform the job. The major advantages of this method include that it does not rely on individual memory and that the process prompts recognition of hazards. For infrequently performed or new jobs, observation may not be practical. With these, one approach is to have a group of experienced workers and supervisors complete the analysis through discussion. An advantage of this method is that more people are involved allowing for a wider base of experience and promoting a more ready acceptance of the resulting work procedure.

Members of the joint occupational safety and health committee should participate in this process.

Initial benefits from developing a JHA will become clear in the preparation stage. The analysis process may identify previously undetected hazards and increase the job knowledge of those participating. Safety and health awareness is raised, communication between workers and supervisors is improved, and acceptance of safe work procedures is promoted.

The completed JHA, or better still, a written work procedure based on it, can form the basis for regular contact between supervisors and workers on health and safety. It can serve as a teaching aid for initial job training and as a briefing guide for infrequent jobs.

It may be used as a standard for health and safety inspections or observations and it will assist in completing comprehensive accident investigations.

K.6.2 What are the Four Basic Steps?

Four basic stages in conducting a JHA are:
- Selecting the job to be analyzed
- Breaking the job down into a sequence of steps
- Identifying potential hazards
- Determining preventive measures to overcome these hazards

K.6.3 What is Important to Know When "Selecting the Job"?

Ideally, all jobs should be subjected to a JHA. In some cases there are practical constraints posed by the amount of time and effort required to do a JHA. Another consideration is that each JHA will require revision whenever equipment, raw materials, processes, or the environment change. For these reasons, it is usually necessary to identify which jobs are to be analyzed. Even if analysis of all jobs is planned, this step ensures that the most critical jobs are examined first.

Factors to be considered in assigning a priority for analysis of jobs include:
- Accident frequency and severity: jobs where accidents occur frequently or where they occur infrequently but result in disabling injuries.
- Potential for severe injuries or illnesses: the consequences of an accident, hazardous condition, or exposure to harmful substance are potentially severe.
- Newly established jobs: due to lack of experience in these jobs, hazards may not be evident or anticipated.
- Modified jobs: new hazards may be associated with changes in job procedures.
- Infrequently performed jobs: workers may be at greater risk when undertaking nonroutine jobs, and a JHA provides a means of reviewing hazards.

K.6.4 How do I Break the Job into "Basic Steps"?

After a job has been chosen for analysis, the next stage is to break the job into steps. A job step is defined as a segment of the operation necessary to advance the work. See examples below.

Care must be taken not to make the steps too general, thereby missing specific steps and their associated hazards. On the other hand, if they are too detailed, there will be too many steps. A rule of thumb is that most jobs can be described in less than ten steps. If more steps are required, you might want to divide the job into two segments, each with its separate JHA, or combine steps where appropriate. As an example, the job of changing a flat tire will be used in this document.

An important point to remember is to keep the steps in their correct sequence. Any step, which is out of order may miss potential hazards or introduce hazards, which do not actually exist.

Each step is recorded in sequence. Make notes about what is done rather than how it is done. Each item is started with an action verb. Appendix A illustrates a format, which can be used as a worksheet in preparing a JHA. Job steps are recorded in the left hand column, as shown below:

Sequence of events	Potential accidents or hazards	Preventive measures
Park vehicle		
Remove spare and tool kit		
Pry off hub cap and loosen lug bolts (nuts)		
And so on.....		

This part of the analysis is usually prepared by watching the worker do the job. The observer is normally the immediate supervisor but a more thorough analysis often happens by having another person, preferable a member of the joint occupational health and safety committee, participate in the observation. Key points are less likely to be missed in this way.

The worker to be observed should be experienced and capable in all parts of the job. To strengthen full co-operation and participation, the reason for the exercise must be clearly explained. The JHA is neither a time and motion study in disguise, nor an attempt to uncover individual unsafe acts. The job, not the individual, is being studied in an effort to make it safer by identifying hazards and making modifications to eliminate or reduce them. The worker's experience can be important in making improvements.

The job should be observed during normal times and situations. For example, if a job is routinely done only at night, the JHA review should also be done at night. Similarly, only regular tools and equipment should be used. The only difference from normal operations is the fact that the worker is being observed.

When completed, the breakdown of steps should be discussed by all the participants (always including the worker) to make that all basic steps have been noted and are in the correct order.

K.6.5 How do I "Identify Potential Hazards"?

Once the basic steps have been recorded, potential hazards must be identified at each step. Based on observations of the job, knowledge of accident and injury causes, and personal experience, list the things that could go wrong at each step.

A second observation of the job being performed may be needed. Since the basic steps have already been recorded, more attention can now be focused on potential hazards. At this stage, no attempt is made to solve any problems, which may have been detected.

To help identify potential hazards, the job analyst may use questions such as these (this is not a complete list):

- Can any body part get caught in or between objects?
- Do tools, machines, or equipment present any hazards?
- Can the worker make harmful contact with objects?
- Can the worker slip, trip, or fall?
- Can the worker suffer strain from lifting, pushing, or pulling?
- Is the worker exposed to extreme heat or cold?
- Is excessive noise or vibration a problem?
- Is there a danger from falling objects?
- Is lighting a problem?
- Can weather conditions affect safety?
- Is harmful radiation a possibility?
- Can contact be made with hot, toxic, or caustic substances?
- Are there dusts, fumes, mists, or vapors in the air?

Potential hazards are listed in the middle column of the worksheet, numbered to match the corresponding job step. For example:

Sequence of events	Potential accidents or hazards	Preventive measures
Park vehicle	1. Vehicle too close to passing traffic 2. Vehicle on uneven, soft ground 3. Vehicle may roll	
Remove spare and tool kit	1. Strain from lifting spare	
Pry off hub cap and loosen lug bolts (nuts)	1. Hub cap may pop off and hit you 2. Lug wrench may slip	
And so on.....	1 ...	

Again, all participants should jointly review this part of the analysis.

K.6.6 How do I "Determine Preventive Measures?"
The final stage in a JHA is to determine ways to eliminate or control the hazards identified. The generally accepted measures, in order of preference, are:

K.6.6.1 Eliminate the Hazard
This is the most effective measure. These techniques should be used to eliminate the hazards:
- Choose a different process
- Modify an existing process
- Substitute with less hazardous substance
- Improve environment (ventilation)
- Modify or change equipment or tools

K.6.6.2 Contain the Hazard
If the hazard cannot be eliminated, contact might be prevented by using enclosures, machine guards, worker booths or similar devices.

K.6.6.3 Revise Work Procedures
Consideration might be given to modifying steps, which are hazardous, changing the sequence of steps, or adding additional steps (such as locking out energy sources).

K.6.6.4 Reduce the Exposure
These measures are the least effective and should only be used if no other solutions are possible. One way of minimizing exposure is to reduce the number of times the hazard is encountered. An example would be modifying machinery so that less maintenance is necessary. The use of appropriate personal protective equipment may be required. To reduce the severity of an accident, emergency facilities, such as eyewash stations, may need to be provided.

In listing the preventive measures, use of general statements such as "be careful" or "use caution" should be avoided. Specific statements, which describe both what action is to be taken and how it is to be performed are preferable. The recommended measures are listed in the right hand column of the worksheet, numbered to match the hazard in question. For example:

Sequence of events	Potential accidents or hazards	Preventive measures
Park vehicle	1. Vehicle too close to passing traffic 2. Vehicle on uneven, soft ground 3. Vehicle may roll	1. Drive to area well clear of traffic. Turn on emergency flashers 2. Choose a firm, level area 3. Apply the parking brake; leave transmission in gear or in PARK; place blocks in front and back of the wheel diagonally opposite to the flat
Remove spare and tool kit	1. Strain from lifting spare	1. Turn spare into upright position in the wheel well. Using your legs and standing as close as possible, lift spare out of truck and roll to flat tire.
Pry off hub cap and loosen lug bolts (nuts)	1. Hub cap may pop off and hit you 2. Lug wrench may slip	1. Pry off hub cap using steady pressure 2. Use proper lug wrench; apply steady pressure slowly.
And so on.....	1. ...	1. ...

K.6.7 How Should I Make the Information Available to Everyone

JHA is a useful technique for identifying hazards so that measures can be taken to eliminate or control them. Once the analysis is completed, the results must be communicated to all workers who are, or will be, performing that job. The side-by-side format used in JHA worksheets is not an ideal one for instructional purposes. Better results can be achieved by using a narrative-style format. For example, the work procedure based on the partial JHA developed as an example in this document might start out like this:

K.6.7.1 Park Vehicle

1. Drive vehicle off the road to an area well clear of traffic, even if it requires rolling on a flat tire. Turn on the emergency flashers to alert passing drivers so that they will not hit you.
2. Choose a firm, level area so that you can jack up the vehicle without it rolling.
3. Apply the parking brake, leave the transmission in gear or PARK, place blocks in front and back of the wheel diagonally opposite the flat. These actions will also help prevent the vehicle from rolling.

K.6.7.2 Remove Spare and Tool Kit

1. To avoid back strain, turn the spare up into an upright position in its well. Stand as close to the trunk as possible and slide the spare close to your body. Lift out and roll to flat tire.

K.6.7.3 Pry Off Hub Cap, Loosen Lug Bolts (Nuts)

1. Pry off hub cap slowly with steady pressure to prevent it from popping off and striking you.
2. Using the proper lug wrench, apply steady pressure slowly to loosen the lug bolts (nuts), so that the wrench will not slip and hurt your knuckles.

K.6.7.4 And So On

Appendix A: Sample form for job hazard analysis worksheet

Job hazard analysis worksheet		
Job:		
Analysis by:	Reviewed By:	Approved by:
Date:	Date:	Date:
Sequence of Events	Potential accidents or hazards	Preventive measures

Appendix B: Sample forms for tasks and job inventory

Tasks with potential exposure to hazardous materials or physical agents		
Analysis by:	Reviewed by:	Approved by:
Date:	Date:	Date:
Sequence of events	Potential accidents or hazards	Preventive measures

Job inventory of hazardous chemicals		
Analysis by:	Reviewed by:	Approved by:
Date:	Date:	Date:
Sequence of events	Potential accidents or hazards	Preventive measures

What is a Job Hazard Analysis? (Job Safety Analysis, OSH Answers Fact Sheets, Reprinted with Permission, n.d.)

K.6.8 Standard operating procedure changing a tire

{insert simple instructions}

1. Car has flat tire

Insert picture that fits this instructions

2. Pull car off of roads

Insert picture that fits the instructions

3. Prepare to remove tire

Insert picture that fits the instructions

Procedure starts over at Step #1.

Appendix L Sample Operator General Observations & Machine/Equipment-Specific Daily Inspection Checklist

(Customize this checklist for each type of machine and equipment)

Date	Time	Signature
Location – Machine/ Equipment		

Description	Yes	No	Comments
Did you attend a shift-review?			
Was proper communication on problems provided by the previous shift operator?			

Note: When conducting the daily inspection of your machine/equipment, you must perform a risk assessment for each item listed using the Risk Guidance Card. Refer to Chapter 8.

Description	1	2	3	Comments
Are you using the proper gloves for the operation?				
Are you using the proper approved knives for the operation?				
Are all machine guards in place?				
Are all machine guards functioning properly?				
Is machine safe from loose objects/tools that could fall into moving parts?				
Is everyone kept a safe distance away from rotating parts?				
Do you have the correct tools for machine-required task?				
Did you walk around your equipment at the beginning of your shift to check for safety and housekeeping issues?				

(Roughton & Crutchfield, 2013)

Appendix M Sample Manager/Supervisor Daily/Weekly/ Monthly Safety Activity Report

Month	Date of report
Department	Manager/Supervisor

Method for improving the safety culture

What have I personally done to communicate and/or train employees on the key elements of the safety management system?

Management leadership

Employee involvement

Risk and hazard identification and assessment

Hazard prevention and control

Education and training

Evaluation of program effectiveness

Daily safety topic/shift review

What percentage of required daily shift reviews were accomplished this week?

Daily topic

1.

2.

3.

4.

5.

6.

7.

One-on-one communication

"How many of my direct reports did I contact this week to discuss safety their efforts?

Employee (List employees met with for one-on-one communications:

Safety walkthrough

Were safety action plans developed for hazards identified?

Number determined this week? _____ How many safety action plans remain open? _____

Hazards identified and safety plan developed for each. If hazards with severe associated risk were identified using the risk guidance card, are these under control or the activity/operation stopped until resolution made? Do you inform leadership of the issue?

If not completed, Why not?

Specific machine/equipment review

What percentage of machine/equipment reviews was completed with employees this week?

Machine/equipment reviewed

Safety meetings

"How many safety meetings were held?" ___ "How many managers/supervisors attended?" _____

1. Weekly

2. Weekly

3. Weekly

4. Wekly/monthly combined

Safety training
What safety training was provided and what topics covered this week?

"Incidents/near miss/loss-producing event investigations
Were incidents, near misses, and any loss producing events and
investigation reports completed and submitted to the safety department
within 24 h?" If no, why? (Note: Report any event immediately while
the investigation is being completed.)

Did I participate in any other loss-producing incident reviews? List
loss-producing events in my department with a brief description of the
injury or damage

Name	Incident description	Root cause conducted	Action plan developed

(Roughton & Crutchfield, 2013)

Appendix N Sample Activities and Results Measurements

The objective of any organization is to continue to expand the focus on
process metrics (leading indicators) as the primary means of measuring the
safety management system performance (i.e., loss-producing events are not
the only measurement).

You want to define and implement a "scorecard" approach, which provides measurements that are a combination of leading indicators and trailing indicators.

For example, reducing the dependence on TCIR as the trailing indicator and using performance level scores.

The following are example activity metrics that can be used to monitor
and assess your safety management system in a positive manner. Modify and
adjust for your organization.

N.1 The leadership team
This category includes support for safety, perception of the safety culture,
goal setting, establishing objectives based on operational procedures, and the
employee perception of credibility.
• Number of times leadership participated in preshift safety meetings.
• Number of physical hazard inspections with leadership involvement.
• Number of times safety action plans were reviewed with employees.

- Percent of actions completed in the safety action plan.
- Percent of projects with predesign safety reviews.
- Percent of employees, supervisors, and manager groups involved in goal setting process.
- Percentage of loss-producing reports reviewed by members of the leadership team.
- Number of safety-related walkthroughs taken by members of the leadership team.
- Percentage of managers with specific safety roles.
- Number of safety goals identified in performance reviews
- Number of safety goals that are met on schedule.
- Percentage of sampled employees who can state organization safety goals and objectives.
- Number of times communication on status of corrective actions is completed.
- Ratio of safety suggestions implemented versus submitted.
- Average length of time feedback is provided on a suggestion, corrective action, etc.
- Percent of safety suggestions by employees that were acted upon.

N.2 Employee involvement

Track each employee's "meaningful" safety-related activities. The intent is to identify the level of involvement of each employee in the safety management system. An idea safety culture will allow employees involved in various safety-related activities. Employees are not expected to be involved in every safety related activity but should have safety assignments based on their skills and experience. For example, if an employee is assigned or volunteering to do hazard surveys, how many were completed in the desired time frame? If not completed, what were the circumstances that prevented completion?

- Number of hazard surveys
- Number of investigations reviewed
- Number of standard operating procedures
- Number of job hazard analysis completed
- Number of safety committee meetings attended
- Number of preshift reviews conducted.
- Number of times safety meetings lead or presentations made
- Number of objectives on action plan controlled by employees

N.3 Hazard recognition and control

Hazard recognition and control activities should track leadership and employee involvement using elements of the safety management system:

- Number of new products/processes analyzed using a hazard identification method.
- Percent of employees involved in hazard identification.

- Percent of employees trained in hazard recognition techniques.
- Percent of employees involved in hazard correction.
- Number of hazard inspections performed.
- Number of hazards identified from the inspections.
- Percent of hazards assessed for severity using the risk guidance card.
- Average time between hazard identification and abatement completion.
- Percent of hazards corrected in a timely manner (timeliness is defined).
- Percent of physical hazards that have been identified, but have not been corrected.
- Percent of tasks that have a job hazard analysis completed, developed/reviewed/revised versus expected.

N.4 Education and Training

- Number/percent of employees receiving new employee orientation training.
- Number/percent employees receiving annual refresher job safety training.
- Number/percent of transferred receiving refresher/area specific safety training.
- Percent safety training performed properly documented.
- Number of employees that receive incident investigation.
- Number of employees trained divided by the total number required to be trained.
- Percentage of employees with ergonomics training.
  (Roughton & Crutchfield, 2013)

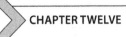
Assessing Training Needs

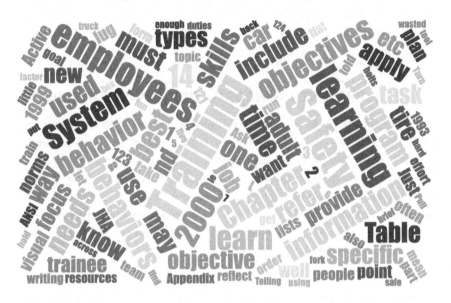

"A picture in the head is worth more than a word in the ear."

—*Richard Gandy*

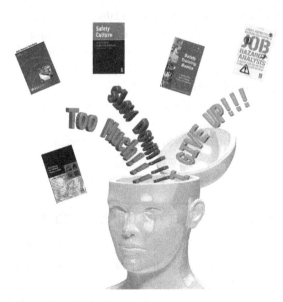

Job Hazard Analysis. http://dx.doi.org/10.1016/B978-0-12-803441-5.00012-X

Chapter Objectives

At the end of the chapter, you will be able to:

- Define an employee-training program.
- Design a training program.
- Discuss various training methods.
- Develop learning objectives.
- Discuss the types of learning.

12.1 PRESENTING INFORMATION IS NOT SUFFICIENT

Organizations have the responsibility to ensure that their employees are trained to achieve its objectives. If the training has been presented properly, each employee should be able to demonstrate knowledge of the fundamentals of their job duties and the safety system. Training is more complicated than simply telling someone how to perform a job. Training is the transfer of knowledge from the instructor to the employee in a way that allows immediate use of the information provided (Roughton & Lyons, 1999; Roughton & Whiting, 2000).

"Telling Ain't Training," Harold Stolovitch

Safety training does not operate in a vacuum and should have support from all levels of the organization. Safety training is unlikely to have a long-term impact on the organization if it does not factor in the forces that will form obstacles to the use of the desired skills. The leadership team should be both coach and mentor to employees in order to reinforce the desired actions presented in safety training (System Safety Training, 2000).

Refer to Appendix O for the following:

- Sample, Safety and Health Training Policy
- Sample Lesson Plan, General Industry Outreach Training Program (10 h)
- ANSI Guidelines for Evaluating Training Programs
- Sample Safety Training Program Audit
- Sample Training Certification

12.2 HOW IS A GOOD TRAINING DEFINED?

Learning theorists generally agree that an individual will learn most efficiently when they are motivated toward a goal that is attainable (Petersen, 1993).

Why, when employees are trained on a topic, do some employees understand the material presented while others do not seem to have a clue as to what was said? It may be because of the initial development of the materials and methods used for its delivery. Trainers need to ask several following questions:

- Could it be the way that the training program was developed?
- Did I deliver training in a logical and consistent manner?
- Did the training atmosphere create a good learning environment?
- Do we know our subject so well that we have a hard time conveying our message?
- Is it that we only have a limited time to present the content?

Too often, safety training is developed to be more difficult than it needs to be, adding too many details and materials in the time allowed. Sometimes training is conducted because it is mandated. The employees respond accordingly, "we are required to attend the class, you are required to talk, and then we go back to work with no follow-up." Sometimes training is provided with the belief that employees want the training when it is actually the trainer who wants to share their knowledge.

12.3 BASIC TRAINING PRINCIPLES

Training requires the customization of information to meet the needs of the intended audience. The presentation of information should be about a topic or concern that benefits the time and effort for its delivery. The broadcast of generic information across a wide geographic and demographic group without an analysis of need results in demeaning both the instructor and employees who realize their time is being wasted (refer to Table 12.1 for definitions of education and training).

12.4 TRAINING PRINCIPLES

Training does not need to be complex or lengthy. Six basic training principles can be used as guidelines:

1. Communicate the purpose of the training. Everyone involved should understand the purpose of the training. The beginning of any training program should focus on WHY the training is important and what personal benefit will be received.
2. Organize the presentation to maximize understanding (refer to Table 12.2 for an example training outline "How to change a tire"). If you are instructing someone, the sequence in which you present the material must match the steps that they must take to accomplish the task. This example was used for developing a JHA in Chapter 11.

Table 12.1 Definition of education and training

Education defined:
- Leads one out of ignorance.
- Anything that affects our knowledge, skills, and attitudes/abilities (KSA's).
- The "WHY" in safety educates the employee about natural occurrences, hazard recognition, awareness and prevention, injury causation, and consequences of exposures (coaching and/or reward) of behavior?
- Primarily increases knowledge and attitudes.

Training:
- One method of education.
- The "How to do" and "What to do" in safety.
- Primarily increases knowledge and skills.
- A specialized form of education that focuses on developing or improving skills, the focus on performance.

Source: Be Trained!: Your guide to OR-OSHA's Safety and Health Training Requirements (n.d.)

Table 12.2 How to change a tire

The following sequences of events are example instructions on how to change a tire on a car.
- Pull off to the side of the road out of traffic.
- Park on level ground and provide safe distance from traffic.
- Apply the parking brake and place the transmission in park if it is an automatic. If the car has a standard transmission, place the shift in first gear or reverse.
- Turn off engine.
- Turn on your hazard warning lights.
- Watch out for oncoming traffic as you exit the car
- Set safety flashers or reflectors five car lengths front and back.
- Pull spare tire and all tools out of the trunk.
- Remove wheel covers.
- Properly place jack under the car. Consult your owners' manual and find where the jack needs to be positioned.
- Jack the car up part way so tire is still touching ground. Raise the car just enough to take the weight off the tire.
- Using the lug wrench, loosen the lug nuts slightly but do not remove.
- Jack up the car so the tire is above ground.
- Remove the lug nuts from the bolts. Place on wheel covers where they will not be lost.
- Remove the flat tire.
- Replace the flat tire with the spare.
- Replace the lug nuts on the bolts and tighten, but not too tight, just enough to hold the tire in place while you lower the car.
- Lower the car until it touches the ground, and then firmly tightens all of the lug nuts.
- Gather everything and put in trunk.
- As soon as possible, have the flat tire repaired and reinstalled.

3. Provide appropriate work practices. Employees should be able to practice and apply new skills and knowledge as soon as possible. Learning is best when immediately practiced and newly acquired skills and knowledge is applied. Instruction time should include information, demonstration, practice, and application. The learning curve (information retention over time) drops quickly in a very short period of time with the details of training forgotten without immediate use.

4. Provide immediate feedback. As employees practice, the instructor needs to determine if training is effective. Practicing a task incorrectly creates the wrong behavior. Feedback for correct behavior enhances motivation and encourages formation of the desirable behavior.

5. Account for individual differences. A successful training program incorporates a variety of learning techniques, that is, written instruction, video/audio-visual, lectures, hands-on, coaching, some fun, etc. Individuals learn at different speeds and the pace of the training should recognize these differences. The attention span and focus of employees should be considered (Figure 12.1). Brief sessions allow the trainee to incorporate

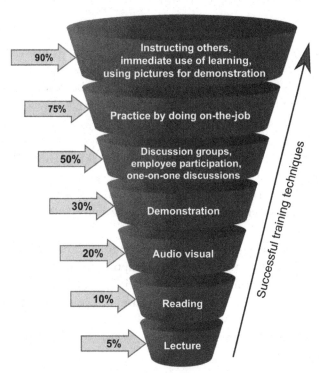

Figure 12.1 *Average Retention Rates. Adapted from Roughton and Crutchfield, N. (2013).*

the information. Long sessions tend to lose the attention of most of participants.

6. Keep the employees involved and active in training. One effective way to learn is by having employee(s) personally instruct each other in a controlled environment. After the initial instruction and practice, the group is divided into teacher/learner teams giving them both a chance to learn (Safety and Health Management – Safety Pays Program, n.d.).

The following five principles of teaching and learning should be followed to maximize program effectiveness:
• Employees should understand the purpose of the training.
• Information should be organized to maximize effectiveness.
• People learn best when they can immediately practice and apply newly acquired knowledge and skills.
• As employees practice, they should receive immediate and detailed feedback.
• People learn in different ways, so an effective program will incorporate a variety of training methods.

Source: Best Practices for the Development, Delivery, and Evaluation of Susan Harwood Training Grants (2010).

The many ingredients for a good training program make the task of blending the required elements challenging. For example, as outlined in Table 12.2, it is considered a relatively simple job; however, a number task and steps are required as well as a basic knowledge of driving, traffic, tool use, and physical skills.

For most trainers, the objective of training is to improve performance or behavior and increase the trainee's knowledge. We tend to do an "information dump and as technical experts we have a tendency to focus on delivering in-depth content which does not always create a good learning environment (Roughton & Lyons, 1999; Roughton & Whiting, 2000).

Instead of an ego-dump, we must get serious about assessing employee's knowledge of the subject before attempting to train. We must validate posttraining to determine retention at various times after training, as we must keep our own ego in check (Roughton & Lyons, 1999; Roughton & Whiting, 2000).

Refer to Table 12.3 for ANSI/ASSE Z490.1-2009 guidelines on training development.

Table 12.3 Overview of the ANSI/ASSE Z490.1-2009 guidelines on training development

ANSI Z490.1-2009, Criteria for Accepted Practices in Safety, Health, and Environmental
Training, is a broad-based voluntary consensus standard covering all aspects of safety training that includes training development, delivery, evaluation, and management of the training function. The criterion in the standard was established based on accepted best practices in the training industry and the safety, health and environmental industries.

What does the standard say about training program elements?
Section 3.2, states that a "safety-training program should include written plans for how training development, delivery, documentation, recordkeeping, and evaluation will be accomplished." Elements should include the following:

1. Training development: Procedures for developing a needs assessment, learning objectives, course design, evaluation strategy, and criteria for course completion.
2. Training delivery: Ensures that the quality of training is delivered by a competent instructor with subject matter expertise in a suitable training environment. Delivery includes planning/preparation, participant safety/comfort, materials, delivery methods, timely feedback.
3. Training documentation and recordkeeping: Provides procedures, forms, and reports that ensure that the quality and maintenance of training delivery and program evaluations, and instructor and trainee certifications.
4. Training evaluation plan: Describes how evaluation of training program design and performance will be accomplished with a continuous improvement approach. Evaluation includes the program, process followed, results, criteria followed, etc. (Training Requirements in OSHA Standards and Training Guidelines, 1998).

(Best Practices for the Development, Delivery, and Evaluation of Susan Harwood Training Grants, 2010)

Source: Criteria for Accepted Practices in Safety, Health, and Environmental Training, Z490.1 (2001).

Refer to Table 12.4 for OSHA training development guideline (Figure 12.2).

Case Study #1

An organization purchased generic safety-training material to better provide a consistent message to multiple locations. One message was on how to safely drive in snow. However, the facility was in Florida where snow is not a problem.

Table 12.4 OSHA training development guideline

The OSHA model has seven elements:
1. Determine if training is needed.
2. Identify training needs.
3. Identify goals and objectives.
4. Develop learning activities.
5. Conducting the training.
6. Evaluating effectiveness.
7. Improving the program.

The model is used to develop and administer safety-training programs that address site- specific issues, fulfill the learning needs of employees, and strengthen the overall safety program.

Source: Training Requirements in OSHA Standards and Training Guidelines (1998).

Case Study #2

In one situation, a supervisor was assigned the task of discussing fork truck safety. The supervisor, as ordered, used a prepared script and presented a 30-min session to his employees. Unfortunately, the time was wasted as no one in the class drove a fork truck, as they were machine operators. When asked, the supervisor's response was: "This is my monthly requirement." He was being measured on the delivery of content not on the training's effectiveness.

12.5 TYPES OF EDUCATION

"We are forced to rely on people, who are why we put so much emphasis on training them."

–Henry Block, H&R Block

Traditionally, one-on-one (face-to-face) meeting, daily, weekly, and monthly safety meetings have been used as types of safety training. "Toolbox talks," "2-min drills," and weekly and monthly meetings are used in construction and other high-hazard industries where the work situation changes rapidly. These activities provide the means for communicating hazards and associated risk that may be present, discuss injuries that have occurred as well as identify environmental changes and procedures (Roughton & Whiting, 2000; Roughton & Lyons, 1999).

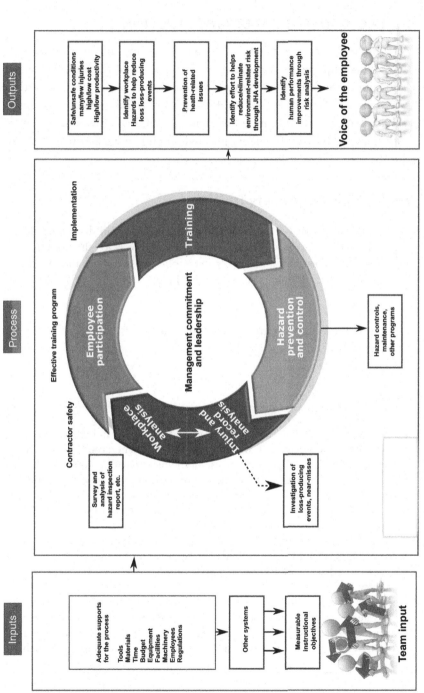

Inputs

Adequate supports
for the process

Tools
Materials
Time
Budget
Equipment
Facilities
Machinery
Employees
Regulations

Other systems

Measurable
instructional
objectives

Team input

Process

Effective training program

Contractor safety

Implementation

Survey and
analysis of
hazard inspection
report, etc.

Employee
participation

Training

Workplace
analysis

Injury and
record
analysis

Management commitment
and leadership

Hazard
prevention
and control

Investigation of
loss-producing
events, near-misses

Hazard controls,
maintenance,
other programs

Outputs

Safe/unsafe conditions
many/few injuries
high/low cost
High/low productivity

Identify workplace
Hazards to help reduce
loss-producing
events

Prevention of
heath-related
issues

Identify effort to helps
reduce/eliminate
environment-related risk
through JHA development

Identify
human performance
improvements through
risk analysis

Voice of the employee

Figure 12.2 *Process Strategy for Analyzing the Workplace.*

12.6 GENERAL SAFETY INSTRUCTION

Employees receive specific safety education and information through various work experiences beginning with a new employee orientation, attending safety meetings, one-on-one with members of the leadership team, etc.) (Managing Worker Safety and Health, n.d.; Training Requirements in OSHA Standards and Training Guidelines, 1998). It is critical to the safety culture that the initial job orientation be comprehensive and that the control of hazards and associated risk made clear.

12.6.1 Conducting Safety Training

"A lesson plan is an instructional prescription, a blueprint describing the activities the instructor and student may engage in to reach the objectives of the course. The main purpose is to prescribe the key events that should occur during the module." (Mager & Pipe, 1983).

Refer to Table 12.5 for an overview of who needs training.
Refer to Appendix L.

Table 12.5 Who needs training

Who needs training?
- New hires, contract/temporary employees, and employees in high-risk areas.
- Leaders should be included in training plan development. Leaders should receive training in hazard recognition, use of the hierarchy of controls, Haddon energy release, risk assessments, incident investigations, and how to provide and reinforce safety training. Training for leaders should emphasize the importance of their role and responsibilities in visibly supporting safety and ensuring that the safety system is used.
- Long-term employees who change a position as a result of a new process or material changes should be provided training prior to startup.
- The entire workforce should be provided periodic refresher training in general safety awareness.
- The safety system should be evaluated when designing the training program. The evaluation can identify the safety system strengths, weaknesses, opportunities and threats (SWOT) for improvement, and the basis for future changes.
- Training records will document and ensure that all employees receive timely training.

Source: Be Trained!: Your guide to OR-OSHA's Safety and Health Training Requirements (n.d.).

"Though it seems hard to believe, instructors are frequently asked to develop courses intended to teach people what they already know, or to use instruction to solve problems that can't be solved by instruction." (Mager & Pipe, 1983).

Refer to Figure 12.3 for a flow diagram outlining Mager's decision tree for improving safety performance.

12.7 CONDUCTING A TRAINING NEEDS ASSESSMENT

A needs assessment is the most important objective when developing a safety-training program. Training programs are often pulled "off of the shelf" with limited effort made to adapt the content to the specific application. A generic training approach may save time and be easy to implement but may fail to ensure that the content matches what the employees need to know (Table 12.6).

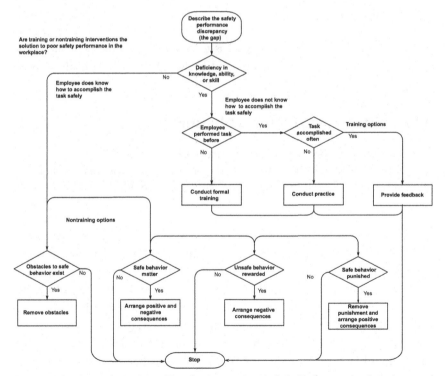

Figure 12.3 *Mager's Decision Tree for Improving Safety Performance. Based on and adapted using Mayer, Robert, Peter Pipe, Analyzing Performance Problems.*

Table 12.6 Types of safety training needs

- Orientation training for new employees, contractors, and temporary employees.
- Standard operating procedures.
- Hazard recognition training.
- Required specific regulatory compliance training.
- Emergency response training and emergency drills.
- Injury and illness prevention program content training.

Source: Best Practices for the Development, Delivery, and Evaluation of Susan Harwood Training Grants (2010).

A three-part organizational analysis is used to determine how to target the training emphasis.

1. Develop a clear understanding of both short- and long-term training goals. What is the organization trying to achieve in its overall safety efforts in general and specifically by each department?
2. Develop and organize an inventory of the company's human and physical resources.
3. Review and analyze the "climate" of the organization. What is the level of energy that the organization has to develop to implement the training process? Are adequate time and budget provided to do the job effectively? (Petersen, 1993)

12.7.1 Establishing Learning Objectives

"Now it's time to describe the instructional outcomes (the need to do's); it's time to construct a verbal word picture that will help guide you in developing the instruction and help guide students in focusing their efforts" (Mager & Pipe, 1983).

A learning objective is a brief, clear statement of what the employee will be able to do as a result of completing the training. The groundwork for the learning objective is laid out through the job analysis that has been completed. The learning objectives should focus only on the tasks to be included in the training session. At times, an entire job should be learned, whereas only a portion of a task within a step needs to be learned in some cases. A learning objective defines how well and under what conditions tasks should be performed to verify that they has been effectively learned (System Safety Training, 2000).

Learning objectives help the instructor to do the following:

- Design, develop, and/or select instructional content and procedures.
- Organize the sessions to involve the employee's own efforts and activities.
- Select the media to use for content presentation and delivery.
- Evaluate or assess the success of instruction.

It is important to express training objectives in specific terms. In addition, it is important to make your objectives measurable. This will focus the content of your course on the objectives.

12.7.2 Guidelines for Writing Learning Objectives

Learning objectives are written from the viewpoint of what the trainee will do, not what the instructor will do.

Right: Employee will be complete a JHA.

Wrong: Instructor will cover the JHA process.

Verbs or action words are used to describe behavior and should be as specific as possible. Words that should be avoided include vague words such as "know," "learn," "comprehend," "study," "cover," and "understand" (System Safety Training, 2000).

Right: The employees will be able to complete a JHA.

Wrong: The employees will learn how to do JHAs.

The desired behavior should be observable and measurable so that the instructor can determine if the task has been learned (System Safety Training, 2000).

Right: The employees will demonstrate their ability to complete a hazard assessment.

Wrong: The employee will know how to conduct a hazard assessment.

Objectives should be given both verbally and in writing so that employees understand the purpose of the training session.

12.7.3 Components of Learning Objectives

There are four components that need to be considered each time a learning objective is developed: Target audience, behavior, conditions, and standards (System Safety Training, 2000).

12.7.4 Target Audience

A critical step in the training assessment is the analysis of the intended audience. The instructor should determine

- the general educational level of the audience,
- their specific job duties,

- their previous training history,
- the class/group's average length of employment,
- the general emotional climate of the organization,
- current behavioral norms, and
- organizational attitudes toward training.

It is vital to determine if employees have mastered any pre-requisite skills and knowledge in order to target the training appropriately (System Safety Training, 2000).

"Upfront" discussions are used to pinpoint the expectations of the employee(s) to be trained. Do they believe that the training will be of benefit to them? Survey employees both informally and through questionnaires where feasibly. Providing a tour of the operation or facility is an opportunity to ask employees' training-related questions and to assess expectations.

A determination should be made as to how much support exist from the leadership team and what are leadership's desired training objectives (System Safety Training, 2000).

The target audience should be considered on the basis of the experience and background of the group. All courses and activities should be designed for the adult learner. One thing that is important is to ensure that courses and activities are designed for the adult learner. The following examples must be considered on the basis of the learning objectives for adult learning.

- Always include goals or objectives that let employees know what is coming.
- Adult learners must be given time to reflect or think about each point of learning. Focus on one thing at a time. They should not have to take a lot of notes when you want them to listen.
- Design in time to reflect or think about each point of learning into the process.
- Include samples, stories, scenarios that apply the learning to something they can relate to.
- Include lists and acronyms. We use a lot of safety acronyms and assume that everyone understands them.
- Flag important information. Use a "parking lot" list to keep ideas fresh in the trainees mind.
- Adults do not effectively learn by simply being told. They must have a chance to digest the material and, whenever possible, apply the learning to something they can relate. Ask questions and involve the trainees.

Table 12.7 Summary of sequencing safety training

- Content: What subjects the training will cover?
- Connecting: How will each topic be related to the workplace? Why is it important?
- Loading: To what depth will each subject be covered?
- Sequencing: In what order will the topics be covered?
- Known to unknown: Common chemicals at home.
- Simple to complex: Simple lockout/tagout procedure.
- General to specific: fall protection systems.
- Theory to practice: Accident investigation.
- Step by step: Any procedure.

Source: An Introduction to Effective Safety Training (n.d.).

Include open-end questions and exercises. Design active audience participation in the learning process whenever possible.

Information more easily enters the long-term memory when it is linked to old memories or can be related to something the learner has experienced.

The short-term memory is linear, works best through lists, and is the only conscious part of the brain.

Giving adult learners an advance organizer, such as workshop goals or objectives, helps them to retain information.

Let them know what is important, what to focus on every time there is a change in points or a new topic to discuss.

The mind pays more attention to what is novel than what is ordinary (Oregon OSHA Workshop Materials, Hazard Identification and Control, n.d.; Roughton & Whiting, 2000) (Table 12.7).

> "Behavior that is primarily aimed at producing a desired result, like attempting to understand the needs of another party and attempting to satisfy those needs, such as the personality and salesmanship that is displayed by a sales representative that leads to the customer opening a new account." (Affective Behavior, n.d.)

12.7.5 Learning Styles

One of the pitfalls of instruction is that instructors tend to develop safety-training programs that accommodate the way the instructor learns best, not the way the employees learn best. For example, if the instructor learns best by reading, a manual may be provided to the employees. The trainee will be expected to master the procedure by reading the manual. If the instructor learns best through experimentation, they tend to throw employees into a situation with little guidance. For a visual learner, they use videos, graphs, and pictures (System Safety Training, 2000).

Passive learners
- Reading manuals/books
- Watching audio-visual presentations
- Hearing a lecture
- Observation demonstrations

Source: An Introduction to Effective Safety Training (n.d.)

Active learners
- Participating in discussions
- Role-playing
- Performing an experiment
- Taking a field trip
- Hands-on learning
- Responding to a scenario
- Making a presentation

Source: An Introduction to Effective Safety Training (n.d.)

Some learners prefer to learn by themselves whereas others prefer to work in groups. Some learners need a lot of organization and learn in small steps sequentially whereas others assimilate whole concepts with a flash of insight or intuition.

Some learners are visual and learn best through videos, drawings, picture, demonstrations, etc., whereas others learn best through words and enjoy reading and slides with words, and lectures (System Safety Training, 2000).

In each case, the instructor needs to understand that there are differences in learning styles that exist. The key is to try and combine as many types of activities and media as possible so that the trainees can have access to the way they learn best and also learn to adapt to other learning styles as applicable. This means that a training session might include a handout for readers, a lecture for listeners, and an experiment for doers, depending on the objective (System Safety Training, 2000).

The key to accommodating learning styles is that all instructional strategies and media are selected as a means to help the employee and not as a convenience for the instructor (System Safety Training, 2000).

12.7.6 Adults Learners

One serious mistake for an instructor is to approach the learner as a parent–child relationship. Instructors may act like a parent lecturing a child. Instructors should understand adult learning principles and view themselves as facilitators of the process (System Safety Training, 2000; Petersen, 1993; Mager & Pipe, 1983).

The following examples are based on adult learning objectives:

- Always begin with goals and objectives that let employees know what the training will cover and its importance to the organization.
- Adult learners need time to reflect or think about each point of learning. The sessions should focus on one thing at a time and participants should not have to take many notes when listening to new material.
- Build time into the process for reflection or thinking about each point of learning.
- Use examples, stories, scenarios, experiences, etc. that participants can relate to the training content. Include lists and acronyms. Many safety acronyms are used with the assumption that they are universally known.
- Highlight and emphasize important information by making use of video, handouts, flipcharts, whiteboards, and interesting media.
- Adults do not effectively learn by simply being told and should have a chance to digest the material and apply the learning to something they can relate.
- Active audience participation in the learning process is essential in adult learning.

During the planning of training sessions one should keep the following characteristics of adult learners in mind. The adult learner wants to know the "big picture." Most adults want satisfactory answers to their questions: "Why is this training important?" and "How can I apply the training?" Function in roles which mean that they are capable of and desirous of participating in decision making about learning.

Adults have specific objectives for learning and generally know how they learn best. Adults have experienced learning situations before and have positive and/or negative consequences about learning.

12.7.7 Course Content Development

Training methods are selected on the basis of the training objectives, the needs assessment, the audience analysis, and intent of the training. A toolbox of various training techniques can then be applied where appropriate to a specific group or audience (Table 12.8).

Table 12.8 Common types of training methods

Case study	Actual or hypothetical situation
Lecture	Oral presentation of material, usually from prepared notes and visual aids.
Role play	Employees improvise behavior of assigned fictitious roles.
Demonstration	Live illustration of desired performance.
Games	Simulations of real-life situations.
Stories	Actual or mythical examples of course content in action.
Discussion	Facilitated opportunity for employees to comment.
Question	Employees question the instructor and receive answers to questions.
Small group	Employees divide into sub-groups for discussion or exercise.
Exercises	Various tasks related to specific course content.
Instruments/job aids	Tools, equipment and materials used on the job.
Reading	Employees read material prior to, during, and/or after the session.
Manuals	Handbooks or workbooks distributed to employees.
Handouts	Selected materials, usually not part of a manual.

Source: An Introduction to Effective Safety Training (n.d.).

After completing training program design, a "pilot run" should be conducted using a small test group. This pilot run works out the kinks and allows the necessary changes to make it flow properly before implementation. The pilot run also evaluates the effectiveness of the overall goals and objectives (Roughton & Whiting, 2000; Roughton & Lyons, 1999).

Lesson Learned #1

The authors have experience unrealistic requests:

For example, requiring training to be completed at 7:00 a.m. on Saturday with no additional pay for employees who have just completed a night shift from 11:00 p.m. to 7:00 a.m. In this case, the potential for effective learning is very low if not nonexistent.

12.8 DOCUMENTATION AND RECORDKEEPING

Maintaining training records is essential to sustaining the training process. A basic form can be used to identify the trainees and instructors, the topics to be covered, materials provided and basic information such as the training date, student evaluation and successful class completion. Training records provide the history of training sessions, participants who completed the sessions, and refresher courses provided. Training documentation curation allows the organization to ensure it has met all of its legal and regulatory mandates (Appendix L) (Roughton & Whiting, 2000; Roughton & Lyons, 1999).

12.9 BEHAVIORS AND LEARNING STYLES

12.9.1 Types of Behavior in Learning Objectives

The next step is to identify the domains of learning, the types of behavior that can be described within an objective. Behaviors are categorized in one of the following domains of learning: cognitive, psychomotor, or affective.

12.9.1.1 Cognitive Behaviors

"Cognitive behaviors" describe observable and measurable ways that the employee can demonstrate that they have gained the knowledge and/or skill necessary to perform a task safely. Most learning objectives describe cognitive behaviors as these behaviors are easy to master while others are much more difficult. In designing safety instruction, trainers move from the simple to the complex to verify that employees have the basic foundation they need before moving to the next level of skills (System Safety Training, 2000).

This does not mean that the basic skills have to be re-taught if the trainer cannot verify acknowledgement through observations, pretests, training records, etc., that prerequisite skills have been mastered. However, training sessions have turned into a disaster because the trainer made the assumption that the employees had mastered basic skills and began the training at too high a level. In contrast, training sessions have bored the employees by being too basic. It is important for trainers to be able to label learning objectives and design training sessions appropriate to the level of cognitive behavior required to perform a task. The following section will describe examples of types of cognitive behaviors (System Safety Training, 2000):

Knowledge-level cognitive behaviors are the easiest to teach, learn, and evaluate. They often refer to rote memorization or identification. Employees often "parrot" information or memorize lists or name objects. Common action words such as: identify, name, list, repeat, recognize, state, match, and define (System Safety Training, 2000).

Comprehension-level cognitive behaviors have a higher level of difficulty than knowledge-level cognitive behaviors because they require the employee to process and interpret information. The employee is not required to apply or demonstrate the behavior. Commonly used action words include verbs such as: explain, discuss, interpret, classify, categorize, cite evidence for, compare, contrast, illustrate, give examples of, differentiate, and distinguish between (System Safety Training, 2000).

Application-level cognitive behaviors move beyond the realm of explaining concepts orally or in writing. They deal with putting ideas into practice and involve a routine process. Employees apply the knowledge they have learned. For example, action words commonly used include the following: demonstrate, calculate, do, operate, implement, compute, construct, measure, prepare, and produce (System Safety Training, 2000).

Problem-solving cognitive behaviors involve a higher level of skills than application-level cognitive behaviors. The easiest way to differentiate between the application level and problem-solving level is to apply application level to a routine activity and problem-solving level to nonroutine activities. Problem-solving skills require analysis (breaking a problem into parts), synthesis (looking at parts of a problem and formulating a generalization or conclusion), evaluating (judging the appropriateness, effectiveness, and/or efficiency of a decision or process and choosing among alternatives).

Examples of action words commonly used include: troubleshoot, analyze, create, develop, devise, evaluate, formulate, generalize, infer, integrate, invent, plan, predict, reorganize, solve, and synthesize (System Safety Training, 2000). This is the behavior that will be used in development of JHAs.

12.9.1.2 Psychomotor Behaviors

Learning new behaviors requires developing new cognitive skills (knowledge, comprehension, application and/or, problem solving) as well as new psychomotor skills that may be required in the application phase of learning.

Psychomotor behaviors pertain to the proper and skillful use of body mechanics and may involve both gross and fine motor skills. Safety-training sessions for psychomotor skills should involve as many of the senses as possible. The trainer must adapt the format involving such physical movements to match the skill level of the learner and the difficulty of the task (System Safety Training, 2000).

The key to teaching psychomotor skills is that the more the learner observes the task, explains the task, and practices the task correctly; the better trainee performs the task.

12.9.1.3 Affective Behaviors

"Affective" behaviors include the attitudes, feelings, beliefs, values, and emotions. Trainers must recognize that affective behaviors influence how efficiently and effectively learners acquire cognitive and psychomotor behaviors. Learning can be influenced by positive factors (success, rewards, reinforcement, perceived value, etc.) and by negative factors (failure, disinterest, punishments, fears, etc.) (Best Practices for the Development, Delivery, and Evaluation of Susan Harwood Training Grants, 2010; Geigle, n.d.). Other affective behaviors (attitudes and emotions) that must be considered go beyond positive or negative motivations toward learning (System Safety Training, 2000).

Training objectives that state affective behaviors are usually much more difficult to observe and measure than cognitive behaviors. Nevertheless, they are critical to the ultimate success of the safety-training program.

A critical factor to remember is that while training can stress the importance of affective behaviors, employees are mostly influenced by the behavioral norms of an organization. Behavioral norms refer to the peer pressures that result from the attitudes and actions of the employees/management as a group. Behavioral norms are the behaviors a group expects its members to display. Before attempting to make changes in an organization, it is important to identify existing norms and their effects on employees (System Safety Training, 2000).

The design of training should incorporate whether the job requires skill-based, rule-base, or knowledge-based performance as discussed in Chapter 2. These types of performance should incorporate the concept noted previously.

12.9.2 Learning Styles

One of the pitfalls of instruction is that trainers tend to develop safety-training programs that accommodate the way the trainer learns best, not the way the employees learn best. For example, if the trainer learns best by reading, a manual may be provided to the employees and the trainee will be expected to master the procedure by reading the manual. If the trainer learns best through experimentation, they tend to throw employees into a situation workshop with little guidance. If a visual learner, they use videos.

It is important to emphasize individual growth and remember that employees have different learning styles with which they are most comfortable. Every employee is different and must be treated as an individual (System Safety Training, 2000).

Some learners prefer to learn by themselves whereas others prefer to work in groups. Some employees need a lot of organization and learn in small steps sequentially whereas others assimilate whole concepts with a flash of insight or intuition. Some employees are visual and learn best through drawings, pictorial transparencies, slides, demonstrations, etc., whereas others learn best through words and enjoy reading transparencies and slides with words, and lectures increased retention results from what we know of split hemisphere learning. Just as different areas of the brain control the body, so does the brain absorb and record different types of information (System Safety Training, 2000).

In each case, the trainer needs to understand that there difference in learning styles that exist. The key is to try and combine as many types of activities and media as possible so that employees can have access to the way they learn best and also learn to adapt to other learning styles as applicable. This means that a training session might include a handout for readers, a lecture for listeners, and an experiment for doers, depending on the objective (System Safety Training, 2000).

The key to accommodating learning styles is that all instructional strategies and media are selected as a means to help the employee and not as a convenience for the instructor. The safety trainer should constantly look for alternate strategies and media so that if one strategy or type of media is ineffective, the safety trainer has multiple strategies from which to select (System Safety Training, 2000).

12.9.3 Conditions

The "condition" component of the objective describes special constraints, limitations, environment, or resources under which the behavior must be demonstrated. Note that the condition component indicates the conditions under which the behavior will be tested, not the conditions under which the behavior was learned (System Safety Training, 2000). The JHA should define the environment in which the job is completed.

SUMMARY

Organizations have the responsibility to ensure that their employees are trained to achieve its objectives and that each employee understands the hazards of their work environment and how to protect themselves from specific hazards.

Safety training does not operate in a vacuum and should have support from all levels of the organization. The organizational climate and behavioral norms are likely to be more powerful than the desired actions and behavior taught in safety-training sessions.

Experienced training professionals continue to fight against the misconception that all operational problems are training problems and that by developing a training program, the organization readily solves all problems. They understand that training is not the answer to all operational problems. Organizational obstacles and behaviors can drive employee behavior toward harmful, at-risk actions.

Training requires the customizing of information presentation to meet the needs of the intended audience. The presentation of information should be about a topic or concern that benefits the time and effort for its delivery.

Training does not need to be complex or lengthy. Six basic training principles can be used as guidelines.

ANSI Z490.1-2009, Criteria for Accepted Practices in Safety, Health, and Environmental.

Training, is a broad-based voluntary consensus standard covering all aspects of safety training that includes training development, delivery, evaluation, and management of the training function.

Traditionally, one-on-one (face-to-face) meeting, daily, weekly, and monthly safety meetings has been used as a type of safety training.

A needs assessment is the most important objective when developing a safety-training program. Training programs are often pulled "off of the shelf" with limited effort made to adapt the content to the specific application.

A three-part organizational analysis is used to determine how to target the training emphasis.

A learning objective is a brief, clear statement of what the employee will be able to do as a result of completing the training. The groundwork for the learning objective is laid out through the job analysis that has been completed. Learning objectives are written from the viewpoint of what the trainee will do, not what the instructor will do.

A critical step in the training assessment is the analysis of the intended audience

One of the pitfalls of instruction is that instructors tend to develop safety-training programs that accommodate the way the instructor learns best, not the way the employees learn best.

One serious mistake for an instructor is to approach the instructor–learner as a parent–child relationship. Instructors may act like a parent lecturing a child. Instructors should understand adult learning principles and view themselves as facilitators of the process.

Training methods are selected on the basis of the training objectives, the needs assessment, the audience analysis, and intent of the training.

Maintaining training records is essential to sustaining the training process.

CHAPTER REVIEW QUESTIONS

1. What responsibility does an organization have regarding training?
2. What are the six basic training principles?
3. What is ANSI Z490.1?
4. Lists the types of safety education?
5. Compare education versus training.
6. What is training needs assessment?
7. What is a learning objective?
8. How is a target audience determined?
9. Discuss the various learning styles?
10. Discuss six types of training methods.

BIBLIOGRAPHY

A Guide to Voluntary Training and Training Requirements. (n.d.). N.C. Department of Labor, Occupational Safety and Health Division (OSHA), Public Domain, Based on and Adapted for Use. Retrieved from http://bit.ly/VPKZg3

Be Trained!: Your guide to OR-OSHA's Safety and Health Training Requirements. (n.d.). Oregon Occupational Safety and Health Division (Oregon OSHA), Public Domain, Permission to Reprint, Modify, and/or Adapt as necessary. Retrieved from http://bit.ly/11dc14h

Best Practices for the Development, Delivery, and Evaluation of Susan Harwood Training Grants. (2010). Occupational Safety and Health Administration (OSHA), Public Domain, Permission to Reprint, Modify, and/or Adapt as necessary. Retrieved from http://1.usa.gov/Z5nKoy

Geigle, S.J. (n.d.). Introduction to OSH Training, Train the Trainer Series. OSHAcademy (TM), Course 703 Study Guide, Permission to Reprint, Modify, and/or Adapt as necessary. Retrieved from http://bit.ly/VAZrxt

Roughton, J., & Lyons, J. (1999). *Training program design, delivery, and evaluating effectiveness: An overview* (pp. 31–33). American Industrial Association, The Synergist.

Roughton, J., & Whiting, N. (2000). *Safety training basics: A handbook for safety training program development*. Government Institutes. Retrieved from http://amzn.to/111dlWB

System Safety Training, Chapter 14. (2000). Federal Aviation Administration (FAA), Public Domain. Retrieved from http://1.usa.gov/VPo9dw

Safety & Health Training. (n.d.). Occupational Safety and Health Management (OSHA), Public Domain, Based on and adapted for Use. Retrieved from http://www.osha.gov/ SLTC/etools/safetyhealth/comp4.html
Safety and Health Management Basics, Module One: Management Commitment. (n.d.). Oregon Occupational Safety and Health Division (Oregon OSHA), Public Domain, Permission to Reprint, Modify, and/or Adapt as necessary. Retrieved from http://bit. ly/Yztx5p
Safety Management Training Course. (n.d.). The Associated General Contractors (AGC) of America. Retrieved from http://www.agc.org/cs/safety_management_training_ course
Training Requirements in OSHA Standards and Training Guidelines. (1998). Occupational Safety and Health Administration (OSHA), Publication 2254, Public Domain. Retrieved from http://1.usa.gov/XFQkYt
Training Support Package (TSP) Lesson Plan, SH 350-70 APP E. (n.d.). Maneuver Center of Excellence Fort Benning, Georgia, Pubic Domain. Retrieved from http:// www.benning.army.mil/mcoe/QASFD/content/pdf/TSP%20lesson%20plan%20 explain.pdf

FURTHER READINGS

Affective Behavior. (n.d.). Retrieved from http://bit.ly/1K7vFGh
An Introduction to Effective Safety Training. (n.d.). Oregon Occupational Safety and Health Division (Oregon OSHA), OR-OSHA 105, Public Domain, Permission to Reprint, Modify, and/or Adapt as necessary. Retrieved from http://bit.ly/WF1Yor
Criteria for Accepted Practices in Safety, Health, and Environmental Training. (2001). American National Standards Institute (ANSI), Secretariat American Society of Safety Engineers (ASSE), Z490.1.
Mager, R.F., & Pipe, P. (1983). Analyzing Performance Problems; or "You Really Oughta Wanna.
Managing Worker Safety and Health. (n.d.). Missouri Occupational Safety and Health Administration (OSHA), Office of Cooperative Programs, Public Domain, Adapted for Use. Retrieved from http://on.mo.gov/15C4FyS
Oregon OSHA Workshop Materials, Hazard Identification and Control. (n.d.). Oregon Occupational Safety and Health Division (Oregon OSHA), Public Domain, Permission to Reprint, Modify, and/or Adapt as necessary. Retrieved from http://bit.ly/1tg4a8A and http://bit.ly/1yIBKVk
Petersen, D. (1993). *The challenge of change: Creating a new safety culture.* Portland, OR: Core-Media Training Solutions.
Roughton, J., & Crutchfield, N. (2013). *Safety Culture: An Innovative Leadership Approach.* In B. Heinemann, (Ed.). MA: Butterworth Heinemann. Retrieved from http://amzn. to/1qoD4oN
Safety and Health Management – Safety Pays Program. (n.d.). Oklahoma Department of Labor - Consultation Services, Safety Pays, Public Domain, Based on and Adapted for Use. Retrieved from http://bit.ly/1GLYtCi

Appendix O Reference Material for Documenting Training Efforts

• Sample, Safety and Health Training Policy
• Sample Lesson Plan, General Industry Outreach Training Program (10 h)

- ANSI Guidelines for Evaluating Training Programs
- Sample Safety Training Program Audit
- Sample Training Certification

This appendix was adapted from the following:

Be trained! Your guide to Oregon OSHA's safety and health training requirements (Be Trained!: Your guide to OR-OSHA's Safety and Health Training Requirements, n.d.)

A Guide to Voluntary Training and Training Requirements (A Guide to Voluntary Training and Training Requirements, n.d.)

Developing OSH Training, Train the Trainer Series (Geigle, n.d.)

Safety & Health Training (Safety & Health Training, n.d.)

Safety and Health Management Basics, Module One: Management Commitment (Safety and Health Management Basics, Module One: Management Commitment, n.d.)

Safety Management Training Course (Safety Management Training Course, n.d.)

Safety Training Basics: A Handbook for Safety Training Program Development (Roughton & Whiting, 2000)

System Safety Training, Chapter 14 (System Safety Training, Chapter 14, 2000)

Training Program Design, Delivery, and Evaluating Effectiveness: An Overview, pp. 31–33 (Roughton & Lyons, 1999)

Training Support Package (TSP) Lesson Plan, SH 350-70 APP E (Training Support Package (TSP) Lesson Plan, SH 350-70 APP E, n.d.)

Best Practices for the Development, Delivery, and Evaluation of Susan Harwood Training Grants (Best Practices for the Development, Delivery, and Evaluation of Susan Harwood Training Grants, 2010)

Training Requirements in OSHA Standards and Training Guidelines, Occupational Safety and Health Administration, OSHA 2254 (Training Requirements in OSHA Standards and Training Guidelines, 1998)

O.1 Sample, Safety and Health Training Policy

O.1.1 Purpose

Training is one of the most important elements in our company's safety program. It provides employees an opportunity to learn their jobs properly, bring new ideas to supervision, reinforce existing ideas and practices, and put the safety program into action.

Everyone in our company will benefit from safety training through fewer workplace injuries, reduced stress, and higher morale. Productivity, profits, and competitiveness will increase as production costs per unit, turnover, and workers' compensation rates lower.

O.1.2 Management commitment

_____ will provide the necessary funds and scheduling time to ensure effective safety training is provided. This commitment will include paid work time for training and training in the language that the employee understands. Both management and employees will be involved in developing the program.

To most effectively carry out their safety responsibilities, all employees must understand (1) their role in the training program, (2) hazards, potential hazards, and consequences of exposure that need to be prevented or controlled, and (3) the ways to protect themselves and others. We will achieve these goals by the following:

- Educating all managers, supervisors and employees on their safety management system responsibilities
- Educating all employees about the specific hazards and control measures in their workplace
- Training all employees on hazard identification, analysis, reporting, and control procedures
- Training all employees on safe work procedures

Our training program will focus on safety concerns that determine the best way to deal with a particular hazard. When a hazard is identified, we will first try to remove it entirely. If that is not feasible, we will then train employees to protect themselves, if necessary, against the remaining hazard. Once we have decided that a safety problem can best be addressed by training (or by another method combined with training), we will follow up by developing area-specific training goals based on those particular needs.

Employees. At a minimum, all employees must know the general safety rules of the organization, site-specific hazards and the safe work practices needed to help control exposure, and the their role in all types of emergency situations. We will ensure all employees understand the hazards to which they may be exposed and how to prevent harm to themselves and others from exposure to specific hazards.

We will commit available resources to ensure that all employees receive safety training during the following:

- Whenever a new employee is hired, a general safety orientation including an overview of company safety rules, and why those rules must be followed.
- Whenever an employee is given a new job assignment conducting formal classroom training, when the supervisor provides specific task training. It is extremely important that supervisors emphasize safety during initial task assignment.
- Whenever new work procedures are begun, during formal classroom training and supervisor on-the-job training.
- Whenever new equipment is installed, if new hazards are introduced.
- Whenever new substances are used, hazard communication program may apply.
- The bottom line, train safety whenever a new hazard is introduced to the employee.

Employees must know they are responsible for complying with all company safety rules, and that most injuries will be prevented by their safe work practices. They must be very familiar with any PPE required for their jobs. They must know what to do in case of emergencies.

Each employee needs to understand that they are not expected to start working on a new assignment until they have been properly trained. If a job places an employee at risk then they will report the situation to their supervisor.

Supervisors. Supervisors will be given special training to help them in their leadership role. They need to be instructed how to look for hidden hazards under their supervision, to insist with the maintenance of the physical protection in their areas, and to reinforce employee hazard training through performance feedback and, when necessary, fair and consistent enforcement.

We will commit necessary resources to ensure supervisors understand the responsibilities and the reasons for the following:
- Detecting and correcting hazards in their work areas before they result in injuries
- Providing physical resources and psychosocial support that promote safe environment
- Providing performance feedback and effective recognition and discipline techniques
- Conducting on-the-job training

Supervisors are considered the primary safety trainers. All supervisors will complete train-the-trainer classes to learn training techniques and how to test employee knowledge and skills. They will also receive training on how to apply fair and consistent recognition and discipline. Supervisor training may be provided by the supervisor's immediate manager, by the safety department, or by outside resources.

Managers. All line managers must understand their responsibilities in the safety program. This may require classroom training and other forms of communication that will ensure that managers understand their safety responsibilities. The subject can be covered periodically as a part of regular management meetings.

Managers will be trained in the following subject areas:
- The elements of a safety-management system, and the positive impact of the various processes in the system can have on corporate objectives.
- Their responsibility to communicate the safety goals and objectives to their employees,
- Their role also includes making clear assignments of safety responsibilities, providing authority and resources to carry out assigned tasks, and holding subordinate managers and supervisors accountable.
- Actively requiring compliance with mandatory safety policies and rules and encouraging employee participation in discretionary safety

activities such as making suggestions and participation in the safety committee.

Training will emphasize the importance of managers' visibly showing their commitment to the safety program. They will be expected to set a good example by scrupulously following all the safety rules themselves.

O.1.3 Recognition and reward

The purpose of an effective system of recognition is to motivate employee participation and build ownership in the safety system. When employees make suggestions that will improve safety training, we will recognize them. When employees make a significant contribution to the success of the company, we will recognize and reward their performance. Employees will submit all suggestions directly to immediate supervisors. Supervisors are authorized to reward employees on the spot when the suggestion substantially improves the training process or content.

O.1.4 Training and accountability

To help make sure our efforts in safety is effective we have developed methods to measure performance and administer consequences. Managers must understand that they have a responsibility to first meet their obligations to our employees prior to administering any discipline for violating safety policies and rules.

Managers and safety staff will be educated on the elements (processes) of the safety accountability system. They will be trained on the procedures to evaluate and improve these elements. Training will focus on improving the safety program whenever hazardous conditions and unsafe or at-risk behaviors are detected. At the same time, we will use effective education and training to establish a strong "culture of accountability."

Safety orientation will emphasize that compliance with safety policies, procedures, and rules as outlined in the safety plan is a condition of employment. Discipline will be administered to help the employee increase desired behaviors, not to in any way punish. Safety accountability will be addressed at every training session.

O.1.5 Types of training

We will also make sure that additional training is conducted as deemed appropriate.

_____ (Responsible individual) will ensure safety training is in full compliance with any OSHA standards.

New employee orientation. The format and extent of orientation training will depend on the complexity of hazards and the work practices needed to control them. Orientation will include a combination of initial classroom and follow-up on-the-job training.

For some jobs, orientation may consist of a quick review of site safety rules; hazard communication training for the toxic substances present at the site; training required by relevant OSHA standards, for example, fire protection, lockout/tagout, etc; and a run-through of the job tasks. This training be presented by the new employee's supervisor or delegated employee.

For larger tasks with more complex hazards and work practices to control them, orientation will be structured carefully. We will make sure that new employees start the job with a clear understanding of the hazards and how to protect themselves and others.

We will follow up on supervisory training with a buddy system, where an employee with experience is assigned to watch over and coach a new employee, either for a set period of time or until it is determined that training is complete.

If the orientation is brief or lengthy, the supervisor will make sure that before new employees begin the job, they receive instruction in responding to emergencies. All orientation training received will be properly documented.

Temporary employees will receive training to recognize our specific workplace's hazards or potential hazards.

Experienced workers will be trained if the installation of new equipment changes their job in any way, or if process changes create new hazards or increase previously existing hazards.

All employees will receive refresher training as necessary to keep them prepared for emergencies and alert to ongoing housekeeping problems.

Personal protective equipment (PPE). Employees needing to wear PPE and persons working in high-risk situations will need special training. Supervisors and employees alike must be instructed in the proper selection, use, and maintenance of PPE. Since PPE sometimes can be cumbersome, employees may need to be motivated to wear it in every situation where protection is necessary. Therefore, training will begin with a clear explanation of why the equipment is necessary, how its use will benefit the wearer, and what its limitations are. Remind your employees of your desire to protect them and of your efforts, not only to eliminate and reduce the hazards but also to provide suitable PPE where needed.

Individual employees will become familiar with the PPE they are being asked to wear. This is done by handling it and putting it on. Training will consist of showing employees how to put the equipment on, how to wear it properly, and how to test for proper fit and how to maintain it. Proper fit is essential if the equipment is to provide the intended protection. We will conduct periodic exercises in finding, donning, and properly using emergency personal protective equipment and devices.

Vehicular safety. All employees operating a motor vehicle on the job (on or off premises) will be trained in its safe vehicle operation, safe loading and unloading practices, safe speed in relation to varying conditions, and proper vehicle maintenance. We will emphasize in the strongest possible terms the benefits of safe driving and the potentially fatal consequences of unsafe practices.

Emergency response. We will train our employees to respond to emergency situations. Every employee in every area will understand the following:
- Emergency telephone numbers and who may use them
- Emergency exits and how they are marked
- Evacuation routes
- Signals that alert employees to the need to evacuate

We will practice evacuation drills at least semi-annually, so that every employee has a chance to recognize the signal and evacuate in a safe and orderly fashion. Supervisors or their alternates will practice counting personnel at evacuation gathering points to ensure that every worker is accounted for.

We will include procedures to account for visitors, contract employees, and service employees such as cafeteria employees. At sites where weather or earthquake emergencies are reasonable possibilities, additional special instruction and drilling will be given.

Periodic safety training. In some areas, complex work practices are necessary to control hazards. Elsewhere, occupational injuries are common. At such sites, we will ensure that employees receive periodic safety training to refresh their memories and to teach new methods of control. New training also will also be conducted as necessary when OSHA standards change or new standards are issued.

Where the work situation changes rapidly, weekly meetings will be conducted needed. These meetings will remind employees of the upcoming week's tasks, the environmental changes that may affect them, and the procedures they may need to protect themselves and others.

Identifying types of training. Specific hazards that employees need to know about should be identified through total site health and safety surveys, job hazard analysis, and change analysis. Company accident and injury records may reveal additional hazards and needs for training. Near-miss reports, maintenance requests, and employee suggestions may uncover still other hazards requiring employee training.

0.1.6 Safety training program evaluation

We will determine if the training provided has achieved its goal of improving employee safety performance. Evaluation will highlight training program strengths and identify areas of weakness that need change or improvement.

_____ (The safety committee/coordinator) will evaluate training through the following methods:
- Observation of employee skills.
- Surveys and interviews to determine employee knowledge and attitudes about training.

- Review of the training plan and lesson plans.
- Comparing training conducted with hazards in the workplace.
- Review of training documents.
- Compare pre- and posttraining injury and accident rates.

   If evaluation determines program improvement is necessary, the safety committee/coordinator will development recommendations.

O.1.7 Certification
   Reviewed by (Signature) Date
   Approved by (Signature) Date

O.2 ANSI guidelines for evaluating training programs
ANSI Z490.1-2001, Section 3.4, recommends evaluating three important elements of a safety-training program (Criteria for Accepted Practices in Safety, Health, and Environmental Training, 2001).

O.2.1 Evaluate training program management
Training works best when it's designed and implemented as an integrated system, rather than a series of unrelated training sessions. Elements to evaluate include the following:
- Responsibility and accountability
- Staffing and budgets
- Facilities and equipment
- Development and delivery
- Documentation and records
- Evaluation processes

O.2.2 Evaluate the training process
Training should be conducted using a systematic process that includes a needs assessment, objectives, course materials, lesson plans, evaluation strategies, and criteria for successful completion. Areas of emphasis include the following:
- Quality (clarity, appropriateness, relevance) of training goals
- Adequacy of the learning environment
- Quality (operational, clarity, relevance) of learning objectives
- Effectiveness of the training process

O.2.3 Evaluate the training results
By evaluating the results of training, it's possible to make improvements to existing plans and gain awareness of the need for new training. Items to evaluate include the following:
- Quality of the strategic training plan of action
- Support for long term (life-long learning)
- Quality of program management and manager competency
- Application of a systems approach that links training program elements
- Identification of completing demand and setting priorities
- Adequate support and funding

O.3 Sample safety training program audit

O.3.1 Introduction

This audit evaluates criteria for safety, health, and environmental training programs, including development, delivery, evaluation, and program management detailed in ANSI/ASSE Z490.1-2001 (Criteria for Accepted Practices in Safety, Health, and Environmental Training, 2001).

O.3.2 Purpose

The purpose of this audit is to measure the degree to which the employer is utilizing accepted practices for safety, health, and environmental training.

O.3.3 Instructions

Completing this audit is primarily a two-step process. First read each question below and the five categories below to conduct an analysis. Next, evaluate each question using a 0–5 point rating system described below to justify your ratings.

Analysis. Analyze each of the following five categories to develop a justification for the rating more accurately determines the rating.

- Standards: Analyze policies, plans, programs, budgets, processes, procedures, appraisals, job descriptions, and rules. Are they informative and directive? Are they clearly and concisely communicated?
- Conditions: Inspect the workplace for hazards that might indicate the effectiveness of training. The absence of hazards indicates effectiveness.
- Behaviors, actions: Observe both employee and manager behaviors and activities. Are they consistent and appropriate? Do they reflect effective safety education and training?
- Knowledge, attitudes: Analyze what employees are thinking by conducting surveys and interviews. Do employees have full knowledge, positive attitudes? High trust and low fear indicate effectiveness.
- Results: Analyze training records that validate knowledge, skills and abilities are effectively applied in the workplace. Continually improving results indicate effectiveness.

Evaluate: Enter your rating to the left of each statement. Use the following guidelines for your rating.

5-Fully met: Analysis indicates that the condition, behavior, or action described is fully met and effectively applied. There is room for continuous improvement, but workplace conditions and behaviors, indicate effective application. (Employees have full knowledge and express positive attitudes. Employees and managers not only comply but also exceed expectations. Effective leadership is emphasized and exercised. Safety policies and standards are kept clear, concise, fair, informative and directive. These policies and standards must be communicated to everyone. Results in this area reflect that continual improvement is occurring.

This area is fully integrated into line management. Line management reflects safe attitude and behavior. Safety is considered a "Value and not a Priority."

3–Mostly met: Analysis indicates the condition, behavior, or action described is adequate, but still there is room for improvement. Workplace conditions, if applicable, indicate compliance in this area. Employees have adequate knowledge; they generally express positive attitudes. Some degree of trust between management and labor exists.

Employees and managers comply with standards. Leadership is adequate in this area. Safety policies and standards are in place and are generally clear, concise, fair, informative and directive. Results in this area are consistently positive, but may not reflect continual improvement.

1–Partially met: Analysis indicates that the condition, behavior, or action is partially met. Application is most likely too inadequate to be effective. Workplace conditions, if applicable, indicate improvement is needed in this area. Employees lack adequate knowledge, express generally negative attitudes. Mistrust may exist between management and labor. Employees and managers fail to adequately comply or fulfill their accountabilities. There is lack of adequate management and leadership in this area. Safety policies and standards are in place and are generally clear, concise, fair, informative and directive. Results in this area are inconsistent, negative, and does not reflect continual improvement.

0–Not Present: Analysis indicates the condition, behavior, or action described in this statement does not exist or occur.

Section 3.0 Training program administration and management

Rating (circle one)	Criteria
0 1 3 5	Safety training is integrated into an overall safety, health, and environmental management system.
0 1 3 5	The training program addresses responsibility and accountability for the training program.
0 1 3 5	The training program identifies and allocates resources available to the trainer and trainee.
0 1 3 5	The training program includes an effective course development process.
0 1 3 5	The training program includes an effective course design process.
0 1 3 5	The training program describes effective course presentation using appropriate techniques.
0 1 3 5	The training program describes appropriate and effective delivery strategies?

O.4 Sample training certification

Training subject	Date	Location

Trainee certification. I have received on-the-job training on those subjects listed (see other side of this sheet):

This training has provided me adequate opportunity to ask questions and practice procedures to determine and correct skill deficiencies. I understand that performing these procedures/practices safely is a condition of employment. I fully intend to comply with all safety and operational requirements discussed. I understand that failure to comply with these requirements may result in progressive discipline (or corrective actions) up to and including termination.

Employee name	Signature	Date

Trainer certification. I have conducted orientation/on-the-job training to the employees(s) listed above. I have explained related procedures, practices and policies. Employees were each given opportunity to ask questions and practice procedures taught under my supervision. Based on each student's performance, I have determined that each employee trained has adequate knowledge and skills to safely perform these procedures/practices.

Trainer	Signature	Date

Training validation. On _____ (date) I have observed the above employee(s) successfully applying the knowledge and skills learned during the training.

Supervisor	Signature	Date

(Page 2 of certification) Sample hazard communication training outline
The following information was discussed with students:
- Overview of the hazard communication program – purpose of the program
- Primary, secondary, portable, and stationary process container labeling requirements
- Discussion of the various sections of the MSDS and their location
- Emergency and spill procedures
- Discussion of the hazards of the following chemicals to which students will be exposed

- Symptoms of overexposure
- Use/care of required personal protective equipment used with the above chemicals
- Employee accountability
  The following procedures were practiced
- Chemical application procedure
- Chemical spill procedures
- Personal protective equipment use
- Emergency first aid procedure
  The following (oral/written) test was administered.

(You may want to keep these tests as attachments to the safety-training plan and merely reference it here to keep this document on one sheet of paper. OSHA recommends at least 25 questions for technically complex training.)

1. What are the labeling requirements of a secondary container? (Name of chemical and hazard warning)
2. When does a container change from a portable to secondary container? (When employee loses control)
3. What are the symptoms of over-exposure to _____? (Stinging eyes)
4. Where is the "right to know" station (or MSDS station) located? (In the production plant)
5. What PPE is required when exposed to_____? (Short answer)

CHAPTER THIRTEEN

Basis Elements of a Safety System

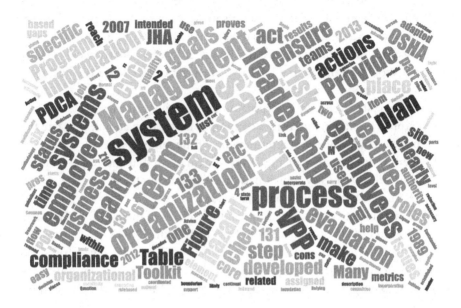

"Unless commitment is made, there are only promises and hopes ... but no plans."

—*Peter Drucker*

Chapter Objectives

At the end of the chapter, you should be able to:

- Identify the core elements of a safety system.
- Discuss the PDCA cycle and how it applies to a safety system.
- Discuss the six basic elements of a safety system.
- Discuss why it is important to select and follow a standard process.
- Discuss the important of employee participation.
- Discuss the differences between the compliance-based and voluntary safety management systems.
- Discuss performance and measurement criteria.
- Discuss how the JHA fits within the overall safety system.

Job Hazard Analysis. http://dx.doi.org/10.1016/B978-0-12-803441-5.00013-1

13.1 GENERAL OVERVIEW OF A SAFETY SYSTEMS

An organization consists of many various processes that need to be coordinated to ensure that an organization's intended goals and objectives are efficiently met. The safety system should function between the organization's boundaries and cut across the departments, divisions, and sections of an organization (Roughton & Crutchfield, 2013). For this to occur, a safety system should clearly define how the organization measures the effectiveness of its actions.

Safety systems should incorporate the following criteria:
- Express the leadership team's commitment to safety and clearly state the policies, objectives, and requirements of the safety system.
- Define the structure of the safety system as well as the responsibilities and authority of key individuals of the leadership team
- Define each element of the safety system.
- Communicate the expectations and objectives of the safety system to all employees (Safety Management System Toolkit, 2007).

The information as presented in Tables 13.1 and 13.2 was based on and adapted from the Safety System Toolkit developed by the Joint Helicopter Safety Implementation Team of the International Helicopter Safety Team.

Table 13.1 Applying the normal business approach to safety system

Business vision/mission	Safety system
Vision/mission about what the organization desires and espouses.	Vision/mission should be aligned with the Business Model.
Corporate goals both long and short term.	Safety goals and related efforts should be aligned with all corporate goals.
Corporate objectives to reach goals.	Safety objectives should be considered as part of the overall corporate objectives and meet similar goals.
Policies and procedures for overall management and administration of the organization.	A safety policy statement and other safety policies and procedures should be presented in a similar format as the business objectives and should be incorporated in business policies and procedures.

Source: Safety Management System Toolkit (2007).

Table 13.2 The business process versus the safety processes

Business processes	Safety processes
Identify noncompliance with policies and procedures, i.e., HR compliance, accounting, operational, quality, etc.	Identify and control hazards and associated risk in addition to compliance with corporate and regulatory policies and procedures
Implement solutions to organizational issues.	Advise and assist implementing solutions on hazard and associated risk reduction and controls such as the JHA process.
Measure performance of the organization	Measure performance of the safety system applying similar metrics as the business systems.
Lessons learned developed and communicated.	Lessons learned developed and communicated.
Repeat the above proves – Plan, Do, Check, and Act.	Repeat the above proves – Plan, Do, Check, and Act. (Figure 13.1).

Source: Safety Management System Toolkit (2007).

13.2 THE PLAN, DO, CHECK, ACT CYCLE FOR LEARNING AND IMPROVEMENT

The simple concept of a "Plan, Do, Check, Act" (PDCA) methodology called the Shewhart cycle (Shewhart, 1980) can be applied to any safety system. The PDCA has been at the core of quality management efforts for many decades. The cycle has been adapted within the framework of voluntary compliance standards such as ANSI/AIHA/ASSE Z10 "Occupational Safety Process" (Occupational Health and Safety Systems, 2012) (Figure 13.1). Refer to Appendix P for examples of "Advanced Safety Management Systems," (Occupational Health & Safety Management Systems, 2012).

The PDCA provides a structure (road map) that is a dynamic format that reveals how a system is not static and is always in continual movement and renewal. The four steps move a system from its beginning development through an action phase that continues for the life cycle of the system:

Step 1: Plan: Define the goals and objectives of the safety system. The goals and objectives will define specific conditions and behaviors desired for the implementation of the of the safety system elements. The

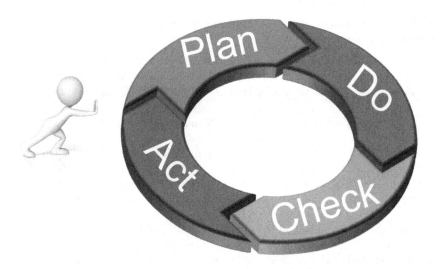

Figure 13.1 *Shewhart – Plan, Do, Check, Act (PDCA) Cycle for Learning and Improvement.*

intended results expected are established in this phase and are discussed with and approved by the leadership team. The Plan ensures that all employees are on board with the desired changes.

Step 2: Do: Begin the implementation of the safety system goals and objectives.

The implementation starts with the leadership team and employee training and communication of the safety system. Step 2 represents a transition from past efforts to a new system using the Plan that defines the actions necessary to reach the goals and objectives.

Step 3: Check: As the new or revised safety system is implemented, feedback from periodic reviews is received that assess if the Plan is still being followed, if resistance to change is present, and any concerns or issues that should be addressed.

Step 4: Act: The findings of the Check phase provide corrective actions for changes and modifications needed. The cycle continues as the Plan is adjusted, "Doing" continues, Checks of the results are made and Acting on corrective actions takes place and so on.

(Shewhart, 1980; Roughton & Crutchfield, 2008; How to Effectively Assess and Improve your Safety and Health Program through Safety and Health Evaluation, n.d.)

For a more advanced process refer to Chapter 15.

13.3 THE COMMON LINK BETWEEN SAFETY SYSTEMS

The two types of safety systems used are:
- Governmental safety-related system programs, both mandated and voluntary guidelines depending on the jurisdiction.
- Voluntary safety management systems developed by national and international recognized standards agencies and professional organizations.

Refer to Appendix P for Comparison of Governmental Safety-Related System Programs and Voluntary Compliance Standards – Governmental Safety-Related Programs (Roughton & Crutchfield, 2013).

Either of the safety system types follow the same six basic core elements that provide the foundation and establish a PDCA cycle. While giving the appearance of being a simple process, each element has additional criteria that can be complex to implement. The six elements are:
- Management leadership
- Employee participation
- Risk and hazard identification and assessment
- Hazard prevention and control
- Education and training
- Performance and measurement

(Injury and Illness Prevention Program (I2 P2), n.d.; Managing Worker Safety and Health, n.d.)

If one part of the system is missing, it represents a serious gap that should be addressed (Figures 13.2 and 13.3) (Roughton & Crutchfield, 2013).

13.4 MANAGEMENT LEADERSHIP

"The job of management is not supervision, but leadership."

—Dr. W. E. Deming

A high level of leadership team commitment and leadership from the top down through all levels of the organization is needed given the complexity that a full safety system requires.

The leadership team commitment is considered the driving force in all successful safety systems. This team provides the vision/mission, direction,

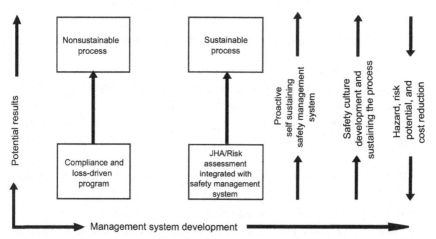

Figure 13.2 *Journey to a Successful Safety Management System with a Sustainable Process Integrated with the Overview of the JHA Development Process.* *Based on and adapted from Roughton & Crutchfield, 2013.*

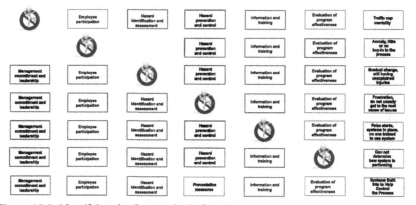

Figure 13.3 *Identifying the Gaps in the Safety System.*

and resources to ensure that the appropriate controls are in place. The leadership team should clearly establish the following:

- Responsibilities for safety-related goals and objectives holding everyone accountable for carrying out their assigned safety responsibilities.
- Providing the authority to make safety related decision, access to relevant information, education, and general resources needed to carry out those safety responsibilities.
- Designating a qualified individual to coordinate the safety system activities, receive and respond to communications and concerns

about safety conditions and, where appropriate, to initiate corrective action.

(Roughton & Crutchfield, 2013; Safety and Health Management Basics, Module Eight: Evaluating The Safety Management Systems, n.d.)

If employees can visibly see that the leadership team places emphasis on the safety efforts as it does on other organizational functions, they will be more likely to follow the example and pattern these efforts in their own activities.

The leadership team can show their support for the safety system in almost all of its activities. For example:

- Incorporating safety reports into planning and managerial meetings and communications.
- Ensure a safety system is selected and customized that matches the organization hazard and risk assessment findings.
- Providing budget and make time available for employee participation in the safety system.
- Personally providing and reviewing the tracking of safety performance metrics, etc.
- Participating in safety committee meetings, reviewing training, JHA development, workplace safety inspections, reviews, etc.
- Personally supporting corrective actions and alternative solutions. (Managing Worker Safety and Health, n.d.)

The overall safety efforts of an organization cannot be the sole responsibility of one person or designated group. A safe work environment develops from the many interactions of all parts or elements of the organization. The objective of the leadership team is to influence and shape the organization in its control programs for hazards and associated risk.

Relying only on rule-based regulatory compliance can create a climate that regards the safety function a "police force" rather than as a mentor who understands the needs of the organization.

Question to ask to determine the status of the safety system include:

- Is there a written safety policy statement for the organization?
- Is the safety policy statement signed by the current leadership team?
- Is the safety policy statement readily available and communicated to everyone in the organization?
- Is there access to the senior leadership team?
- Is everyone in the organization aware of their specific safety-related responsibilities?
- Are all employees evaluated on their individual safety performance?

- Does the leadership team communicate with all employees in the organization regularly about their commitment to safety?
- Does the leadership team participate in site inspections to reinforce their commitment of safety practices and behaviors?
- Is there a process in place that addresses contractor/temporary employee safety?
- Does the leadership team provide the resources needed (budget, time, equipment, materials, etc.) to enhance the safety efforts?

(Building an Effective Health and Safety Management System, 1989; Roughton & Crutchfield, 2008)

Refer to Figure 13.4 for a typical "Overview of the OSHA Voluntary Protection Program Process."

13.5 EMPLOYEE PARTICIPATION

Getting employees involved in the developing and sustaining of the safety system is particularly important for creating ownership and buy-in. Employee participation in the development of the safety system will help to ensure that it fits within the existing organizational culture.

Many opportunities can be used to get employees involved in the safety process that include: involvement in the development of hazard assessments, area and site inspections, review of preventative maintenance, assisting in training and mentoring, participate in emergency response teams, identifying potential loss-producing events, participating in the JHA process, etc. The scope of opportunities is based on how much flexibility the leadership team can balance in time and budget.

> "Effectively engaging workers to actively participate in health and safety requires thoughtful planning and implementation processes/policies that will build an atmosphere of trust" (Occupational Health and Safety Systems, 2012).

Employee participation closely follows the leadership team's commitment. Most employees want to do the right thing with regard to their assigned duties and tasks. Ensuring employee participation should be as diverse as possible. The following areas can become avenues for enhanced participation:

- Ensure that two-way communications are in place and rapid response is provided on any reports and recommendations. The system should allow

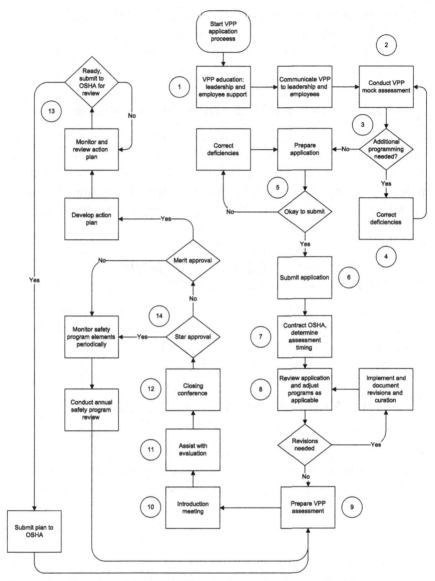

Figure 13.4 *Overview of the OSHA Voluntary Protection Program Process.*

immediate correction of issues and allow employees to make recommendations as appropriate.

- Provide easy and practical access to safety-related information with quick and reliable communications methods that do not filter or block concerns about identified hazards.

- Provide techniques that allow each individual to assess specific perceived risk and hazard identification with a practical method to prioritize issues. Refer to the risk guidance card as discussed in Chapter 8.

13.6 DEFINING ROLES AND RESPONSIBILITIES

Clearly defined and well-communicated safety roles and responsibilities for all levels of the organization are critical in the beginning phases of developing a safety system. These outline all expectations about performance and accountability among the leadership team, employees, contractors, and site visitors (Building an Effective Health and Safety Management System, 1989).

13.7 HAZARD AND RISK ASSESSMENT IDENTIFICATION AND ANALYSIS

Hazard and risk identification and analysis are the core functions of a safety. It is important to proactively assess and identify the specific hazards that may be built into jobs and activities (Building an Effective Health and Safety Management System, 1989).

13.8 HAZARD PREVENTION AND CONTROL

Effective planning and design of the workplace and job requirements are an ongoing concern as technology, the workplace, materials, equipment, and operations are constantly under change. The safety system would include specific actions that act as the organization's early warning system for potential problems. As part of an overall risk assessment, the design of any work order system should be reviewed to ensure that it can prioritize request for corrective actions.

13.9 INFORMATION AND TRAINING

The gathering of information and training materials is the linchpin that holds the safety system together. Establishing a structured method to gather and maintain information and data increases the leadership team and the employee ability to influence and design safety performance requirements.

Employee training and education programs should be designed and implemented to ensure that all employees demonstrate and understand that they are fully aware of the hazards and associated risk inherent in the operations (Chapter 12).

13.10 PERFORMANCE AND MEASUREMENT

The safety system should have a feedback loop that communicates to the leadership team the status of the various programs and systems. The safety system should be revised as gaps or deficiencies are identified by comprehensive audits and evaluations. The organization should keep a schedule of audits and inspections and ensure evaluations are not delayed or ignored.

Safety system audits are focused on all aspects of its administration and the scope and effectiveness of control systems in place. The audit should include:
- The comprehensiveness and scope of the safety system and its fit to the organization. Is the system current with existing operational needs.
- Determination of resource levels and expertise currently available.
- The nature and types of communications used.
- Scope and depth of employee participation.
- The continued use of risk assessments.
- Status of hazard and risk controls.
- Patterns and trends of system improvements and loss-producing events.

Safety performance measurements should be able to generate information or data that clearly provides valid evidence on the effectiveness of the safety system.

13.11 PROS AND CONS OF A STANDARDIZED SAFETY SYSTEM

The pros of implementing a safety system can include, but not limited to, the following:
- Structure a system that can be integrated with all other management processes and not just become a standalone program.
- Focus the leadership team and employees, so that is everyone is on the same page.

- Provide benchmarks to highlight achievements and progress by use of formats developed from the experience of other organizations with similar hazards and risk.
- Provide communications on the status of the system and encourage discussion, corrective action, and problem solving.

The cons of a safety system include areas that should be constantly monitored. The safety system may have problems if:
- It is not implemented properly and appears to be a "canned" approach that cannot be integrated with other management processes.
- Its scope is too narrowly implemented and viewed as a series of programs and not as a process.
- It allows a false sense of security to develop if the process is not routinely audited and its elements not implemented correctly, conscientiously, and consistently.
- An honest, comprehensive and routine appraisal system is not in place to ensure that "pencil whipping" (false documentation) is not occurring.
- It may be perceived as too time consuming. If the traditional methods of safety program success are dependent on such data as OSHA recordability (TCIR) and loss events are low then the attitude may be "we don't need to do this."

13.12 OTHER AREAS FOR CONSIDERATION

If your organization is just starting off with evaluating safety system and is not ready for implementation of a robust system, the VPP is the first logical step.

Bear in mind that the VPP is a program and not a process – need to expand.

13.12.1 Voluntary Protection Program

One method for complying with OSHA mandates and one type of safety management system is to become an OSHA Voluntary Protection Program (VPP) member. Refer to Table 13.3 for a summary of what it takes to certify under the VPP process. Refer to Figure 13.4 for a flow diagram of the OSHA Voluntary Protection Program. This diagram summarizes the information as listed in Table 13.3 and help you to apply for and successful obtain VPP status.

Table 13.3 Voluntary protection process implement process

Preapplication stage
1. VPP education: Management and employees
2. Communicate VPP to all employees
   a. Management's roles and responsibilities
   b. Employees roles, responsibilities, and rights
   c. Union's roles, responsibilities, and rights
3. VPP Mock evaluation/assessment
   a. Process deficiencies identified and corrected
      - Major deficiencies – 6–12 months
      - Major deficiencies – up to 6 months
      - Major deficiencies – up to 3 months

Application stage
4. Correct process deficiencies
   a. 3 months
   b. 6 months
   c. 12 months
   d. Longer as applicable
5. Prepare application
   a. Applications to read like a "Resume"
   b. Every item in application to have documented proof/verification.
6. Submit application
   a. Three-ring binder with tabs by subject
   b. Make 5 copies
   c. Send certified mail.

Postapplication stage
7. Contact OSHA office
   a. Determine evaluation date
   b. Determine team
   c. Determine who receive application
8. Review process
   a. Implement revisions
   b. Document revisions
9. Prepare for VPP Evaluation
   a. Provide conference room
   b. Provide computer
   c. Organize documents
   d. Prepare list of all employees for interviews
   e. Provide VPP team members escorts for plant walk around.

(Continued)

Table 13.3 Voluntary protection process implement process *(cont.)*

Evaluation Stage

10. Introduction meeting
    a. Introduce OSHA VPP team
    b. Let OSHA VP team discuss the logistics of this evaluation
    c. Present overview or organization
       - Management structure
       - Safety and health process
       - Safety team members
    d. Request daily briefing and draft pre-approval report
11. Evaluation
    a. Provide all document in conference room
    b. Provide escorts
    c. Provide lunch
12. Closing conference
    a. CELEBRATE that it is over
13. Postevaluation stage
    a. Merit (with plan) approval
       - Develop plan of action (POA)
       - Monitor and review progress
       - Document POA and activities
       - Submit POA proof
       - Provide for VPP evaluation
14. Star approval
    • Monitor safety and health process quarterly
    • Conduct annual VPP safety and health process review and revise as needed
    • Prepare for VPP evaluation.

Source: Roughton & Crutchfield (2008).

SUMMARY

An organization consists of many various processes that need to be coordinated to ensure that an organization's intended goals and objectives are efficiently met. The safety system should function between the organization's boundaries and cut across the departments, divisions, and sections of an organization.

The simple concept of a "Plan, Do, Check, Act" (PDCA) methodology called the Shewhart cycle can be applied to any safety system. The PDCA has been at the core of quality management efforts for many decades.

The leadership team commitment is considered the driving force in all successful safety systems. This team provides the vision/mission, direction, and resources to ensure that the appropriate controls are in place.

Relying only on rule based regulatory compliance can create a climate that regards the safety function a "police force" rather than as a mentor who understands the needs of the organization.

Getting employees involved in the developing and sustaining of the safety system is particularly important for creating ownership and buy-in. Employee participation in the development of the safety system will help to ensure that it fits within the existing organizational culture.

Clearly defined and well-communicated safety roles and responsibilities for all levels of the organization are critical in the beginning phases of developing a safety system.

Hazard and risk identification and analysis are the core functions of a safety. It is important to proactively assess and identify the specific hazards that may be built into jobs and activities.

The gathering of information and training materials is the linchpin that holds the safety system together.

 CHAPTER REVIEW QUESTIONS

1. Explain the concepts of the Plan-Do-Check-Act (PDCA) Cycle.
2. What are the six basic core safety process elements?
3. Discuss why Leadership support is essential.
4. What is the purpose of a safety system?
5. How does the Plan-Do-Check-Act (PDCA) apply to a safety system? Provide several examples.
6. Compare and contrast the Plan-Do-Check-Act (PDCA) and the Define, Measure, Analyze, Improve, and Control (DMAIC) system.
7. What are the benefits of using a standardized safety system?
8. Identify the pros and cons of a standardized safety system. Provide some examples from your experience.

BIBLIOGRAPHY

Building an Effective Health and Safety Management System. (1989). Partnerships in Health and Safety program, Partnerships in Injury Reduction (Partnerships), Reprinted/Modified and/or adapted with Permission. Retrieved from http://bit.ly/WsHteC

Guide to Developing Your Workplace Injury and Illness Prevention Program with Checklists for Self-inspection. (n.d.). State of California, Department of and Industrial Relations, Public Domain, Based on and Adapted for Use. Retrieved from http://bit.ly/Xewi5m

How to Effectively Assess and Improve your Safety and Health Program through Safety and Health Evaluation. (n.d.). Oregon Occupational Safety and Health Division (Oregon OSHA), OR-OSHA 116, Public Domain, Permission to Reprint, Modify, and/or Adapt as necessary. Retrieved from http://bit.ly/106AhmR

ILO-OSH, Overview and History, Module 2, Lesson 1. (2001). North Carolina Safety University. Retrieved from http://bit.ly/XOTbMM
Injury and Illness Prevention Program (I2 P2). (n.d.). Occupational Safety and Health Administration (OSHA), Public Domain, Based on and Adapted for Use. Retrieved from http://1.usa.gov/IIszWK
ISO 31000, Risk Management – Principles and Guidelines. (2009). International Organization or Standardization. Retrieved from http://bit.ly/Uobg8J
Managing Worker Safety and Health. (n.d.). Illinois OSHA Onsite Safety & Health Consultation Program, Public Domain,Based on and Adapted for Use. Retrieved from http://bit.ly/WTsneh
Occupational Health & Safety Management Systems. (2012).The American Society of Safety Engineers,ANSI/AIHA/ASSE Z10. Retrieved from http://bit.ly/1MsT6MG
Occupational Health and Safety Management standard (OHSAS 18001). (2007). Praxiom Research Group Limited,Translated into Plain English.
Occupational Health and Safety Systems. (2012).The American Industrial Hygiene Association,ANSI/AIHA Z10.
Occupational Safety and Health Management. (2006). Canadian Standards Association, CSA standard, Z 1000-06.
Program Evaluation Profile (PEP),Adapted for Use. (1996). Occupational Safety and Health Administration (OSHA). Retrieved from http://1.usa.gov/VuKM1C
Roughton, J., & Crutchfield, N. (2008). Job hazard analysis: A guide for voluntary compliance and beyond. Chemical, Petrochemical & Process. Elsevier/Butterworth-Heinemann. Retrieved from http://amzn.to/VrSAq5
Roughton, J., & Crutchfield, N. (2013). Safety culture: An innovative leadership approach. (B. Heinemann, Ed.). Butterworth Heinemann. Retrieved from http://amzn.to/1qoD4oN
Safety and Health Management Basics, Module Eight: Evaluating The Safety Management Systems. (n.d.). Oregon Occupational Safety and Health Division (Oregon OSHA), Online Course 100, Public Domain, Permission to Reprint, Modify, and/or Adapt as necessary. Retrieved from http://bit.ly/UVLJj0
Safety Culture Act. (n.d.). State of Montana Department of Labor & Industry, Public Domain. Retrieved from http://1.usa.gov/ohJMKR
Safety Management System Toolkit. (2007). Developed by the Joint Helicopter Safety Implementation Team of the International Helicopter Safety Team,The International Helicopter Safety Symposium, Montréal, Québec, Canada. Retrieved from http://bit.ly/YaSCOg
Shewhart, W.A. (1980). Economic control of quality of manufactured product. Republished by BookCrafters, Inc., Cleslesa, Michagan.
Voluntary Protection Program (DOE-VPP). (n.d.). Department of Energy, Public Domain. Retrieved from http://1.usa.gov/14ob6Rt
Voluntary Protection Protection (VPP). (n.d.). Occupatonal Safety and Health Administration (OSHA), Public Domain, Based on and Adapted for Use. Retrieved from http://1.usa.gov/T0j6EW

Appendix P Examples of advanced safety management systems
The following are examples of voluntary advanced safety management systems that we thought may be useful.These systems have the same basic formats and use similar concepts in their structure. By researching and studying

the underlined fundamentals of these recognized voluntary standards, you can review your current system in your organization and determine the best approach for moving towards a more structured, advanced, and industry recognized safety management system.

Occupational health and safety management, ANSI Z10-2012

"The purpose of the standard is to provide organizations with an effective tool for continual improvement of their and safety performance. Although Z10 is a guidance standard, implementation is not required by OSHA, the use of these guidelines is expected to improve occupational health and safety among American organizations."
Management leadership and employee participation
• Occupational health and safety policy
• Responsibility and authority
• Employee participation
Planning
• Identify and prioritize OHSMS issues
• Develop objectives for risk control based on prioritized OHSMS issues
• Formulate implementation plans to accomplish prioritized objectives.
Implementation and operation
• Hierarchy of controls
• Design review and management of change
• Procurement and contractors
• Emergency preparedness
• Education, training, competence
Evaluation and corrective action
• Monitoring, measurement, assessment, incident investigations, audits
• Corrective action
Management review
• Annual review of OHSM

Source: Occupational Health and Safety Systems (2012).

CSA Z1000-06 Occupational health and safety management

• "CSA Z1000-06 Occupational Health and Safety Management, is intended to reduce or prevent injuries, illnesses and fatalities in the workplace by providing companies with a model for developing and implementing an occupational health and safety management system" (Occupational Safety and Health Management, 2006).

Source: Occupational Health and Safety Systems (2012).

Overview of occupational health and safety management, Z1000-06

OHS Safety management system
- Responsibility, accountability, and authority.
- Management representatives.
- Worker participation.
- OHS policy.

Planning
- Review.
- Legal and other requirements.
- Hazard and risk identification and assessment.
- OHS objectives and targets.

Implementation
- Preventative and protective measures.
- Emergency prevention, preparedness, and response.
- Competence and training.
- Communication and awareness.
- Procurement.
- Contracting.
- Management of change.

Documentation
- Control of documents.
- Control of records.

Evaluation and corrective action
- Monitoring and measurement.
- Incident investigation and analysis.
- Internal audits.
- Preventive and corrective action.

Management review
- Continual improvement.
- Review input.
- Review output.

Source: Occupational Safety and Health Management (2006).

Occupational health and safety management standard (OHSAS 18001)

The British Standard has established formal consensus criteria for occupational health and safety management systems.

"OHSAS 18001 has been developed to be compatible with the ISO 9001 (Quality) and ISO 14001 (Environmental) management systems standards, in order to facilitate the integration of quality, environmental and occupational health and safety management systems by organizations, should they wish to do so.

The (OHSAS) specification gives requirements for an occupational health and safety (OH&S) management system, to enable an organization to control its OH&S risks and improve its performance. It does not state specific OH&S performance criteria, nor does it give detailed specifications for the design of a management system."

General requirements
- Establish an OHSMS for your organization

Planning requirements
- Analyze OH&S hazards and select controls
- Respect legal and nonlegal OH&S requirements
- Establish OH&S objectives and programs

Implementation requirements
- Establish responsibility and accountability
- Ensure competence and provide training
- Establish communication and participation
- Establish OH&S communication procedures
- Establish OH&S participation and consultation
- Control your organization's OH&S documents
- Implement operational OH&S control measures
- Establish an OH&S emergency management process

Checking requirements
- Monitor and measure your OH&S performance
- Evaluate legal and nonlegal compliance
- Evaluate compliance with legal requirements
- Evaluate compliance with nonlegal requirements
- Investigate incidents and take remedial action
- Investigate your OH&S incidents
- Take corrective and preventive action
- Establish and control OH&S records
- Conduct internal audits of your OHSMS

Review requirements
- Review the performance of your OHSMS

Source: Occupational Health and Safety Management standard (OHSAS 18001) (2007).

ISO 31000 – risk management

"This standard provides principles, framework, and a process for managing risk. It can be used by any organization regardless of its size.

Organizations using it can compare their risk management practices with an internationally recognised benchmark, providing sound principles for effective management and corporate governance."

Establish context
Communication and consultation
Risk assessment
- Risk assessment
- Risk analysis
- Risk evaluation
Risk treatment
Monitoring and review

Source: ISO 31000, Risk Management – Principles and Guidelines (2009).

Occupational safety and health (OSH) management systems, ILO-OSH 2001 guidelines

"The International Labor Organization (ILO) is a specialized agency of the United Nations (UN) with a primary goal to promote opportunities for women and men to obtain decent and productive work in conditions of freedom, equity, security, and human dignity. The ILO developed its voluntary guidelines on occupational safety and health (OSH) management systems in 2001: ILO-OSH 2001 Guidelines."

Policy
- Occupational safety and health policy
- Worker participation

Organizing
- Responsibility and accountability
- Competence and training
- Occupational safety and health management system documentation
- Communication

Planning and implementation
- Initial review
- System planning, development, and implementation
- Occupational safety and health objectives
- Hazard prevention
  - Prevention and control measures
  - Management of change
  - Emergency prevention, preparedness, and response
  - Procurement
  - Contracting

Evaluation
- Performance monitoring and measurement
- Investigation of work-related injuries, ill health, diseases and incidents, and their impact on safety and health performance
- Audit
- Management review

Action for improvement
- Preventive and corrective action
- Continual improvement

Source: ILO-OSH, Overview and History, Module 2, Lesson 1 (2001); Roughton & Crutchfield (2013).

Comparison of Governmental Safety-Related System Programs

Proposed I2P2	Voluntary protection program (VPP)	Department of energy voluntary protection program (DOE-VPP)	California model injury and illness prevention programs	OSHA performance evaluation profile (cancelled)	Building an effective health and safety management system, partnerships in injury reduction, Alberta
Management leadership	Management leadership	Management commitment	Management commitment/assignment of responsibilities	Management leadership and employee participation	Management leadership and organizational commitment
Employee participation	Employee participation	Employee involvement	Safety communications		
Hazard identification and assessment	Hazard identification and assessment	Worksite analysis	Hazard assessment and control	Workplace analysis	Hazard identification and assessment
Hazard prevention and control	Hazard prevention and control	Hazard prevention and control	Safety planning, rules and work procedures	Hazard prevention and control	Hazard control
Information and training	Information and training	Safety and health training	Safety and health training	Safety and health training	Worker competency and training

(Continued)

Comparison of Governmental Safety-Related System Programs (cont.)

Proposed I2P2	Voluntary protection program (VPP)	Department of energy voluntary protection program (DOE-VPP)	California model injury and illness prevention programs	OSHA performance evaluation profile (cancelled)	Building an effective health and safety management system, partnerships in injury reduction, Alberta
Evaluation of program effectiveness	Evaluation of program effectiveness				
			Accident investigation	Accident and record analysis	Incident reporting and investigation
				Emergency response	Emergency response planning
					Worksite inspections
					Program administration

Source: Roughton & Crutchfield (2013).

Voluntary compliance standards - governmental safety-related programs

If your organization is not prepared to develop a robust safety management system at this time then the Occupational Safety and Health Administration's (OSHA) voluntary protection program (VPP) program is a good stated point.

The following section provides some insight on various safety management programs in order to help you make a more informed decision on what type of management system you and your organization will want to adopt. The list below provides examples of several standardized governmental-related guidelines safety management systems:

Various states and provinces may have their own suggested or mandated safety management systems. Examples of a state or province system are
- The mandated California OSHA Injury and Illness Prevention Program Title 8-§3203
- Building an effective health and safety management system partnerships in injury reduction, Alberta
- The mandated Montana Safety Culture Act

An older model of an OSHA safety management system that was proposed and offers a good process audit format is the program evaluation profile (PEP), proposed in an earlier effort to develop a safety management program (Program Evaluation Profile (PEP), Adapted for Use, 1996).

California OSHA injury and illness prevention program title 8-§3203

"In California every employer is required by law (Labor Code Section) to provide a safe and healthful workplace for his/her employees. Title 8 (T8), of the California Code of Regulations (CCR), requires every California employer to have an effective Injury and Illness Prevention Program in writing that must be in accord with T8 CCR Section 3203 of the General Industry Safety Orders."

These following elements are required:

- Management commitment/assignment of responsibilities;
- Safety communications system with employees;
- System for assuring employee compliance with safe work practices;
- Scheduled inspections/evaluation system;
- Accident investigation;
- Procedures for correcting unsafe/ unhealthy conditions;
- Safety and health training and instruction; and
- Recordkeeping and documentation.

Source: Guide to Developing Your Workplace Injury and Illness Prevention Program with Checklists for Self-inspection (n.d.).

OSHA proposed injury and illness prevention plan (I2P2)

An example of a proposed regulatory mandated safety process is the US Occupational Safety and Health Administration's (OSHA) proposed Injury and Illness Prevention Plan. The proposal has been under review for a number of years and if implemented, the rule will "require employers to develop and implement a program that minimizes worker exposure to safety and health hazards" (Injury and Illness Prevention Program (I2 P2), n.d.).

Voluntary protection program (VPP)

VPP has been in effect and has been effective based on OSHA studies in establishing in-depth compliance based programs.

"The VPP recognize employers and workers in the private industry and federal agencies who have implemented effective safety and health management systems and maintain injury and illness rates below national Bureau of Labor Statistics averages for their respective industries.
In VPP, management, labor, and OSHA work cooperatively and proactively to prevent fatalities, injuries, and illnesses through a system focused on: hazard prevention and control; worksite analysis; training; and management commitment and worker involvement. To participate, employers must submit an application to OSHA and undergo a rigorous onsite evaluation by a team of safety and health professionals.
Union support is required for applicants represented by a bargaining unit. VPP participants are re-evaluated every three to five years to remain in the programs. VPP participants are exempt from OSHA programmed inspections while they maintain their VPP status."

Source: Voluntary Protection Protection (VPP) (n.d.).

Department of Energy VPP Elements

"The Department of Energy Voluntary Protection Program (DOE-VPP) promotes safety and health excellence through cooperative efforts among labor, management, and government at the Department of Energy (DOE) contractor sites. DOE has also formed partnerships with other Federal agencies and the private sector for both advancing and sharing its Voluntary Protection Program (VPP) experiences and preparing for program challenges in the next century. The safety and health of contractor and federal employees are a high priority for the Department."

Source: Voluntary Protection Program (DOE-VPP) (n.d.).

Building an effective health and safety management system

This is a health and safety management system provided by Partnerships in Injury Reduction, Alberta that involves the introduction of processes designed to help reduce Injuries.

"Successful implementation of the system requires management commitment to be vested in the system, effective allocation of resources, and a high level of employee participation. The scope and complexity of a Health and Safety management system will vary according to the size and type of workplace."

Source: Building an Effective Health and Safety Management System (1989).

Montana Safety Culture Act

"The Safety Culture Act enacted by the 1993 Montana State Legislature encourages workers and employers to come together to create and implement a workplace safety philosophy. It is the intent of the act to raise workplace safety to a preeminent position in the minds of all Montana's workers and employers. Listed …are the six requirements all employers must meet, and the additional three requirements employers with more than five employees must meet, to comply with the Montana Safety Culture Act (MSCA)…from the Department of Labor and Industry offered as guidelines for implementation of the MSCA."

Source: Safety Culture Act (n.d.).

Program evaluation profile

The program evaluation profile (PEP) (Program Evaluation Profile (PEP), Adapted for Use, 1996) was intended to have been used as a safety and health program evaluation for the employer, employees, and OSHA. The PEP was to provide a method to score an organization's safety program. A numerical score was to provide an indicator of where program weaknesses were apparent (Program Evaluation Profile (PEP), Adapted for Use, 1996; Roughton & Crutchfield, 2013).

Becoming a Curator for the Safety System

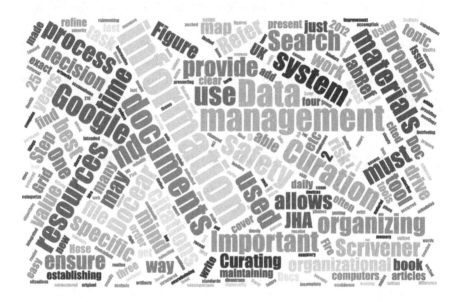

"Model it – you need to try to imagine what it would be like if you did it"

—Seth Godin Marketer

Chapter Objectives

At the end of the chapter, you should be able to:

- Discuss the importance of the JHA information curator.
- Define and discuss curation.
- Discuss various concepts to organize JHA information.
- Discuss several tools that might be used in organizing JHA information.

Job Hazard Analysis. http://dx.doi.org/10.1016/B978-0-12-803441-5.00014-3

14.1 CURATING SAFETY

In recent years, a major shift has occurred with the unlimited access to information that has changed what we do and how we manage our jobs. Massive amounts of information are readily available and can be overwhelming (Pink, 2012). This simply means that we must become curators to organize the information that accumulates.

The use of smart phones, tablets, computers, and other devices has opened up the search capabilities available to leaders and employees. This shifts the emphasis to not just providing material but ensuring that the information is accurate and from reliable resources.

14.2 USING AND CURATING INFORMATION

To accomplish any specific task, three areas must be considered:
- The gathering of pertinent and verifiable information.
- Organizing ("Curation") of the information
- Retrieving, selecting, and presenting the information.

These three areas must be structured in such a manner that the information is clear and concise and allows the intended audience to not just receive the information but be able to use the information.

If asked to explain a standard, write a memo on a safety-related topic, complete a standards review, and/or write a summary report, how would you begin? How would the findings be presented? When asked to present safety system information to others, how do you prepare and review the information to keep it informative, timely, and of value to anyone expected to use it?

Content curation is not about collecting and bookmarking web links or becoming an information pack rat, it is more about putting gathered information into a context that is filed, organized, annotated, and can be readily developed for presentation. Content curators provide a customized, vetted selection of the best and most relevant resources on a very specific topic or theme.

According to Bhargava's work as cited in (Kanter, n.d.) "a content curator continually seeks, makes sense of, and shares the best and most relevant content on a particular topic online. Content curators have integrated this skill into their daily routine" (Kanter, n.d.).

Lesson Learned #1

Too often, entire documents are lost because of the lack of a curation system and "reinventing the wheel" is an ongoing problem with organizations. Curation provides a method to reduce the loss of organizational memory as time passes, new personnel come in and experienced personnel leave. A comprehensive system should be present to maintain information.

14.3 THE IMPORTANCE OF BECOMING AN INFORMATION CURATOR

Given daily work schedules packed with many meetings, activities, and management duties, one of the last things usually considered is how to organize and categorize safety system information for easy access in the future or when needed by others. The issue faced has shifted from being the sole source of limited information to being the "curator" of properly selected and organized information.

"Curation – The act of curating, of organizing and maintaining of a collection of artworks or artifacts" (Curation, n.d.). The term curation is now used to cover the gathering, organizing, and maintaining of all types of information.

"Making decision based on incomplete, inaccurate, or wrong information can have disastrous consequences. Decision making knowledge workers need to have access to the right information and need to have confidence in that information. Data curation can be a vital tool to ensure knowledge workers have access to accurate, high-quality, and trusted information that can be reliably tracked to the original source, in order to ensure its credibility" (Curry & O'Riain, n.d.).

By establishing a curation process for safety system resources and history, information resources can be used to establish more effective action plans, job improvement goals and objectives. The JHA process should have a built-in method to ensure they are updated and kept current as changes are made in the workplace.

> The ANSI/AIHA/ASSE Z10, advocates that a process must be established to create and maintain documents and records.
>
> The document and record control process is to show that these have been created and maintained in order to
> 1. "Implement an effective OHSMS:
> 2. Demonstrate or assess conformance with the requirements of this standard."
> (Occupational Health and Safety Systems, 2012)

14.4 RESEARCHING AND CURATING INFORMATION

Resources to support JHA conclusions and recommendations must be clearly defined. It is critical that all selected resources be referenced to show how conclusions about risk severity and exposures were developed. Any document or procedure developed for the organization must clearly provide an outline for selected concepts and the exact wording of references used.

Citations and referencing is important for any type of written documentation, especially those for regulatory and best practices criteria. Citations and references provide the reader additional and more detailed discussions points and provide a way to evaluate the accuracy of JHA descriptions, analysis, and conclusions.

Lesson Learned #2

When writing several books, organizing and reviewing collected data was an enormous task. Citations, references, figures, appendix, tables, etc. had to be tracked with changes in chapters detailed. Dropbox was used to create digital "binders" that allowed the exchange data and maintain the book structure.

Essentially, Dropbox provided a form of the internal computer public drive used by organizations. Having worked with both, it was found that an understanding of how information is exchanged in an organization is critical to the safety system and the JHA process.

When utilizing any resource for internal or external publications, the key is to ensure that all resources are referenced and cited demonstrating directly quoted information to show the difference between ideas and the exact words of the resource(s).

Lesson Learned #3

An issue encountered within organizations is that situations exist where safety related information is spread across many departments.

Human resources may have a form used for new hire orientation with some basic training provided. Operations may have other detailed work instructions with specific step-by-step procedures that are similar to the JHA but without the hazard or risk assessment. Quality control has its own applications, in particular if the product must meet some specific standard mandated by its industry or regulatory agencies. Each of these examples can, over the years, include safety-related criteria that used different nomenclature, wording, and criteria.

The challenge is being able to bring together the various documents and ensure they are aligned to use the same safety, hazard, and risk nomenclature.

It has been said "if you cannot find it, it does not exist!" It may be the best of safety articles or risk related information, but if you cannot put your hands or eyes on it, then it is only a figment of your imagination (Roughton & Crutchfield, 2013).

 ## 14.5 HOW TO APPLY MANAGEMENT MATRIX TO CURATION

Urgency is now the expected norm and no longer reserved for special cases and becomes a "fire hose" of information that can alter and overwhelm the researcher Figure 14.1. A consistent discipline must be developed for consistently managing resources and data (Figure 14.2).

Dwight D. Eisenhower, known for his decision making, is alleged to have used the following statement about making decisions: "What is important is seldom urgent, and what is urgent is seldom important." His strategy for taking action and organizing his tasks was simple and can be applied to the curation process. This statement parallels the Covey time management grid, which is an effective method of organizing specific priorities (Covey, 1990) (Figure 14.3).

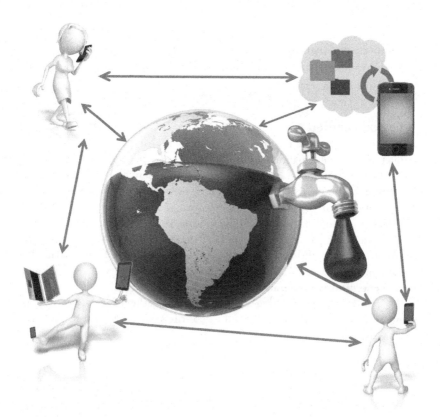

Figure 14.1 *Multiple Sources of Communication and Information.*

The use of a four quadrants matrix based on the Eisenhower or Covey matrix can assist in both determining priorities as well as what should be curated.

- Quadrant I: Urgent and important activities and information. These include activities or data that are important or constantly needed. These are relevant for the task at hand and add value to the organization.
- Quadrant II: Not Urgent and Important activities. Long-term strategizing and development or data that may be important at a later time. These activities have a due date for completion or are somewhat relevant for the task at hand and add some value to the organization.
- Quadrant III: Urgent and Not Important activities. Time pressured distractions. This information or activity is not important. However, you may be asked to support requested information or an activity, but this information and/or an activity is of little relevancy and adds little value to the organization. These type of information or an activity can be delegated to others to get accomplished.

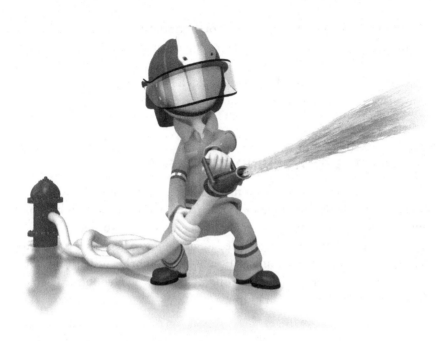

Figure 14.2 *Fire Hose of Information.*

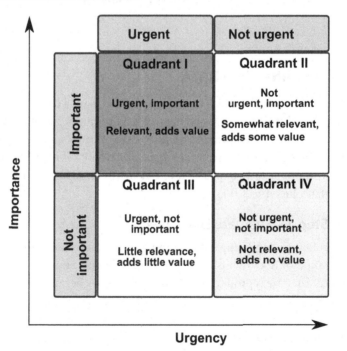

Figure 14.3 *Applying a Management Decision Matrix to Duration. Based on and adapted from Covey, 1990.*

- Quadrant IV: Not Urgent and Not Important activities or information that creates little or no value to the organization (Savara, n.d.; The Time Management Grid, Covey's Time Management Grid, 2014; Time Management for a Small Business, n.d.; The Eisenhower method of time management, n.d.; Covey, 1990; Thomas, 2012; Koort, n.d.).

14.6 THE IDEA BEHIND THE MATRIX

When utilizing this type of matrix, begin by making an inventory of all collected information no matter how relevant it is believed to be. Once collected, review each piece of information and place into one of the four quadrants by priority. Once categories are defined, the list of items will provide a clear picture of what information has highest priority. This "up front" decision process combined with an ongoing review will continue to refine the information requiring curation.

"After figuring out what really matters and which issues need to be addressed, you need to find the time to deal with these tasks" (Koort, n.d.).

14.7 MANAGING DATA

The following checklists have been adapted from a data management-planning checklist from the University of Edinburgh Research Data Management Guidance. They provide questions that can be used to address and how data will be shared (Research Data Management Guidance, Permission to reprint, modify, and adapt for use, Creative Commons Attribution 2.5 UK: Scotland License, 2011).

14.7.1 Step 1 – Evaluate Data Needs

Questions before beginning establishing a data management process:
- What type of documents, materials, and information will be produced?
  - Will they be reproducible? (How will copies be managed?)
  - What would happen if they got lost or became unusable later?
- Who will be the audience for your documents, materials, and information and how will they use them now, and in the long run?
- Who controls the documents, materials, and information?

- Will there be any sharing requirements?
- Is any budget needed to gather and maintain the documents, materials, and information?
- How much documents, materials, and information will be generated and how often will they change?
- How long will these items be retained? For example, 5 years, up to 10 years, or permanently.
- Are there tools or software needed to create/process/visualize the documents, materials, and information?
- What directory and file naming convention will be used?
- What file formats will be used? Are they long-lived?
- What project and identifiers will be assigned?
- Is there good project and data/information documentation? (How will they be inventoried or catalogued?)
- Are there any special privacy or security requirements? For example, personal data, high-security data, proprietary?
- What will be the storage and backup strategy?
- When and where will the documents, materials, data, and information be published?
- Is there an organizational guideline or standard for sharing/integration?

Adapted from Research Data Management Guidance, (Research Data Management Guidance, Permission to reprint, modify, and adapt for use, Creative Commons Attribution 2.5 UK: Scotland License, 2011).

14.7.2 Step 2 – Establish a Plan

A data management plan describes the creating, organizing, documenting, storing, and sharing data. The plan would cover protection and confidentiality, preservation, and curation. It provides a framework that supports the safety management system documents, materials, and information.

- What documents, materials, and information will be created or collected for the safety management system?
- What organizational policies and procedures will apply to the documents, materials, and information?
- What management practices (backups, storage, access control, archiving) will be used.
- What facilities and equipment will be required (hard disk space, backup server, and repository).
- Who will own and have access to the documents, materials, and information.

- Who will be responsible for each aspect of the safety management data?
- How will use of documents, materials, and information be enabled and long-term preservation ensured to maintain the history of the safety management system?

Adapted from Research Data Management Guidance (Research Data Management Guidance, Permission to reprint, modify, and adapt for use, Creative Commons Attribution 2.5 UK: Scotland License, 2011) (Figure 14.4).

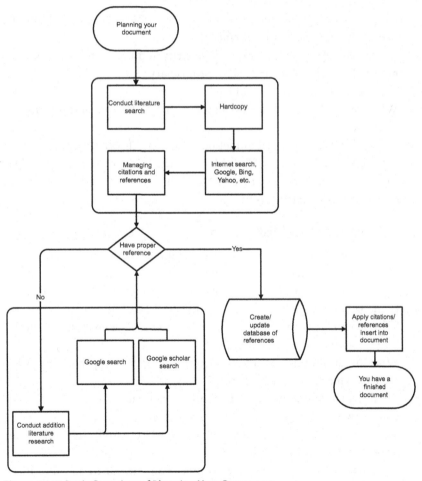

Figure 14.4 *Basic Overview of Planning Your Document.*

14.8 AN APPROACH TO ORGANIZING INFORMATION

Curation methods are dependent on personal preference, organizational protocols, and storage capability. A wide range of methods and concepts are available and beyond the scope this book. In addition, the organization may have a "knowledge manager" and/or developed procedures for storage and retrieval of information. If not, use the system you find most efficient for your purposes.

The following software was found beneficial for collecting, developing, and/or organizing collection of information (Figure 14.5):

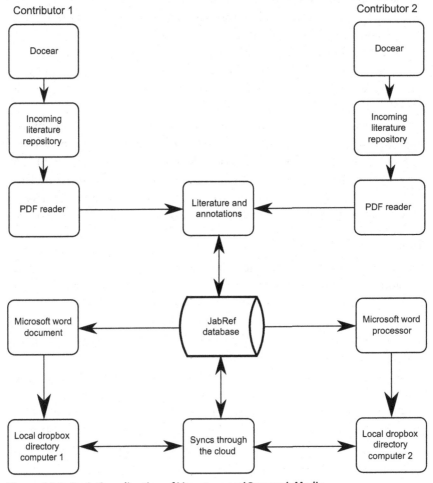

Figure 14.5 *Basic Coordination of Literature and Research Media.*

- Scrivener
- Docear
- JabRef
- Google Scholar
- Google Search
- Google Doc
- Dropbox
- Microsoft OneNote

14.8.1 Scrivener

Safety professionals are normally not considered "writers". However, considerable time can be spent on manuals, procedures, policies, etc. To get the best benefits of the information, this particular software is relatively inexpensive and a great tool for document development.

Writing a research paper, any long document, or just creating a company manual requires a lot of research and collection of documentation to ensure that enough information is available for citing and referencing the completed work (Scrivener, 2015).

Scrivener is a content-generation tool and a word processor and project management tool. It allows the writer to concentrate on composing and structuring long and hard to manage documents (Scrivener, 2015). The software is a collection of tools in one application to help organize information that is placed in selected folders on a computer. For example, Scrivener allows the user to outline and structure ideas, notes, and viewing of resources.

14.8.2 Docear

Docear is an "academic literature suite," which allowed increased structuring and sharing of information, which aided greatly in managing book content. If used properly, Docear is one method that can provide an excellent framework to tie the safety system elements and its information together so that they can be tracked and accessed effectively and efficiently (Docear, n.d.).

Docear allowed information to be placed into a single application that established a digital library and mind maps. It includes an academic search engine, file manager, mind mapping, note taking tool, and reference manager. Build into Docear is "Docear4word," an add-on for Microsoft Word that allows inserting into documents citations and bibliographies (Docear-4Word, n.d.; Mindmap, n.d.).

Documents are saved into a "literature repository" sub-directory Using Docear, documents are then imported into a mind map. The mind map provides a graphic picture showing all the documents in the literature repository for ease of organization. Any document can be directly opened from the mind map.

If the document is in a pdf format, annotations (highlights, comments) can be made and are then displayed in the mind map along with the document (Docear, Details & Features, n.d.).

14.8.3 JabRef

"JabRef "is an open source bibliography reference manager and provides a way to collect and manage a bibliography file (JabRef Reference Manager, n.d.).

14.8.4 Google Scholar

Google Scholar provides a way to search for scholarly literature across many disciplines and sources such as articles, books, abstracts, etc.

14.8.5 Google Scholar Citations

Google Scholar citations provides a simple way for authors to be able to use the proper citations for resources as posted in literature reviews in several formats (MLA, APA, Chicago styles). (Google Scholar, n.d.).

14.8.6 Google Advance Search

Google Advance Search provides specific search terms to narrow down and refine a search statement. Refer to Appendix Q for "Google Advanced Search Features for Related Criteria."

14.8.7 Google Drive (Doc)

Google Docs is similar to Microsoft Word. One of the best features is that Google Docs will save information automatically online to Google Drive Cloud. This allows access to information from anywhere with Internet access and allow sharing it with others (Cantrell, 2014; Goggle Doc, n.d.).

14.8.8 Dropbox

Dropbox is a "cloud "file storage and retrieval application that allows quick and easy sharing of files and documents. It is essentially a "public drive" to move information between computers (Dropbox, n.d.).

SUMMARY

In recent years, a major shift has occurred with the unlimited access to information that has changed what we do and how we manage our jobs. Massive amounts of information are readily available and can be overwhelming.

Content curation is not about collecting and bookmarking web links or becoming an information pack rat, it is more about putting gathered information into a context that is filed, organized, annotated, and can be readily developed for presentation.

Resources to support JHA conclusions and recommendations must be clearly defined. It is critical that all selected resources be referenced to show how conclusions about risk severity and exposures were developed.

Urgency is now the expected norm and no longer reserved for special cases and becomes a "fire hose" of information that can alter and overwhelm the researcher.

When utilizing this type of matrix, begin by making an inventory of all collected information no matter how relevant it is believed to be. Once collected, review each piece of information and place into one of the four quadrants by priority.

Curation methods are dependent on personal preference, organizational protocols, and storage capability.

CHAPTER REVIEW QUESTIONS

1. Discuss the importance of becoming an information curator.
2. Define and discuss Curation.
3. Discuss various concepts to organize information.
4. Discuss several tools that might be used in organizing information.
5. Discuss how a mind map is used.

BIBLIOGRAPHY

Cantrell, J. (2014). Scrivener, Microsoft Word, and Google Docs. Retrieved from http://bit.ly/1dOqNLo

Covey, S. R. (1990). *The 7 habits of highly effective people: Powerful lessons in personal change.* New York: A Fireside Book, Simon and Schuster, Inc, pp. 151. Retrieved from http://amzn.to/WsCA5g.

Curation. (n.d.). Wiktionary, a Wiki-Based Open Content Directory. Retrieved from http://bit.ly/VQ95KJ

Curry, E. & O'Riain, S. (n.d.). *The role of community-driven data curation for enterprises.* Digital Enterprise Research Institute, National University of Ireland, Galway, Ireland. Retrieved from http://bit.ly/W8TQ1O

Docear. (n.d.). Retrieved from http://bit.ly/Ypx4Pv

Docear, Details & Features. (n.d.). Docear, Details & Features. Retrieved from http://bit.ly/WcROh2

Docear4Word. (n.d.). Docear. Retrieved from http://bit.ly/13gar5F

Dropbox. (n.d.). Retrieved from http://bit.ly/YpvKwe

Goggle Doc. (n.d.). Google. Retrieved from http://bit.ly/YR8C8i

Google Scholar. (n.d.). Google. Retrieved from http://bit.ly/W4iu3S

JabRef Reference Manager. (n.d.). Retrieved from http://bit.ly/13g6D4w

Kanter, B. (n.d.). Content Curation Primer. Licensed under a Creative Commons Attribution 3.0 United States License. Retrieved from http://bit.ly/XFtmWz

Koort, K. (n.d.). *A simple handbook for achieving maximum at work*. weekdone.com.

Mindmap. (n.d.). Wikipedia, the free encyclopedia. Retrieved from http://bit.ly/Y2JJWE

Occupational Health and Safety Systems. (2012). The American Industrial Hygiene Association, ANSI/AIHA Z10.

Pink, D.H. (2012). *To sell is human: The surprising truth about moving others*. New York: Riverhead Books. Retrieved from http://books.google.com/books?id=q2uuuAAACAAJ

Research Data Management Guidance, Permission to reprint, modify, and adapt for use, Creative Commons Attribution 2.5 UK: Scotland License. (2011). Edinburgh University Data Library. Retrieved from http://www.ed.ac.uk/is/data-management

Roughton, J., & Crutchfield, N. (2013). In B. Heinemann (Ed.), *Safety culture: An innovative leadership approach*. Butterworth Heinemann, Retrieved from http://amzn.to/1qoD4oN.

Savara, S. (n.d.). Time Management Matrix by Stephen Covey–Urgent vs Important. Blog Post. Retrieved from http://bit.ly/1BwgCQs

Scrivener. (2015). Literature & Latte Ltd. Retrieved from http://bit.ly/1ALXenZ

The Eisenhower method of time management. (n.d.). ProcessPolicy.com. Retrieved from http://bit.ly/1SIt22n

The Time Management Grid, Covey's Time Management Grid. (2014). US Department of the Interior, U.S. Geological Survey. Retrieved from http://on.doi.gov/1FIhe9A

Thomas, M. N. (2012). *Personal productivity secrets*. Hoboken, NJ: John Wiley & Sons, Inc.

Time Management for a Small Business. (n.d.). US Small Business Administration (SBA), Financial Education Curriculum, Instructor Guide, Public Domain.

OTHER RESOURCES FOR CONSIDERATION

The following books offer ideas and thoughts on organizing. An Amazon book search will provide a wealth of books on the topic.

"*Getting things done: The art of stress-free productivity*" by David Allen.

"*Taming the paper tiger at home*" by Barbara Hemphill.

"*File…don't pile: A proven filing system for personal and professional use*" by Pat Dorff.

Appendix Q Google Advanced Search Features – Narrowing the Search Terms

Q.1 Explicit phrase
- "Safety Culture"

Q.2 Exclude words
- "-" (dash) sign in front of the word – job hazard analysis

Q.3 Site specific search

- site:www.osha.gov

Q.4 Similar words and synonyms

Use the "~" in front of the word –
- "job hazard analysis" ~ job hazard analysis

Q.5 Specific document types

Looking for documents related to job hazard analysis
- "job hazard analysis" filetype:ppt
- "job hazard analysis" filetype:doc

Q.6 This OR That

The OR has to be capitalized
- job hazard analysis OR JHA

Q.7 Word definitions

Example:
- define: job hazard analysis

CHAPTER FIFTEEN

Effectively Managing a JHA Process using Six Sigma

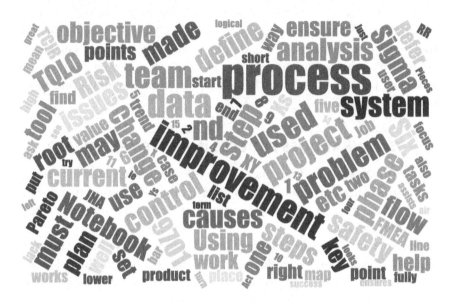

Begin with the end in mind,"

—Steven Covey

Chapter Objectives

At the end of the chapter, you should be able to:

- Discuss the basic framework used by Six Sigma.
- Discuss the process improvement criteria.
- Identify what DMAIC stands for and how it can be used.
- Discuss the XY Matrix and how it can be used with the JHA.
- Discuss various tools used in Six Sigma.
- Cite the levels of Six Sigma and what they mean.

Job Hazard Analysis. http://dx.doi.org/10.1016/B978-0-12-803441-5.00015-5

15.1 BRIEF SIX SIGMA OVERVIEW

Six Sigma's main objective is to help improve a process so that a problem does not recur. The pressures of the work environment tend to drive individuals to find and use short-term solutions or taking "short cuts" that increase the risk potential for product defects, employee injury, or damage.

Six Sigma is a system that attempts find the root cause of organizational problems instead of accepting them as the "norm" or using ineffective short-term solutions. Its philosophy is that process improvement can be made by reducing variation. As the JHA looks at removing the variation in various job tasks and steps, it becomes a beneficial tool to use and adopt within Six Sigma.

15.2 WHAT DOES PROCESS IMPROVEMENT MEAN?

A process improvement mentality requires a different way of thinking about an organization and how it operates. It requires viewing an operation as a system of processes that require various programs to define and explain what must be done.

Improving a process is more than updating procedures or administrative controls. To relate this to developing a JHA process, consider the following:
- What is the best way to learn about the process so that the appropriate sub-elements can be identified for improvement?
- What resources are required to complete improvement efforts?
- Are the individuals with the necessary skills available and trained who can help process improvement?
- Is a team of difference skills and expertise needed and what type of approach using a team can be used to accomplish improvements?
- How can the improved process be institutionalized in the organization?

Many current mandates take time and resources away from process improvement. For example, the Occupational Safety and Health Administration (OSHA) record keeping requirements use downstream data and measures success by using Total Case Incident Rate (TCIR). A high TCIR is indicative of something wrong with the current work environment. The TCIR is a post-loss indicator and should be considered only one of many pieces of data collected about a process under review.

"Process improvement" is simply making things work better and not just for trying to manage through all types of crises. It is a way of looking at how a process can be changed to work more efficient. It also attempts to design a process that includes reducing the potential for human error as well as failures.

A logical problem-solving approach should be used to define the root causes of problems. If the root cause is not identified, then problems will re-occur as long as the process is used. Without looking for the base causes, situations can be made worse when changes are made without fully understanding of how the process components interrelate.

The benefit of improving a process is that a standardized approach is developed and used to evaluate how well an organization performs. The organization can, in turn, have a better chance of learning how to operate in a more efficient manner.

15.3 BEGINNING THE SIX SIGMA PROCESS

Six Sigma begins with problem identification, a search for the cause and modifies the process to reduce variation by changing and/or removing activities or methods that contribute no value to the system. A team approach develops a list of factors called "critical X's." In the JHA process, these critical X's are a list of the steps determined to have high-risk potential and/or injury history. Once critical X's are identified, the gap between what is actually happening and what is desired to happen in the process is determined. The team examines all factors affecting the specific process similar to how the JHA is developed. Modifications and changes are made and implemented using a structured process that be measured.

15.4 IMPROVING THE PROCESS USING THE SIX SIGMA METHODOLOGY

The most important and the most essential element of any process is to ensure that the leadership team and employees buy into what is to be accomplished. The leadership team must ensure that the necessary education and training effectively assists process improvement efforts.

15.5 A BASIC SIX SIGMA PROCESS IMPROVEMENT MODEL

DMAIC is at the heart of Six Sigma. DMAIC is an acronym defining the five phases of Six Sigma: Define, Measure, Analyze, Improve, and Control (Figure 15.1). DMAIC is a problem-solving method using

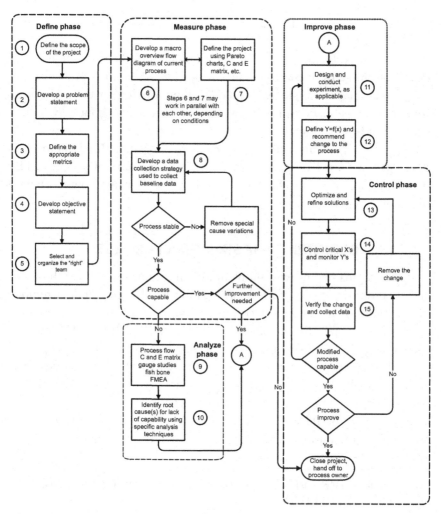

Figure 15.1 *Basic Six Sigma Process Model Process. Based on and adapted from Breakthrough Management Group, Inc. (n.d.); Handbook For Basic Process Improvement Public Domain, (n.d.); Roughton & Crutchfield (2013).*

specific tools to turn a persistent problem that cannot be measured into a statistical-based problem, generate a statistically based solution, and then convert the statistical solution into a practical application. Refer to Appendix R for a "Six Sigma Case Study" and "Selected Six Sigma Tools" that will utilize Six Sigma methodology to enhance the safety system.

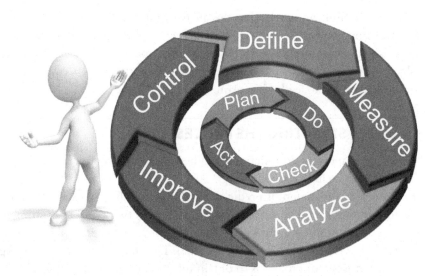

Figure 15.2 *Overview of the Relationship Between the Define, Measure, Analyze, Improve, and Control (DMAIC) and the Plan, Do, Check, Act (PDCA) Processes.*

15.6 DEFINE, MEASURE, ANALYZE, IMPROVE, AND CONTROL

The DMAIC is a more advanced approach than the traditional PDCA and helps to define a project in more detail (Figure 13.1) (Figure 15.2).

The following sections will provide a summary of the 15 DMAIC steps used in conducting a Six Sigma review of a safety system.

15.7 DEFINE PHASE

The purpose of the Define phase is to develop a problem statement, the requirements and the objectives of the project. The objectives of this phase are to focus on critical issues with the problem statement, establish a defined project strategy, and list "customer" requirements. The customer is the user of the process, i.e., employees. The Define phase includes obtaining the leadership team support, buy-in, budget, and approval to define and continue the project.

15.8 STEP 1, DEFINE THE SCOPE OF THE PROJECT

When an organization undertakes Six Sigma improvement projects, the areas designated for improvement must be clearly identified and decisions made on which issues are most critical to the operation.

Step 1 begins with selecting the areas to improve – injury reductions, product improvement, inventory management, etc. A well-defined scope is established that will validate the business issues under review. The scope and objective can be established by a designated team, the process owner, and/ or a member of the leadership team.

15.9 SELECTING THE PROCESS

The important considerations to be taken into account when selecting a process include the following:

- Process improvement is predicated on understanding what is important to the customer. Every work environment has two types of customers, internal customers (employees) and external customers (product, services, buyers, contractors, vendors, etc.). The starting point in selecting an improvement process is to obtain information from the customer regarding their likes or dislikes about the current process (safe operation), by asking the question: What do you want to see as an end result? (The Process Improvement Notebook, TQLO Publication No. 97-01, n.d.).
- Each project is clearly defined. As the project moves forward, other issues that become visible can be identified and put on a "parking lot" list and then addressed at a later time. The key is to ensure that the project is clearly defined and focused. One of the most common mistakes made is to try to resolve too many issues at one time. It is critical to ensure that the steps involved in meeting the objective are located inside the boundaries of the desired established requirements. Define the project sets the appropriate boundaries and include a start and end point. (The Process Improvement Notebook, TQLO Publication No. 97-01, n.d.).

Once a project is identified, a thorough investigation of the current scope of the issues determines the feasibility of the project and the needs of the organization. Knowing the importance of the problem establishes a well-defined process improvement objective. The definition of the objective should answer: "What improvement do we want to accomplish?"

The objective is frequently determined by listening (most importantly) to customers during the discovery phase. A questionnaire and/or use interviews can identify primary metrics (what is to be measured as well as what is being measured) to set goals and benchmark improvements to defined issues (The Process Improvement Notebook, TQLO Publication No. 97-01, n.d.).

A "Pareto" diagram or a series of Pareto diagrams are used to identify one or more factors which may occur frequently and need further investigation. This analysis would be based on preliminary data collected and could be injury data from various operations or areas within a facility. The objective is to validate with data the justification for what area(s) need to be improved.

> A Pareto chart is used to graphically summarize and display the relative importance of the differences between groups of data (Simon, n.d.).
>
> The Pareto chart will rank issues from the largest to the lowest using a bar chart that show highest on the left in descending order from left to right.

Trend chart: The Trend chart helps to visualize the trend of defects over a specific period of time. It is uses a line graph that shows time period selected on the x-axis and items measured on the y-axis (number of injuries, rates, etc.).

Process flow chart: A process flow chart is designed to help define how the current process functions and elements in sequence. It shows how the flow of steps in the current process combines to affect the outcome (The Process Improvement Notebook, TQLO Publication No. 97–01, n.d.). Flow diagrams have been used throughout this book to show how they can be used to graphically present a process. A flow diagram, if develop correct, provide a great overview of any type of concept.

> A flowchart is a graphical representation of a process, depicting inputs, outputs, and units of activity. It represents the entire process at a high or detailed level (depending on the use) or level of observation, allowing analysis for optimization of the workflow.
>
> They can represent an entire process from start to finish, showing inputs, pathways, action or decision points, and data collection point. They serve as an instruction manual or a tool for facilitating detailed analysis and optimization of workflow project (Flowchart, n.d.).

15.10 STEP 2, DEVELOPING A PROBLEM STATEMENT

The problem statement consists of the basic "what, when, where, how much and how do we know" (The Process Improvement Notebook, TQLO Publication No. 97–01, n.d.). The question is: What is to be measured and in what format?

It is similar to "root cause" investigations conducted for injury and damage incidents. The problem statement is not usually set in stone in the initial stage of the project, as it can be redefined as new project specification limits are identified. Once baseline data is collected, the problem statement can be further defined. At this point the problem statement will shift from "We do not know what we want to do" to "We know exactly what we want to do." At this stage a data-driven system begins to develop that will help understanding on how the selected process works.

For any improvement effort to be successful, the project team must start with a clear definition of "What is the problem?" and "what can be expected from the existing process." As an example:

- Repairing a seal on a high-pressure piece of equipment currently takes 6 h. Management would like to reduce the time required, but is concerned that the quality of the product will suffer if the process is changed. The team believes that the repair time can be reduced to 4 h by improving the process of how the seal is replaced. The objective can be stated as: "High-pressure air compressor fourth stage seals are repaired in 4 h or less, with no increase in the mean time between failures for the repaired parts."

A well-defined problem statement guides the team to proceed in a logical manner. The key is to write a description of the process, for example, "The process by which we change the high-pressure air compressor seal can be modified to change the seal in 4 h with no consequential performance to the equipment." Specify the end result objective of the process improvement effort.

15.11 STEP 3, DEFINE THE APPROPRIATE METRIC – HOW WILL THE SAFETY SYSTEM BE MEASURED?

Defining the appropriate measurement (metrics) to track the progress of the project is as important as the process. This step determines the types of metrics required – business-related (costs, defects, etc.), hazard/risk related injury data or other types. The team must understand primary and secondary ways of monitoring improvements using the data.

A decision must be made to determine if the project requires measurable objectives such as consequential metrics – a business or process measurement that allows tracking of any negative impacts on the implementation of solutions on a given project. Consequential metrics are used to measure unintended consequences of potential changes (The Process Improvement

Notebook, TQLO Publication No. 97-01, n.d.). The key is to improve a process and not have unintended consequences that will increase hazards or risk as well as require more time, budget, or resources then the initial problem.

15.12 STEP 4, DEVELOP OBJECTIVE STATEMENT

It is important to know and understand the desired end result and keep in focus what is to be achieved. In the case of safety, it might be a specific type of injury reduction through improved hazard and risk controls.

For example, "Put an "evergreen" (a living method) process in place that can stand the test of time in an ever changing organizational environment."

15.13 STEP 5, SELECT AND ORGANIZE THE "RIGHT" TEAM

Identifying and selecting the "right" people to serve on the team ensures that the resources for the improvement project are effectively used. The team will need to allocate time, determine the budget and materials needed. It will set reporting requirements and the overall schedule. This step establishes the team's level of authority over process changes and is formalized in a written charter.

The applicable tools during the Define phase include the following:

Project and team charter development

Creating a team charter and identifying the key personnel who will champion (mentor) the project ensures that the problem statement is clearly defined, problem/defect definitions are developed and that a written charter and deliverables for the project are established (The Process Improvement Notebook, TQLO Publication No. 97-01, n.d.).

Team charters include the business case analysis such as problem and goal statements (injury and/or damage reduction), project scope, benchmarks/milestones, and the roles and responsibilities of the team. One key element in the team charter is a plan for communicating information to leadership team on the status of each stage of the project (Waddick, n.d.).

Collection of baseline data can through use of a well-defined questionnaire. As example with regard to a hazard/risk control improvement project, a questionnaire can be distributed to employees with description of an injury type. The employee can describe their perception of the issues that related to the injury and provide feedback on what almost happened (near misses or injuries).

Questionnaires require in-depth coordination to ensure that reading skills, language skills, the process to be used to distribute and collect the surveys are defined. You need to determine if hardcopy and/or computers can offer security controls in regards to confidentiality. The design of the survey must allow it to be analyzed efficiently and quickly (The Process Improvement Notebook, TQLO Publication No. 97-01, n.d.).

Employees working in the process under review can potentially identify activities that require extra physical and mental effort to accomplish, are designed inefficiently with redundant or unnecessary steps, hazardous at-risk events, and/or are subject to frequent breakdowns or other delays (Chapter 4).

Problems (injuries, damage, defects) are symptoms of process failure, and it is the deficiencies in the process that must be identified for improvement.

15.14 MEASURE PHASE

The purpose of the Measure phase is to develop an understanding of the current conditions of the process problems and issues by identifying numerical data that provides the best measurement of the current performance. This data is used to establish baseline measurement used to track and measure the project progress. The measurements developed must be relevant to identify and measure the source of "variation" in the process. Variation is a measurement of the fluctuation over time of the data. It is essential in determining process improvement.

The Measure phase includes:
- Identifying the specific performance requirements.
- Mapping the process to define Inputs (X's) and Outputs (Y's). Mapping is conducted at each process step identifying the relevant outputs and all the potential Inputs and how they are connected to each other.
- Generating a list of existing and potential measurements needed (gathering the right data.)
- Validating that a problem exists based on the measurements, for example, at-risk events. Analyzing the measurement system, the capability of the system, and establishing a process capability baseline is necessary for any process improvement. As example, the TCIR for one year has limited value. Over a multiyear period, a graph would show it is increasing

or decreasing. A statistical review would determine its variation over time using calculated control limits. Is the variation each year such that without some change in the system, the level of TCIR might well be expected to continue or are there wild swings in rates signifying specific events are occurring?

- Identifying where errors in the measurement system can occur. For example, the job task perception may have been built on wrong assumptions about what is being done.
- Measuring the inputs, processes and outputs, and collecting the data to identify the process parameters.
- Refining the problem statement or objective (that was initially developed in the Define phase). The problem statement and/or objective will need to be modified and/or updated as the project unfolds. What was thought to be the problem may now be only part of a greater issue or problem (The Process Improvement Notebook, TQLO Publication No. 97-01, n.d.).

Applicable tools used during the Define phase include the following:

- Fishbone diagram: The fishbone diagram is a powerful tool and is used to demonstrate the relationships between inputs and outputs (The Process Improvement Notebook, TQLO Publication No. 97-01, n.d.) (Chapters 9, 10, and 11).

The fishbone is a tool that can be used to solve specific problems by identifying and defining the causes of an effect and logically organizing them by branches. "A tool used to solve quality problems by brainstorming causes and logically organizing them by branches. Also called the Cause & Effect diagram and Ishikawa diagram."
(Fishbone, n.d.)

- Process mapping: A process map is used to understand the current process. This will enable the team to graphically define the hidden causes of variation (The Process Improvement Notebook, TQLO Publication No. 97-01, n.d.).

The process map is also a hierarchical method for displaying a visual illustration of how a transaction is processed. Process Mapping comprises a stream of activities that transforms a defined input or set of inputs into a pre-defined set of outputs.
(Process, n.d.)

- Cause & effect matrix: The cause and effect matrix or XY matrix (not to be confused with the fishbone diagram) is used to quantify how significantly each input may affect the desired output (The Process Improvement Notebook, TQLO Publication No. 97-01, n.d.). An overview of the XY matrix is provided for an overview of the process of categorizing and comparing the probability and the severity of risk. Severity and probability potential hazards use a different format shown in Chapter 8 (The Process Improvement Notebook, TQLO Publication No. 97-01, n.d.).
- Gauge repeatability & reproducibility (R&R): The gauge repeatability & reproducibility is another powerful tool that can be used to analyze the variation of the process and the measurement systems so to minimize any unreliability in the measurement systems (The Process Improvement Notebook, TQLO Publication No. 97-01, n.d.). This can be used to calibrate individuals to ensure that everyone sees the same thing consistently.

> Characterizing measurement error is one of the most important but over-looked and misunderstood concept of the Six Sigma process. Gage R&R is used in many forms to assess the measurement precision (spread) (Gage R&R, n.d.).

When developing a project use steps 6 & 7 interchangeably, i.e., they may work in parallel as they may inter-react with each other, depending on conditions.

15.15 STEP 6, DEVELOP A MACRO MAP OF CURRENT PROCESS

In step 6, the team begins to see a picture of the process and is able to ask questions on how the process actually works. The overall process can then be reviewed and using a flow diagram begin assessing how it can be improved by removing redundant or unnecessary steps or task that create hazards, human error potential, etc. This step can be a real eye-opener for leadership team, as the project team prepares to take actions for improving the process. The key is to develop a macro overview flow diagram of current process using organizational charts, network maps, and overview flow diagram of the current safety system.

The flow diagram assists the team in spotting areas of concern or problem areas within the process flow. The review answers the questions:

- What steps and tasks or decision points redundant. The team may find that steps and tasks contain unnecessary inspections, out of date procedures, changes in technology, techniques implemented no longer needed, latent human error potential that has been designed into the process, etc.

- Where are resources not utilized efficiently? The team may find a weak link in the process that they can bolster by adding or removing one or more steps or tasks. Where hazards and associated risk are present are the current controls, PPE, equipment, etc. effective?

Caution – before making any changes to the process based on the "as-is" flowchart, the following questions are asked for each step of the process. Before trying to improve a process, determine if the entire process is valid:

- Does each event work in parallel rather than in sequence?
- Do specific events have to be completed before another event can be started, or can two or more events be performed at the same time?
- What would happen if a series of events are eliminated? Would the output of the process remain the same? What would be the difference? Would the revised output be acceptable or would it be unacceptable due to being incomplete or would the process have too many defects?
- Would eliminating an event achieve the process risk improvement objective?
- Are the events being performed by the appropriate individual? Who else is involved?
- Is the event a work-around (quick fix, "just-do-it") because of poor training or administrative programs inserted into the process to attempt to prevent recurrence of problem or other related issues?
- Is the event a single repeated action, or is it part of the whole system, which can be eliminated?
- Does the event add value to the process?

If the answer to these questions indicate opportunities for improvement through elimination, consideration should be given to doing away with the event. If an event or decision block can be removed without degrading the process or increasing hazards and associated risk, resources might be recovered to be used elsewhere in the organization.

Eliminating redundant or unnecessary events provide an added benefit of decreasing at-risk events. As an example, the current process might imply reaching into a piece of equipment to unjam a piece of material resulting in periodic hand injuries. By removing the at-risk event and its potential for harm (modifying a process to eliminate the need to reach into equipment).

After making preliminary changes to the process, a flow diagram of the new simplified process is completed and compared to the current process. A "sanity" check is then made:

- Is the simplified process acceptable to the business operation? Is it an improvement that removed or reduced risk?
- Does the process continue to be in compliance with applicable company procedures, policies, regulatory requirements, etc.?

If the answer to these questions is "yes," and the customer agrees with the change, and if the team has the authority to make changes, then the simplified process change should be implemented as soon as possible. A new flow diagram is developed that will show the process as the new standard.

Before the proposed change is put in place, everyone (employees, the leadership team, engineering, maintenance, etc.) working in the process must be trained on the new process. The habitual behavior of the organization must be changed to ensure that the new process does not revert back to the traditional way of operating. If a drift is found in the ongoing measurements then other forces are at work that must be identified and reviewed.

Steps 1 through 6 have taken the team through a process simplification phase of process improvement.

15.16 STEP 7, DEFINE THE PROJECT WITH PARETO CHARTS, XY MATRIX, ETC

The goal of this step is to develop a full understanding of the process before any changes are made. The key is not to change any task(s) before it is fully understood what impact a change could do to the system. At this point a detailed fishbone, process map, trend line, XY matrix, risk assessments are used by team to further define the current situation by answering the following questions:

- Does the flowchart show exactly how things are currently being done?
- If not, what needs to be added or modified to make it as close as possible to an "as-is" picture of the process?
- Have all employees in the process been involved and provided their input concerning the process steps and the sequence of events?
- Are other individual (nondepartmental) involved in the process or a similar process? What did they have to say about how the process that really works?

- After gathering this information, once again it may be necessary to re-write the project objective as discussed in Step 1.

As the project moves forward, the team develops new flow diagrams to document the team understanding on how the system actually functions and if the problem statement remains correct.

To develop an accurate flow diagram, the defined work areas is observed for use of the correct work flow and each step and task reviewed as it is actually performed. If employees involved in the project are new to the area they are going to evaluate a number of observations of activities is necessary before a fully understanding of the process.

15.17 STEP 8, DEVELOPING A DATA COLLECTION STRATEGY

Developing a strategy for collecting the baseline data is essential to understand the process, as the baseline measurement is used for comparison as changes to the process are made. This step begins the evaluation of the process against the objectives of the project established in Steps 1 and 2. The tools used, detailed in Step 6, guide the team to determine who should collect data and where, as well as how the process data should be collected. This data collection should be focused on preloss activities and objectives that are used to reduce hazards, associated risk, etc. (Chapter 14).

15.18 ANALYZE PHASE

In the Analyze phase, data is collected so that hypotheses about the root causes of variations in the process measurements can be generated and validated. It is at this stage that issues are analyzed using statistical methods and further inquiry. This analysis includes:

- Generating an hypothesis about possible root causes of variation and potential critical Inputs (Critical X's)
- Identifying the vital few root causes and critical inputs that have the most significant impact
- Validating specific hypotheses by performing the appropriate analysis.

In the Analyze phase, specific qualitative and quantitative methods and tools are used to isolate key factors that are critical to understanding the causes of defects (injuries). The most applicable tools at this phase include the following:

- 5 Why's: Asking 5 Why's is a powerful tool that can be used to help understand the root causes of defects in a process, and to highlight incorrect assumptions about causes.

> The 5 Why's typically refers to the practice of asking "WHY", five times, why the failure occurred in order to get to the root cause/causes of the failure (5 Why's, n.d.).

- Tests for normality: Tests for normality are statistical methods (Descriptive Statistics, Histograms) used to determine if the data collected is normal or abnormal so as to be properly analyzed by other tools.
- Correlation/regression analysis: These tools help to identify the relationship between inputs and outputs or the correlation between two different sets of variables.
- Analysis of variances (ANOVA): ANOVA is an inferential statistical technique designed to test for significance of the differences among two or more sample means.
- Failure mode and effect analysis (FMEA): An FMEA allows the user to identify improvement actions to prevent defects from occurring.

> The FMEA is used to rank & prioritize the possible causes of failures as well as develop and implement preventative actions, with responsible persons assigned to carry out these actions (Failure Mode and Effects Analysis (FMEA), n.d.).

- Hypothesis testing: Hypothesis testing is a series of tests to help identify sources of variability using historical or current data and to provide objective solutions to questions which are traditionally answered subjectively. The bottom line, a need to understand exists if assumptions are to be proven or disproven, based on the data and proper testing for validity.

15.19 STEP 9, REFINE TOOL USE (PROCESS FLOW, XY MATRIX, GAUGE STUDIES, FISHBONE, FMEA)

When a special cause variation is determined to be reducing the effectiveness and efficiency of the process, it is isolated and investigated to better understand the root causes and take action to remove it. If it is determined that the special cause was clearly temporary and one time in nature, no action may be required beyond understanding the reason for this temporary event.

If potential special cause variation is not reviewed and improvement activities are continued, the process may be neither stable nor predictable in the future. This lack of stability and predictability may cause additional problems to occur, preventing the achievement of the process improvement objective.

Once the process has been stabilized by removing or controlling special cause variations, the data collected in Step 8 is used again. Individual data points are used produce a bar graph called a histogram. The collected data, the original baseline, and the specification limits (if applicable) are plotted, and a decision is made on if the process is capable of being improved. Questions to ask are:

- Are unusual patterns noted in the plotted data?
- Does the bar graph show multiple tall peaks and steep valleys? This may be an indication that other processes or sources may be influencing the studied process.
- Do all of the data points fall inside the upper and lower specification limits (if applicable)? If not, the process may not be capable or in control.
- If all of the data points fall within the specification limits, is the data grouped closely enough to the target value? While the process is capable or in control, it may not be producing satisfactory results.
- If no specification limits for the process have been set, is the shape of the histogram, a bell curve (normal curve)? After examining the shape, a decision is made that the curve shape is satisfactory and if the data points are close enough to the target value.

The Six Sigma process establishes a scientific methodology for conducting process improvements. The process has no limitations on how many times the team can attempt to improve the process incrementally.

The analysis of the safety system provides insights on what is and what is not working, where gaps in communication exists, concerns, and issues with the implementation.

15.20 STEP 10, IDENTIFY ROOT CAUSE(S) FOR LACK OF CAPABILITY USING SPECIFIC ANALYSIS

Identify root cause(s) of underlying problems in the implementation: Issues with leadership team and employee involvement, materials, data gathering, lack of specific data gathering analysis, and communications. Where the right goals, activities, correct authorities, adequate budgets, etc. in place to support the safety system? What obstacles are preventing the full application of any of the elements of the safety system?

15.21 TECHNIQUES

Steps 1–9 were concerned with gaining an understanding of the process and documenting its results. The analysis cycle begins by using the cause-and-effect diagram, XY matrix, brainstorming, FMEA, Gauge Studies, and other tools to generate possible reasons why the process fails to meet the desired objective.

Once possible root causes are determined, additional data is collected to determine how many of these causes actually affect the desired results. The key is to follow the data and make decisions based on the data as to what improvements to make.

At various intervals, a reality check and reviewing the data is completed. Does the data make sense? Has the data been collected and organized properly? Have the right analysis tool been selected and used? Can a simple change based on the issues at hand be made?

15.22 IMPROVE PHASE

The Improve phase focuses on developing ideas on how to remove sources of variation in the process. This phase begins testing and standardizing potential solutions. Once how specific inputs affect the outputs are understood, a strategy on how to control the process can be developed. This phase involves the following:

- Identifying ways to remove causes (common and special) of variation
- Verifying critical inputs
- Establishing operating parameters (upper and lower specification limits.)
- Optimizing critical Inputs and/or reconfiguring the relevant process to help in reducing defects.

The most applicable tools to be used at this phase include:

- Process mapping: Process mapping helps to detail the new process identified for improvements (Process, n.d.).
- Process capability analysis (CPK): Process capability analysis helps the user to understand if the process is capable of maintaining the control(s) that have been identified. CPK is used to test the capability of a process after improvement actions have been implemented to ensure that

real improvement has been obtained in preventing defects. Capability analysis is a graphical or statistical tool that visually or mathematically compares actual process performance to the performance standards established by the customer.

15.23 STEP 11, DESIGN AND CONDUCT AN EXPERIMENT, AS APPLICABLE

The safety system is tested by looking at the overall system. After the analysis, the first question to ask: "Is the safety system model selected correct for your organization?" Begin by looking at the measurements being used: activities, two minutes drill, risk guidance card use as discussed in Chapter 8.

Design of Experiment (DOE) is a structured, organized method for determining the relationship between factors (Xs) affecting a process and the output of that process (Y). It is a planned set of tests used to define the optimum settings necessary to obtain the desired output and validate improvements.

> The DOE refers to experimental methods used to quantify indeterminate measurements of factors and interactions between factors statistically through observance of forced changes made methodically as directed by mathematically systematic tables (Design of Experiments – DOE, n.d.).

In this step, an experiment is designed to check for understanding of the capability of the project to assess which change will be most effective. Once a DOE is conducted, a plan is designed for implementing changes based on the possible reasons for the process's inability to meet the objectives set for it. The improvement plan may be as simple as revising the steps created after initial changes were completed.

15.24 STEP 12, DEFINING THE Y= F(X) OF THE PROCESS

(Y is a function and outcome of X.). These are several Six Sigma-related tools that can be used. These tools look at the relationships between elements of the safety system process. If a risk guidance card is used, does it impact on the avoidance, reduction, and control of hazards? If no relationship can be defined, then the use of the risk card must be further reviewed (Chapter 7).

15.25 CONTROL PHASE

The Control phase is the last phase of the Six Sigma methodology and is used to establish a standard measuring system and control plan to ensure the process is capable of maintaining performance and corrections can be made as needed. The Control phase includes:
- Validating the measurement systems
- Verifying the process long-term capability
- Developing and implementing a control plan to ensure that the same issues do not reoccur.

The most applicable tools for the Control phase are:
- Control plans: A control plan is a single document or set of documents that detail the actions identified during the project. This could include schedules and responsibilities needed to control the key process input variables at the optimal settings.
- Process flow chart(s) with documented control points: This is a single chart or series of charts that visually display the new operating processes and details the appropriate control points.
- Statistical process control (SPC) charts: SPC charts help to track a process by plotting data over time taking into account the lower and upper specification limits of the capability of the process.
- Check sheets: Check sheets enable systematic recording and compilation of data from historical sources, or observations as they happen, so that patterns and trends can be clearly detected and shown (The Process Improvement Notebook, TQLO Publication No. 97–01, n.d.).

15.26 STEP 13, OPTIMIZING AND REDEFINING SOLUTIONS

In this step, solutions that have been developed are optimized and refined (The Process Improvement Notebook, TQLO Publication No. 97–01, n.d.). As the process is going to change when the planned improvements are implemented, a review of the original plan is made to ensure that it is still capable of providing the data needed to assess process performance. If the determination is made that the data collection plan should be modified, the same methodologies are used as in Step 5.

This will be a continuous process as changes in the organization's business climate or conditions are constantly ongoing. The safety system offers a structure but can never be considered permanent.

15.27 STEP 14, CONTROL CRITICAL X'S AND MONITOR Y'S

Test the changed process and collect data to verify if the X's identified are controlled.

By mapping the safety system process, the relationships are defined that allow a review of the flow of communication and activity. The implementation of a safety system is not simple. It requires an understanding of as many of the interrelationships of an organization as possible. The potential for successful implementation of a safety system is increased if the sequence of safety system elements is defined.

15.28 STEP 15, VERIFY THE CHANGE AND COLLECT DATA

As mentioned in Step 7, a series of analytical methods to determine process stability are used. If the process is stable, a control plan is established. If not, the process is returned to its former state and another change is planned.

In some situations, a small-scale test may not be feasible. If that is the case, everyone involved in the process must be informed about the nature and expected effects of the change and conduct training adequate to support a full-scale test.

Any changes should be implemented on a limited basis before applied to the entire organization. If the organization is working on a shift basis, the process change could be tried on one shift while the other shifts continue as before. Whatever method used, the goal is to prove the effectiveness of the change, avoid failure, and maintain the organization's support.

The information developed in Step 9 provides the outline for the test plan. During the test, it is important to collect appropriate data so that the results of the change can be evaluated. The following actions are taken in conducting the test to determine whether the change actually resulted in process improvement:

- Finalize the test plan.
- Prepare the data collection sheets.
- Train everyone involved in the test.
- Distribute the data collection sheets.
- Change the process to test the improvement.
- Collect and collate the data.

If the data collected in Step 11 show that process performance is worse, return to Step 8 and try to improve the process again. The process must be stable before going on to the next step (The Process Improvement Note-book, TQLO Publication No. 97–01, n.d.).

15.29 POSITIVE CHANGES TO ORGANIZATIONAL CULTURE

With a Six Sigma focus, an organization's culture can start to shift to one with a systematic approach to problem solving and a proactive attitude among all employees. Successful Six Sigma implementation success can contribute to the overall sense of pride of the employees.

Six Sigma transforms the way an organization thinks and works on major issue. This is accomplished through the following areas:

- Designing processes to have the best and most consistent outcomes from the beginning.
- Investigating and conducting studies to identify the cause of variation and how the variations can interact with each other.
- Using "just-the-facts" with data (analysis and reasoning) to find and support the root causes of variations, instead of educated guesses or intuition. Experience is a great source of information and is very useful in many respects. However, when this knowledge is repeatedly used to fix problems that continue, it represents a "bandage approach". The problem is briefly fixed but no permanent controls are put in place to prevent recurrence.
- Focusing on process improvement as key to excellence in safety, quality, customer satisfaction, and/or services.
- Encouraging employees to be proactive about preventing potential problems instead of waiting for problems to occur and then react.
- Providing a broad participation in problem solving by getting more employees involved in finding causes, solutions for problems.
- Learning and sharing new knowledge in terms of best practices.
- Making decisions based on data collected and analysis, not "gut" reaction. This does not mean it will negatively impact a company's ability to make quick decisions. In contrast, by applying the DMAIC principles, the decision makers are more likely to have the data they need to make a well-informed decision.
- "Just-do-its" are identified during the Six Sigma process and implemented. These issues are usually and only require implementation. For example, a new tool can be substituted and the problem is corrected.

"Just the facts, Ma'am"

–TV episode Detective Sergeant Joe Friday

SUMMARY

In Six Sigma, a process is represented in terms of $Y = f(X's)$, in which the Outputs (Y) are determined by Input variables (X), known as critical X's. If we suspect that there is a relationship between an outcomes, an example could be a hand injury (Y) and potential cause being sticking a hand into a running machine (X's), we must collect and analyze data by using Six Sigma tools and techniques to prove the hypothesis.

If we want to change the outcome, we need to focus on identifying and controlling the causes of the at-risk events (hand into machine), rather than checking the outcomes (hand injury.) When we have collected enough data and have a good understanding of the critical X's (where, where, who, how) then we can more accurately predict Y. Otherwise, we continue to focus our effort on activities like inspection, auditing, testing, and reworking that may or may not reveal the underlying problem of why hand are being stuck into equipment.

Many organizations have recurring problems associated with injuries, shipping products to customers, which do not meet specifications, etc. causing the customer to be unhappy. By reducing the various defect rates, an organization will be able to consistently reduced employee injuries and damage, ship products to customers within specifications and increase customer satisfaction.

By lowering defect rates or injuries, an organization can eliminate medical cost as well as the inefficient use of employee knowledge that could assist in defect reduction. This savings reduces the cost of goods manufactured and/or sold for each unit of output, injuries, (lost workdays), and adds significantly to bottom-line.

CHAPTER REVIEW QUESTIONS

1. What does DMAIC stand for?
2. What is the purpose of the Define phase?
3. What is the purpose of the Measure phase?
4. What is the purpose of the Analysis phase?
5. Where is the focus of the Improve phase?
6. Why is the Control phase important?
7. How is the XY Matrix used in developing the Risk assessment?

BIBLIOGRAPHY

5 Why's. (n.d.). iSixSigma. Retrieved from http://bit.ly/1wU7iDu

Breakthrough Management Group, Inc. (n.d.). Black Bait Training Manual, Define Phase, Black Bait DAMIC Methodology, (pp 17–21), 1999–2004, 31.

Design of Experiments – DOE. (n.d.). iSixSigma. Retrieved from http://bit.ly/1xkkgsZ

Failure Mode and Effects Analysis (FMEA). (n.d.). iSixSigma. Retrieved from http://bit.ly/1IqiGy6

Fishbone. (n.d.). iSixSigma. Retrieved from http://bit.ly/14v46Gn

Flowchart. (n.d.). iSixSigma. Retrieved from http://bit.ly/1NgzR7n

Gage R&R. (n.d.). iSixSigma. Retrieved from http://bit.ly/1fwxBxG

Handbook For Basic Process Improvement Public Domain, (n.d.), US Navy

Process. (n.d.). iSixSigma. Retrieved from http://bit.ly/1su8noK

Roughton, J., & Crutchfield, N. (2013). In B. Heinemann (Ed.), *Safety culture: An innovative leadership approach.* Butterworth Heinemann, Retrieved from http://amzn.to/1qoD4oN.

Simon, K. (n.d.). Purpose of a Pareto Chart. Retrieved from http://bit.ly/1LyR2jw

The Process Improvement Notebook, TQLO Publication No. 97-01. (n.d.). Department of the Navy, Total Quality Leadership Office, Public Domain. Retrieved from http://1.usa.gov/Y7U2ZX

Waddick, P. (n.d.). Six Sigma DMAIC Quick Reference. iSixSigma. Retrieved from http://bit.ly/17DukIM

Appendix R Six Sigma Case Study

A couple of years ago, one of the authors had a real eye opener in regards to training when he was involved in creating a Six Sigma Black Belt Certification Safety Project. The team consisted of leaderships and employees who spent a considerable time deciding on how to conduct a safety-related project using Six Sigma tools. Several team members were "Nay Sayers," and thought that could not be done.

The team asked the question, "Why were the majority of injuries hand-related?" The team begins to search for ways to reduce potential at-risk hand usage. Several months of defining the project and establishing a baseline from general observation developed a picture of the issues. The data from the observations identified that 80% of the employees in the study were putting themselves at-risk while using their hands.

The team asked questions about the current training. The core question became: "Why were not safety-related topics getting through to employees?" In comparison, if any supervisor was asked about a quality issue, they would know exactly what are the issues and could probably discuss many years of production history. The project included determining way to improve the learning retention rates of employees with regard to hand safety.

However, ask a supervisor how many injuries their team had in the last six months and they would have a hard time discussing any facts concerning the injury. If they were asked about their biggest safety issue, use of personal protective equipment (PPE) was their primary issue.

A Six Sigma tool, the "Gauge R&R" (Repeatability and Reproductively (R&R)) study, is used to determine if excessive variability existed in the measurement system. In this project, it was used to assess the instruction to employee variability, as the training was not being retained by the employee.

A Gauge R&R study was conducted using three supervisors and three employees who had knowledge of the production process. A major gap existed between what the supervisors thought regards to trained employees versus what the employee actually retained. The safety message was not getting through to employees.

A Design of Experiment (DOE) was used to determine the effectiveness of four training methods. The DOE incorporated a series of pictures within four training methods with the objective to determine the effectiveness of each specific technique or method. The four training method were:
• Supervisor gave written information to employee to read.
• Supervisor gave written information and pictures to employee to read.
• Supervisor verbally gave information to employee.
• Supervisor verbally gave information with pictures to employee.

Based on the results of the DOE, a new Gauge R&R study was conducted using the same employees and same method. The results of the second R&R concluded that seventy one percent (71.4%) of the employees could identify at-risk behaviors when the Supervisor verbally gave information with pictures. This was a 35% improvement from the first gauge study.

It was determined that supervisor training did not address the fundamentals of one-on-one communication. Training assumed that a high level overview was enough, essentially "I read and you listen."

Several insights were learned from the project that included the following:
• Do not overlook the fundamental need for direct experience (hands on).
• All parties involved must change behaviors if a process is to be improved.
• Data must drive the decision-making process. In this project, it was not just training but the method of communication and training that was critical. Proper training will increase the knowledge and skills and improve the retention needed to fully understand workplace hazards.

Refer to Chapter 12 for a more detailed discussion on training methods.

Appendix R Selected Six Sigma Tools to Help Enhance the Safety System

The JHA process should be the focal point of a safety system. Through hazard identification, employee participation, understating behaviors, and training, core knowledge develops. Implementing a structured JHA that incorporates Cause and Effect Diagrams, risk assessment, establishing priorities using the XY Matrix, and data analysis provide the fine details of how the job really gets done. Knowledge, focus, understanding, and implementation drive efforts.

R.1 Cause and effect matrix

The cause and effect matrix or the XY matrix correlates a process of Y's or critical output factors associated with X's, called the critical input factors. Through a series of rankings, you can generate a score for each X, which can be sorted to establish a priority. This matrix can be used in many situations, especially where there is limited data from the process. As with any type of prioritization, developing a matrix is subjective. Using a well-defined XY matrix allows a team to intelligently prioritize hazards in a logical and more succinct manner. The XY matrix can be used to establish a metric to measure a safety system. The XY matrix can be a critical forward thinking process to help quantify hazards in a more defined manner.

R.2 Developing the matrix

Developing the XY matrix is as simple as having the JHA team develop a detailed process map (flowchart) for the job steps and task being reviewed. This can be developed from the fish bone cause and effect diagram as discussed in Chapter 10. This process map will provide a logical flow as the team starts to quantify the risk of hazards found in the process. Once this is done, the team must agree on operational definitions as to the different way ranking will be recorded. By using a set of definitions developed by the team, you will have a consistent method that can use be used as a guide.

R.3 Brainstorming

Once the process map of the process has been developed, the team can start a brainstorming session to identify the critical X's and Y's of the hazards identified through observation, data collections, etc. (Figure R.1).

The brainstorming is used to ensure that all of the tasks have been captured and that risk levels have been assigned. Try to be as specific as possible, when listing the tasks (critical X's.) In other words, do not just list "tire," use a specific simple definition such as "change a flat tire." This will be consistent with the JHA. The team can use a flipchart for the process mapping and brainstorming.

To complete the assessment, a spreadsheet can be used to calculate the scores. The following is the sequence of events in developing an XY matrix:

- Determining the outputs or "Y's" created by the process is first step. This could be based on past experience, probability, severity, frequency, etc. List the Y's in no particular order in the cells of the spreadsheet along the top. Include all outputs that are necessary to stop an injury (Figure R.2).
- Next use a scale of 1–10 with 10 being the most critical to the process and 1 being the least critical to the process. This is the list of parameters

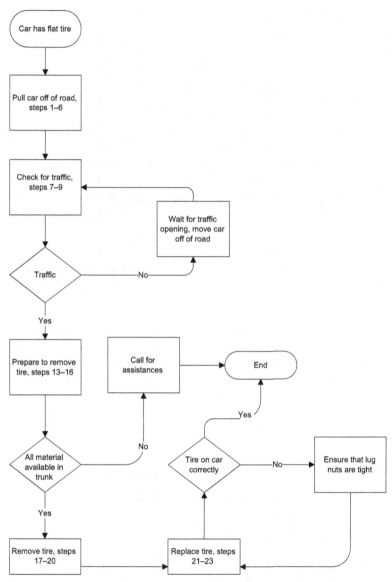

Figure R.1 *Process Flow Diagram of Changing a Tire Based on XY Matrix (Simplified).*

that closely fit your specific conditions. These ranking are independent of each other and they are not required to be in a sequential order. In other words, it is not necessary to use a ranking such as: 10, 9, 8, 7, etc. You can have Y's with the same ranking. It is up to the team and how you have defined the process. Ensure that whatever criteria is used that it

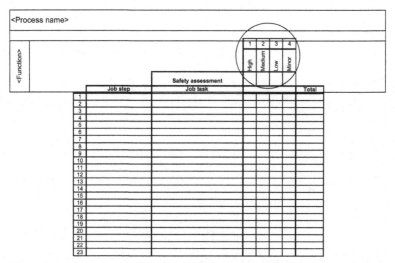

Figure R.2 *List the Inputs (Y's) to the Process XY Matrix for Assessing Job Steps and Task.*

is consistently applied through out the project. In our example, we will use High (10), Medium (7), Low (5), and Minor (1). These rankings are used as a weighting factor only as the scores for X are calculated later (Figure R.3).

• Once you have determined the outputs (Y's,) the next step is to determine a list of inputs, critical X's. List the X's in no particular order down the left column of the spreadsheet.

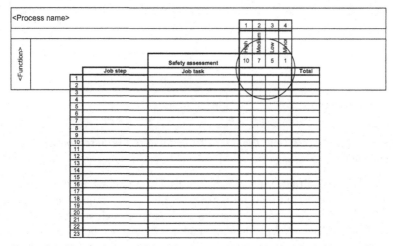

Figure R.3 *List the Inputs (Y's) to the Process XY Matrix and Assigning Ranking.*

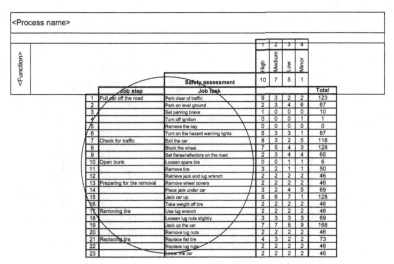

Figure R.4 *List the Process Job Steps and Inputs (Job Task) XY Matrix for Assessing Job Steps and Task.*

Once all of the X's are listed, the team starts the brainstorming. It is important that the team adhere to brainstorming techniques. "All ideas are considered," "No debating of ideas," etc. If a team member has no opinion, ideas, or lacks experience, they should pass. Giving an opinion may create a bias to others. Just as we have established the Y's prioritization, the X's will also be ranked in the matrix (Figure R.4).

- Rank the X's based on the Y's. The spreadsheet ranking will be calculated in the following manner. Look at the row "Park clear of the traffic." In the example, we used the scoring as High (9), Medium (3), Low (2), and Minor (2). When the assessment has been completed the scores will be calculated as follows: $10 \times 9 + 7 \times 3 + 5 \times 2 + 1 \times 2$ which sums to 123. This is the unbiased weighted score that we have developed as a team (Figure R.5).
- Now that you have completed the assessment, you can sort in descending order the list so that all of the X's with the highest scores are on the top of the spreadsheet (Figure R.6).

This provides a weighted risk assessment of the tasks. You can quickly look at the list and know which tasks have the highest risk.

R.4 Reality check

Once the matrix is completed, the team should do a reality check to see if the scores make sense, based on the nature of the job, steps, and tasks.

Since this is a subjective measurement, you need to look at the scores in a subjective manner. Trust your data. This can be verified once further data is collected and adjustments can then be made.

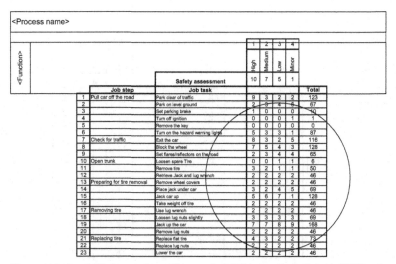

Figure R.5 *Rank the Inputs According to their Effect on Each Output XY Matrix.*

<Process name>

<Function>

#	Job step	Job task	High 10	Medium 7	Low 5	Minor 1	Total
1	Pull car off the road	Park clear of traffic	9	3	2	2	123
2		Park on level ground	2	3	4	6	67
3		Set parking brake	1	0	0	0	10
4		Turn off ignition	0	0	0	1	1
5		Remove the key	0	0	0	0	0
6		Turn on the hazard warning lights	5	3	3	1	87
7	Check for traffic	Exit the car	8	3	2	5	116
8		Block the wheel	7	5	4	3	128
9		Set flares/reflectors on the road	2	3	4	4	65
10	Open trunk	Loosen spare Tire	0	0	1	1	6
11		Remove tire	3	2	1	1	50
12		Retrieve Jack and lug wrench	2	2	2	2	46
13	Preparing for tire removal	Remove wheel covers	2	2	2	2	46
14		Place jack under car	3	2	4	5	69
15		Jack car up	5	6	7	1	128
16		Take weight off tire	2	2	2	2	46
17	Removing tire	Use lug wrench	2	2	2	2	46
18		Loosen lug nuts slightly	3	3	3	3	69
19		Jack up the car	7	7	8	9	168
20		Remove lug nuts	2	2	2	2	46
21	Replacing tire	Replace flat tire	4	3	2	2	73
22		Replace lug nuts	2	2	2	2	46
23		Lower the car	2	2	2	2	46

Safety assessment

Figure R.6 *XY Matrix for Assessing Job Steps and Task, Identify the Critical Inputs from The Totals Column.*

While the matrix is a simple process, it will take time to assemble the right team, collect the data (steps and task), brainstorm the data, and rank each task.

This exercise is worth the effort as you now have a JHA process that incorporates a risk and hazard assessment.

FINAL WORDS: WHERE DO WE GO FROM HERE?

"Genius is 1% Inspiration And 99% Perspiration."

– Thomas Alva Edison

If the intent of an organization is to develop and maintain a safety culture that intent must begin with a full understanding of the hazards and associated risks hidden within how things get done. Without a comprehensive understanding of jobs, their steps and tasks, major gaps in the safety system will be present.

We have found there is no magic solution or easy path to maintain a safety system or a job hazard analysis (JHA) process. Organizations are in constant change unless there is a strong and resilient safety culture. For this reason, developing a safety system and JHA process takes a great deal of patience, effort, and a coordinated team approach. The value of the JHA process must be constantly reinforced with a consistent message and a flexible approach that takes into account the nature of ongoing organizational change.

In Chapter 1, "Why focus on the Job Hazard Analysis," we noted hearing that a safety system was not "rocket science". Usually this comment come from individuals with limited knowledge of what it take to develop and implement any process, much less a safety process. If their statement was true, then all organizations would be able to establish multiple processes that operate with minimal effort or administration. For better or worse, a safety process is a complex specialized system that must operate within an even more complex organizational structure.

You may be asking the question – Why are you qualified to write about the job hazard analysis process?

Our professional careers have, over the years, allowed us to work in different capacities, a number of different industries and deal with many challenges. Our professional skills were developed primarily through direct experience and involvement in attempting to make an impact on our organizations.

We learned is how to organize and focus on the essential actions that appeared to have the most value when making recommendations or taking

Job Hazard Analysis: http://dx.doi.org/10.1016/B978-0-12-803441-5.00027-1

actions designed to reduce or control loss-producing situations. We considered our efforts as a continuous journey of discovery and personal development.

We had a concern that the methods and techniques used in safety systems were falling behind the technology and concepts used in organizations. In particular, the JHA needed to be updated to incorporate not just how to analyze a job, but to make that analysis more efficient. This effort lead to seeing the need for understanding how social media could be used to enhance productivity. In turn, the need to understand communications and networking became apparent as a "fire hose" flow of information was now available. To be effective, we needed to learn how to adapt to the current electronic and social media technology and they are changing the organizational landscape.

"Intelligence is the ability to adapt to change."

– Stephen Hawking

BUILDING ON THE BASICS

Several years ago, we met while at a safety meeting and began to compare and discuss various ideas and concepts that we were using and quickly became friends. We came from very different career paths, manufacturing and risk management. We quickly found that we had similar interest in the same subject – improving the safety systems used in the work environment. Both of us have lived the experience, from both the inside and outside of organizations.

We did not want to just improve safety-related programs but we wanted to find new and creative approaches to improve the overall process of a safety system. After a healthy debate on methods, experiences, and concepts, collaboration began on a number of different projects to bring a consistent approach to developing and presenting our ideas and concepts to various industry groups.

We have both observed good and bad implementation of the elements outlined in a safety process, safety program design, its administration, and leadership. We found that our differences in perspective allowed us to create diverse points of view based on our personal and professional experience, lessons learned, and insights. Since our collaboration begin, we have developed several projects together, the first being this book.

During our research, we began to realize that for a JHA process to have a better chance at being successfully implemented, a more comprehensive approach was needed beyond just completion of the traditional format. The JHA had to be integrated into the overall safety system and take into account the culture of the organization and how it made decisions and met its operational goals.

We wanted this book to be more than simply a retooling of traditional JHA efforts. A wider array of tools, concepts, and techniques was needed for use by the leadership team. In order to accomplish this, the need for a level of understanding of the basic concepts of problem solving through cause and effect, risk management, human performance improvement (HPI), internal/external networking, organizational politics, and safety systems was essential. A safety system does not operate in a vacuum and this knowledge aids in building a stronger foundation for safety efforts in the work environment.

The JHA process begins with the understanding that organizations are adaptive and complex structures that have varying levels of resilience. Many organizations have a tendency to operate in a reactive mode making change as conditions dictate or experience shows that changes are needed. In many, change is made after loss-producing conditions create a crisis or unacceptable conditions. The objective of a JHA process is to reduce the potential of finding hazards only after a job has begun and a loss-producing event has happened. The JHA process builds an increased resilience into the organizations as hazards and associated risk are controlled before the job is begun.

Safety or lack of a safe environment is the result of the dynamics of an ever-changing organizational environment. It can be compared to a jungle ecosystem, a hostile environment of constant changes that requires learning how to read the environment, and to learn how to adapt to each situation as appropriate. Flexibility in approach is necessary as conditions change, if the potential for success even in the short run is to be possible.

The essential key, flexibility, lets the safety system adjusts as needed to the organizational environment and its culture. As with navigating through a dense jungle, a map is needed, a direction set, and a compass used to stay on course. A safety system acts as both the compass and map by which the progress is determined, allowing for adjusting actions as appropriate to meet the demands of the organization.

The JHA process provides a way to gauge the scope and depth of the obstacles encountered, the hazards and risk present that must be controlled if the intended goals and objectives for a safe work environment are to be reached. JHAs can be used as a problem–solving tool useful in assessing the potential for loss–producing events. Each job element has inherent hazards that have varying levels of risk (severity and probability). JHA provides a structure that allows these elements to be analyzed and the desired proper controls better defined.

Safety professionals and those individuals tasked with administrating the safety system are at the core of the organization. They become the "go to" person for many problems and issues beyond safety related issues. They are the ones that must interpret and explain hazards and associated risk to both the leadership team and employees. They must manage multiple specific programs and ensure that those programs are readily understood and fit into the overall organization.

Frankly, this puts them in a most exciting profession that lets one gain insights on all aspects of the dynamics of an organization. For those who desired to remain in a life–long learning and personal development mode, one can't do much better.

APPENDIX 1

Job Hazard Analysis

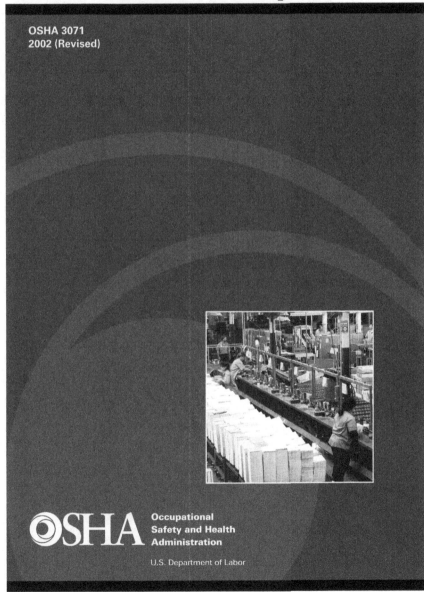

OSHA 3071
2002 (Revised)

⊙SHA Occupational
Safety and Health
Administration

U.S. Department of Labor

Job Hazard Analysis. http://dx.doi.org/10.1016/B978-0-12-803441-5.00016-7

Job Hazard Analysis

U.S. Department of Labor
Occupational Safety and Health Administration
OSHA 3071
2002 (Revised)

Contents

i

Who needs to read this booklet?

This booklet is for employers, foremen, and supervisors, but we encourage employees to use the information as well to analyze their own jobs and recognize workplace hazards so they can report them to you. It explains what a job hazard analysis is and offers guidelines to help you conduct your own step-by-step analysis.

What is a hazard?

A hazard is the potential for harm. In practical terms, a hazard often is associated with a condition or activity that, if left uncontrolled, can result in an injury or illness. See Appendix 2 for a list of common hazards and descriptions. Identifying hazards and eliminating or controlling them as early as possible will help prevent injuries and illnesses.

What is a job hazard analysis?

A job hazard analysis is a technique that focuses on job tasks as a way to identify hazards before they occur. It focuses on the relationship between the worker, the task, the tools, and the work environment. Ideally, after you identify uncontrolled hazards, you will take steps to eliminate or reduce them to an acceptable risk level.

Why is job hazard analysis important?

Many workers are injured and killed at the workplace every day in the United States. Safety and health can add value to your business, your job, and your life. You can help prevent workplace injuries and illnesses by looking at your workplace operations, establishing proper job procedures, and ensuring that all employees are trained properly.

One of the best ways to determine and establish proper work procedures is to conduct a job hazard analysis. A job hazard analysis is one component of the larger commitment of a safety and health management system. (See page 15 for more information on safety and health management systems.)

What is the value of a job hazard analysis?

Supervisors can use the findings of a job hazard analysis to eliminate and prevent hazards in their workplaces. This is likely to result in fewer worker injuries and illnesses; safer, more effective work methods; reduced workers' compensation costs; and increased worker productivity. The analysis also can be a valuable tool for training new employees in the steps required to perform their jobs safely.

For a job hazard analysis to be effective, management must demonstrate its commitment to safety and health and follow through to correct any uncontrolled hazards identified. Otherwise, management will lose credibility and employees may hesitate to go to management when dangerous conditions threaten them.

What jobs are appropriate for a job hazard analysis?

A job hazard analysis can be conducted on many jobs in your workplace. Priority should go to the following types of jobs:

- Jobs with the highest injury or illness rates;

- Jobs with the potential to cause severe or disabling injuries or illness, even if there is no history of previous accidents;

- Jobs in which one simple human error could lead to a severe accident or injury;

- Jobs that are new to your operation or have undergone changes in processes and procedures; and

- Jobs complex enough to require written instructions.

Where do I begin?

1. **Involve your employees.** It is very important to involve your employees in the hazard analysis process. They have a unique understanding of the job, and this knowledge is invaluable for finding hazards. Involving employees will help minimize oversights, ensure a quality analysis, and get workers to "buy in" to the solutions because they will share ownership in their safety and health program.

2. **Review your accident history.** Review with your employees your worksite's history of accidents and occupational illnesses that needed treatment, losses that required repair or replacement, and any "near misses" — events in which an accident or loss did not occur,
   but could have. These events are indicators that the existing hazard controls (if any) may not be adequate and deserve more scrutiny.

3. **Conduct a preliminary job review.** Discuss with your employees the hazards they know exist in their current work and surroundings. Brainstorm with them for ideas to eliminate or control those hazards.

   If any hazards exist that pose an immediate danger to an employee's life or health, take immediate action to protect the worker. Any problems that can be corrected easily should be corrected as soon as possible. Do not wait to complete your job hazard analysis. This will demonstrate your commitment to safety and health and enable you to focus on the hazards and jobs that need more study because of their complexity. For those hazards determined to present unacceptable risks, evaluate types of hazard controls. More information about hazard controls is found in Appendix 1.

4

4. **List, rank, and set priorities for hazardous jobs.** List jobs with hazards that present unacceptable risks, based on those most likely to occur and with the most severe consequences. These jobs should be your first priority for analysis.

5. **Outline the steps or tasks.** Nearly every job can be broken down into job tasks or steps. When beginning a job hazard analysis, watch the employee perform the job and list each step as the worker takes it. Be sure to record enough information to describe each job action without getting overly detailed. Avoid making the breakdown of steps so detailed that it becomes unnecessarily long or so broad that it does not include basic steps. You may find it valuable to get input from other workers who have performed the same job. Later, review the job steps with the employee to make sure you have not omitted something. Point out that you are evaluating the job itself, not the employee's job performance. Include the employee in all phases of the analysis—from reviewing the job steps and procedures to discussing uncontrolled hazards and recommended solutions.

Sometimes, in conducting a job hazard analysis, it may be helpful to photograph or videotape the worker performing the job. These visual records can be handy references when doing a more detailed analysis of the work.

5

How do I identify workplace hazards?

A job hazard analysis is an exercise in detective work. Your
goal is to discover the following:

• What can go wrong?

• What are the consequences?

• How could it arise?

• What are other contributing factors?

• How likely is it that the hazard will occur?

To make your job hazard analysis useful, document
the answers to these questions in a consistent manner.
Describing a hazard in this way helps to ensure that your
efforts to eliminate the hazard and implement hazard controls
help target the most important contributors to the hazard.

Good hazard scenarios describe:

• Where it is happening (environment),

• Who or what it is happening to (exposure),

• What precipitates the hazard (trigger),

• The outcome that would occur should it happen
  (consequence), and

• Any other contributing factors.

A sample form found in Appendix 3 helps you organize
your information to provide these details.

Rarely is a hazard a simple case of one singular cause
resulting in one singular effect. More frequently, many

6

contributing factors tend to line up in a certain way to create the hazard. Here is an example of a hazard scenario:

In the metal shop (environment), while clearing a snag (trigger), a worker's hand (exposure) comes into contact with a rotating pulley. It pulls his hand into the machine and severs his fingers (consequences) quickly.

To perform a job hazard analysis, you would ask:

- **What can go wrong?** The worker's hand could come into contact with a rotating object that "catches" it and pulls it into the machine.

- **What are the consequences?** The worker could receive a severe injury and lose fingers and hands.

- **How could it happen?** The accident could happen as a result of the worker trying to clear a snag during operations or as part of a maintenance activity while the pulley is operating. Obviously, this hazard scenario could not occur
if the pulley is not rotating.

- **What are other contributing factors?** This hazard occurs very quickly. It does not give the worker much opportunity to recover or prevent it once his hand comes into contact with the pulley. This is an important factor, because it helps you determine the severity and likelihood of an accident when selecting appropriate hazard controls. Unfortunately, experience has shown that training is not very effective in hazard control when triggering events happen quickly because humans can react only so quickly.

- **How likely is it that the hazard will occur?** This determination requires some judgment. If there have been "near-misses" or actual cases, then the likelihood of a recurrence would be considered high. If the pulley is exposed and easily accessible, that also is a consideration. In the example, the likelihood that the hazard will occur is high because there is no guard preventing contact, and the operation is performed while the machine is running. By following the steps in this example, you can organize your hazard analysis activities.

The examples that follow show how a job hazard analysis can be used to identify the existing or potential hazards for each basic step involved in grinding iron castings.

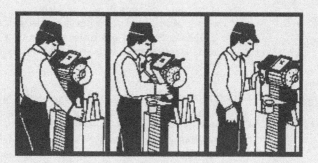

Grinding Iron Castings: Job Steps

Step 1. Reach into metal box to right of machine, grasp casting, and carry to wheel.

Step 2. Push casting against wheel to grind off burr.

Step 3. Place finished casting in box to left of machine.

Example Job Hazard Analysis Form

Job Location: Metal Shop	*Analyst:* Joe Safety	*Date:*

Task Description: Worker reaches into metal box to the right of the machine, grasps a 15-pound casting and carries it to grinding wheel. Worker grinds 20 to 30 castings per hour.

Hazard Description: Picking up a casting, the employee could drop it onto his foot. The casting's weight and height could seriously injure the worker's foot or toes.

Hazard Controls:

1. Remove castings from the box and place them on a table next to the grinder.

2. Wear steel-toe shoes with arch protection.

3. Change protective gloves that allow a better grip.

4. Use a device to pick up castings.

Job Location:	*Analyst*:	*Date*:
Metal Shop	Joe Safety	

Task Description: Worker reaches into metal box to the right of the machine, grasps a 15-pound casting and carries it to grinding wheel. Worker grinds 20 to 30 castings per hour.

Hazard Description: Castings have sharp burrs and edges that can cause severe lacerations.

Hazard Controls:

1. Use a device such as a clamp to pick up castings.

2. Wear cut-resistant gloves that allow a good grip and fit tightly to minimize the chance that they will get caught in grinding wheel.

Job Location:	Analyst:	Date:
Metal Shop	Joe Safety	

Task Description: Worker reaches into metal box to the right of the machine, grasps a 15-pound casting and carries it to grinding wheel. Worker grinds 20 to 30 castings per hour.

Hazard Description: Reaching, twisting, and lifting 15-pound castings from the floor could result in a muscle strain to the lower back.

Hazard Controls:

1. Move castings from the ground and place them closer to the work zone to minimize lifting. Ideally, place them at waist height or on an adjustable platform or pallet.

2. Train workers not to twist while lifting and reconfigure work stations to minimize twisting during lifts.

**Repeat similar forms
for each job step.**

11

How do I correct or prevent hazards?

After reviewing your list of hazards with the employee, consider what control methods will eliminate or reduce them. For more information on hazard control measures, see Appendix 1. The most effective controls are engineering controls that physically change a machine or work environment to prevent employee exposure to the hazard. The more reliable or less likely a hazard control can be circumvented, the better. If this is not feasible, administrative controls may be appropriate. This may involve changing how employees do their jobs.

Discuss your recommendations with all employees who perform the job and consider their responses carefully. If you plan to introduce new or modified job procedures, be sure they understand what they are required to do and the reasons for the changes.

What else do I need to know before starting a job hazard analysis?

The job procedures discussed in this booklet are for illustration only and do not necessarily include all the steps, hazards, and protections that apply to your industry. When conducting your own job safety analysis, be sure to consult the Occupational Safety and Health Administration standards for your industry. Compliance with these standards is mandatory, and by incorporating their requirements in your job hazard analysis, you can be sure that your health and safety program meets federal standards. OSHA standards, regulations, and technical information are available online at www.osha.gov.

12

Twenty-four states and two territories operate their own OSHA-approved safety and health programs and may have standards that differ slightly from federal requirements. Employers in those states should check with the appropriate state agency for more information. A list of applicable states and territories and contact information is provided on page 32.

Why should I review my job hazard analysis?

Periodically reviewing your job hazard analysis ensures that it remains current and continues to help reduce workplace accidents and injuries. Even if the job has not changed, it is possible that during the review process you will identify hazards that were not identified in the initial analysis.

It is particularly important to review your job hazard analysis if an illness or injury occurs on a specific job. Based on the circumstances, you may determine that you need to change the job procedure to prevent similar incidents in the future. If an employee's failure to follow proper job procedures results in a "close call," discuss the situation with all employees who perform the job and remind them of proper procedures. Any time you revise a job hazard analysis, it is important to train all employees affected by the changes in the new job methods, procedures, or protective measures adopted.

When is it appropriate to hire a professional to conduct a job hazard analysis?

If your employees are involved in many different or complex processes, you need professional help conducting your job hazard analyses. Sources of help include your insurance company, the local fire department, and private consultants with safety and health expertise. In addition, OSHA offers assistance through its regional and area offices and consultation services. Contact numbers are listed at the back of this publication.

Even when you receive outside help, it is important that you and your employees remain involved in the process of identifying and correcting hazards because you are on the worksite every day and most likely to encounter these hazards. New circumstances and a recombination of existing circumstances may cause old hazards to reappear and new hazards to appear. In addition, you and your employees must be ready and able to implement whatever hazard elimination or control measures a professional consultant recommends.

14

OSHA Assistance, Services, and Programs

How can OSHA help me?

OSHA can provide extensive help through a variety of programs, including assistance about safety and health programs, state plans, workplace consultations, Voluntary Protection Programs, strategic partnerships, training and education, and more.

How does safety and health program management assistance help employers and employees?

Effective management of worker safety and health protection is a decisive factor in reducing the extent and severity of work-related injuries and illnesses and their related costs. In fact, an effective safety and health program forms the basis of good worker protection and can save time and money—about $4 for every dollar spent—and increase productivity.

To assist employers and employees in developing effective safety and health systems, OSHA published recommended *Safety and Health Program Management Guidelines,* (*Federal Register* 54(18):3908–3916, January 26, 1989). These voluntary guidelines can be applied to all worksites covered by OSHA.

The guidelines identify four general elements that are critical to the development of a successful safety and health management program:

- Management leadership and employee involvement;

- Worksite analysis;

- Hazard prevention and control; and

- Safety and health training.

15

The guidelines recommend specific actions under each
of these general elements to achieve an effective safety and
health program. The *Federal Register* notice is available
online at www.osha.gov.

What are state plans?

State plans are OSHA-approved job safety and health
programs operated by individual states or territories instead
of Federal OSHA. The *Occupational Safety and Health
Act of 1970 (OSH Act)* encourages states to develop and
operate their own job safety and health plans and permits
state enforcement of OSHA standards if the state has an
approved plan. Once OSHA approves a state plan, it funds
50 percent of the program's operating costs. State plans
must provide standards and enforcement programs, as
well as voluntary compliance activities, that are at least as
effective as those of Federal OSHA.

There are 26 state plans: 23 cover both private and
public (state and local government) employment, and
3 (Connecticut, New Jersey, and New York) cover only the
public sector. For more information on state plans, see
the listing at the end of this publication, or visit OSHA's
website at www.osha.gov.

How can consultation
assistance help employers?

In addition to helping employers identify and correct
specific hazards, OSHA's consultation service provides free,
onsite assistance in developing and implementing effective
workplace safety and health management systems that
emphasize the prevention of worker injuries and illnesses.

Comprehensive consultation assistance provided by OSHA includes a hazard survey of the worksite and an appraisal of all aspects of the employer's existing safety and health management system. In addition, the service offers assistance to employers in developing and implementing an effective safety and health management system. Employers also may receive training and education services, as well as limited assistance away from the worksite.

Who can get consultation assistance and what does it cost?

Consultation assistance is available to small employers (with fewer than 250 employees at a fixed site and no more than 500 corporatewide) who want help in establishing and maintaining a safe and healthful workplace.

Funded largely by OSHA, the service is provided at no cost to the employer. Primarily developed for smaller employers with more hazardous operations, the consultation service is delivered by state governments employing professional safety and health consultants. No penalties are proposed or citations issued for hazards identified by the consultant. The employer's only obligation is to correct all identified serious hazards within the agreed-upon correction time frame.

Can OSHA assure privacy to an employer who asks for consultation assistance?

OSHA provides consultation assistance to the employer with the assurance that his or her name and firm and any information about the workplace will not be routinely reported to OSHA enforcement staff.

17

Can an employer be cited for violations after receiving consultation assistance?

If an employer fails to eliminate or control a serious hazard within the agreed-upon time frame, the Consultation Project Manager must refer the situation to the OSHA enforcement office for appropriate action. This is a rare occurrence, however, since employers request the service for the expressed purpose of identifying and fixing hazards in their workplaces.

Does OSHA provide any incentives for seeking consultation assistance?

Yes. Under the consultation program, certain exemplary employers may request participation in OSHA's Safety and Health Achievement Recognition Program (SHARP). Eligibility for participation in SHARP includes, but is not limited to, receiving a full-service, comprehensive consultation visit, correcting all identified hazards, and developing an effective safety and health management system.

Employers accepted into SHARP may receive an exemption from programmed inspections (not complaint or accident investigation inspections) for a period of 1 year initially, or 2 years upon renewal.

For more information concerning consultation assistance, see the list of consultation offices beginning on page 36, contact your regional or area OSHA office, or visit OSHA's website at www.osha.gov.

What are the Voluntary Protection Programs?

Voluntary Protection Programs (VPPs) represent one part of OSHA's effort to extend worker protection beyond the minimum required by OSHA standards. VPP—along with onsite consultation services, full-service area offices, and OSHA's Strategic Partnership Program (OSPP)—represents a cooperative approach which, when coupled with an effective enforcement program, expands worker protection to help meet the goals of the *OSH Act.*

How does VPP work?

There are three levels of VPP recognition: Star, Merit, and Demonstration. All are designed to do the following:

- Recognize employers who have successfully developed and implemented effective and comprehensive safety and health management systems;

- Encourage these employers to continuously improve their safety and health management systems;

- Motivate other employers to achieve excellent safety and health results in the same outstanding way; and

- Establish a relationship between employers, employees, and OSHA that is based on cooperation.

How does VPP help employers and employees?

VPP participation can mean the following:

- Reduced numbers of worker fatalities, injuries, and illnesses;

- Lost-workday case rates generally 50 percent below industry averages;

- Lower workers' compensation and other injury- and illness-related costs;

- Improved employee motivation to work safely, leading to a better quality of life at work;

- Positive community recognition and interaction;

- Further improvement and revitalization of already-good safety and health programs; and a

- Positive relationship with OSHA.

How does OSHA monitor VPP sites?

OSHA reviews an employer's VPP application and conducts a VPP Onsite Evaluation to verify that the safety and health management systems described are operating effectively at the site. OSHA conducts Onsite Evaluations on a regular basis, annually for participants at the Demonstration level, every 18 months for Merit, and every 3 to 5 years for Star. Each February, all participants must send a copy of their most recent Annual Evaluation to their OSHA regional office. This evaluation must include the worksite's record of injuries and illnesses for the past year.

Can OSHA inspect an employer who is participating in the VPP?

Sites participating in VPP are not scheduled for regular, programmed inspections. OSHA handles any employee complaints, serious accidents, or significant chemical releases that may occur at VPP sites according to routine enforcement procedures.

Additional information on VPP is available from OSHA national, regional, and area offices, listed beginning on page 27. Also, see **Outreach** at OSHA's website at www.osha.gov.

How can a partnership with OSHA improve worker safety and health?

OSHA has learned firsthand that voluntary, cooperative partnerships with employers, employees, and unions can be a useful alternative to traditional enforcement and an effective way to reduce worker deaths, injuries, and illnesses. This is especially true when a partnership leads to the development and implementation of a comprehensive workplace safety and health management system.

What is OSHA's Strategic Partnership Program (OSPP)?

OSHA Strategic Partnerships are alliances among labor, management, and government to foster improvements in workplace safety and health. These partnerships are voluntary, cooperative relationships between OSHA, employers, employee representatives, and others such as trade unions, trade and professional associations, universities, and other government agencies. OSPPs are the newest member of OSHA's family of cooperative programs.

What do OSPPs do?

These partnerships encourage, assist, and recognize the efforts of the partners to eliminate serious workplace hazards and achieve a high level of worker safety and health. Whereas OSHA's Consultation Program and VPP entail one-on-one relationships between OSHA and individual worksites, most strategic partnerships seek to have a broader impact by building cooperative relationships with groups of employers and employees.

What are the different kinds of OSPPs?

There are two major types:

- Comprehensive, which focuses on establishing comprehensive safety and health management systems at partnering worksites; and

- Limited, which helps identify and eliminate hazards associated with worker deaths, injuries, and illnesses, or have goals other than establishing comprehensive worksite safety and health programs.

OSHA is interested in creating new OSPPs at the national, regional, and local levels. OSHA also has found limited partnerships to be valuable. Limited partnerships might address the elimination or control of a specific industry hazard.

What are the benefits of participation in the OSPP?

Like VPP, OSPP can mean the following:

- Fewer worker fatalities, injuries, and illnesses;

- Lower workers' compensation and other injury- and illness-related costs;

- Improved employee motivation to work safely, leading to a better quality of life at work and enhanced productivity;

- Positive community recognition and interaction;

- Development of or improvement in safety and health management systems; and

- Positive interaction with OSHA.

For more information about this program, contact your nearest OSHA office or go to the agency website at www.osha.gov.

Does OSHA have occupational safety and health training for employers and employees?

Yes. The OSHA Training Institute in Des Plaines, IL, provides basic and advanced training and education in safety and health for federal and state compliance officers, state consultants, other federal agency personnel, and private-sector employers, employees, and their representatives.

Institute courses cover diverse safety and health topics including electrical hazards, machine guarding, personal protective equipment, ventilation, and ergonomics. The facility includes classrooms, laboratories, a library, and an audiovisual unit. The laboratories contain various demonstrations and equipment, such as power presses, woodworking and welding shops, a complete industrial ventilation unit, and a sound demonstration laboratory. More than 57 courses dealing with subjects such as safety and health in the construction industry and methods of compliance with OSHA standards are available for personnel in the private sector.

In addition, OSHA's 73 area offices are full-service centers offering a variety of informational services such as personnel for speaking engagements, publications, audiovisual aids on workplace hazards, and technical advice.

Does OSHA give money to organizations for training and education?

OSHA awards grants through its Susan Harwood Training Grant Program to nonprofit organizations to provide safety and health training and education to employers and workers in the workplace. The grants focus on programs that will educate workers and employers in small business (fewer than 250 employees), train workers and employers about new OSHA standards or high-risk activities or hazards. Grants are awarded for 1 year and may be renewed for an additional 12 months depending on whether the grantee has performed satisfactorily.

OSHA expects each organization awarded a grant to develop a training and/or education program that addresses a safety and health topic named by OSHA, recruit workers and employers for the training, and conduct the training. Grantees are also expected to follow-up with people who have been trained to find out what changes were made to reduce the hazards in their workplaces as a result of the training.

Each year OSHA has a national competition that is announced in the *Federal Register* and on the Internet at www.osha-slc.gov/Training/sharwood/sharwood.html. If you do not have access to the Internet, you can contact the OSHA Office of Training and Education, 1555 Times Drive, Des Plaines, IL 60018, (847) 297–4810, for more information.

24

Does OSHA have other assistance materials available?

Yes. OSHA has a variety of materials and tools available on its website at www.osha.gov. These include eTools, Expert Advisors, Electronic Compliance Assistance Tools (e-CATs), Technical Links, regulations, directives, publications, videos, and other information for employers and employees. OSHA's software programs and compliance assistance tools walk you through challenging safety and health issues and common problems to find the best solutions for your workplace. OSHA's comprehensive publications program includes more than 100 titles to help you understand OSHA requirements and programs.

OSHA's CD-ROM includes standards, interpretations, directives, and more and can be purchased on CD-ROM from the U.S. Government Printing Office. To order, write to the Superintendent of Documents, U.S. Government Printing Office, Washington, DC 20402, or phone (202) 512–1800. Specify *OSHA Regulations, Documents and Technical Information on CD-ROM (ORDT)*, GPO Order No. S/N 729-013-00000-5.

What other publications does OSHA offer?

OSHA offers more than 100 documents, including brochures, fact sheets, posters, pocket cards, flyers, technical documents, and a quarterly magazine. These documents are available online at www.osha.gov or by calling (202) 693–1888.

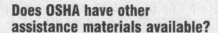

What do I do in case of an emergency or if I need to file a complaint?

To report an emergency, file a complaint, or seek OSHA advice, assistance, or products, call (800) 321–OSHA or contact your nearest OSHA regional or area office listed beginning on page 27. The teletypewriter (TTY) number is (877) 889–5627.

You can also file a complaint online and obtain more information on OSHA federal and state programs by visiting OSHA's website at www.osha.gov.

For more information on grants, training, and education, write: OSHA Training Institute, Office of Training and Education, 1555 Times Drive, Des Plaines, IL 60018; call (847) 297–4810; or see Outreach on OSHA's website at www.osha.gov.

26

OSHA Regional and Area Offices

OSHA Regional Offices

Region I
(CT,* ME, MA, NH, RI, VT*)
JFK Federal Building, Room E340
Boston, MA 02203
(617) 565–9860

Region II
(NJ,* NY,* PR,* VI*)
201 Varick Street, Room 670
New York, NY 10014
(212) 337–2378

Region III
(DE, DC, MD,* PA,* VA,* WV)
The Curtis Center
170 S. Independence Mall West
Suite 740 West
Philadelphia, PA 19106-3309
(215) 861–4900

Region IV
(AL, FL, GA, KY,* MS, NC,*
SC,* TN*)
Atlanta Federal Center
61 Forsyth Street, SW, Room 6T50
Atlanta, GA 30303
(404) 562–2300

Region V
(IL, IN,* MI,* MN,* OH, WI)
230 South Dearborn Street
Room 3244
Chicago, IL 60604
(312) 353–2220

Region VI
(AR, LA, NM,* OK, TX)
525 Griffin Street, Room 602
Dallas, TX 75202
(214) 767–4731 or 4736 x224

Region VII
(IA,* KS, MO, NE)
City Center Square
1100 Main Street, Suite 800
Kansas City, MO 64105
(816) 426–5861

Region VIII
(CO, MT, ND, SD, UT,* WY*)
1999 Broadway, Suite 1690
Denver, CO 80202-5716
(303) 844–1600

Region IX
(American Samoa, AZ,*
CA,* HI, NV,* Northern
Mariana Islands)
71 Stevenson Street, Room 420
San Francisco, CA 94105
(415) 975–4310

Region X
(AK,* ID, OR,* WA*)
1111 Third Avenue, Suite 715
Seattle, WA 98101-3212
(206) 553–5930

*These states and territories operate their own OSHA-approved
job safety and health programs (Connecticut, New Jersey and
New York plans cover public employees only). States with
approved programs must have a standard that is identical to,
or at least as effective as, the federal standard.

27

OSHA Area Offices

Birmingham, AL
(205) 731–1534

Mobile, AL
(251) 441–6131

Anchorage, AK
(907) 271–5152

Little Rock, AR
(501) 324–6291(5818)

Phoenix, AZ
(602) 640–2348

San Diego, CA
(619) 557–5909

Sacramento, CA
(916) 566–7471

Denver, CO
(303) 844–5285

Greenwood Village, CO
(303) 843–4500

Bridgeport, CT
(203) 579–5581

Hartford, CT
(860) 240–3152

Wilmington, DE
(302) 573–6518

Fort Lauderdale, FL
(954) 424–0242

Jacksonville, FL
(904) 232–2895

Tampa, FL
(813) 626–1177

Savannah, GA
(912) 652–4393

Smyrna, GA
(770) 984–8700

Tucker, GA
(770) 493–6644/6742/8419

Des Moines, IA
(515) 284–4794

Boise, ID
(208) 321–2960

Calumet City, IL
(708) 891–3800

Des Plaines, IL
(847) 803–4800

Fairview Heights, IL
(618) 632–8612

North Aurora, IL
(630) 896–8700

Peoria, IL
(309) 671–7033

Indianapolis, IN
(317) 226–7290

Wichita, KS
(316) 269–6644

Frankfort, KY
(502) 227–7024

Baton Rouge, LA
(225) 389–0474 (0431)

Braintree, MA
(617) 565–6924

Methuen, MA
(617) 565–8110

Springfield, MA
(413) 785–0123

Linthicum, MD
(410) 865–2055/2056

Bangor, ME
(207) 941–8177

Portland, ME
(207) 780–3178

August, ME
(207) 622–8417

Lansing, MI
(517) 327–0904

Minneapolis, MN
(612) 664–5460

Kansas City, MO
(816) 483–9531

St. Louis, MO
(314) 425–4249

Jackson, MS
(601) 965–4606

Billings, MT
(406) 247–7494

Raleigh, NC
(919) 856–4770

Omaha, NE
(402) 221–3182

Bismark, ND
(701) 250–4521

Concord, NH
(603) 225–1629

Avenel, NJ
(732) 750–3270

Hasbrouck Heights, NJ
(201) 288–1700

Marlton, NJ
(856) 757–5181

Parsippany, NJ
(973) 263–1003

Carson City, NV
(775) 885–6963

Albany, NY
(518) 464–4338

Bayside, NY
(718) 279–9060

Bowmansville, NY
(716) 684–3891

New York, NY
(212) 337–2636

North Syracuse, NY
(315) 451–0808

Tarrytown, NY
(914) 524–7510

Westbury, NY
(516) 334–3344

Cincinnati, OH
(513) 841–4132

Cleveland, OH
(216) 522–3818

Columbus, OH
(614) 469–5582

Toledo, OH
(419) 259–7542

Oklahoma City, OK
(405) 278–9560

Portland, OR
(503) 326–2251

Allentown, PA
(610) 776–0592

Erie, PA
(814) 833–5758

Harrisburg, PA
(717) 782–3902

Philadelphia, PA
(215) 597–4955

Pittsburgh, PA
(412) 395–4903

Wilkes–Barre, PA
(570) 826–6538

Guaynabo, PR
(787) 277–1560

Providence, RI
(401) 528–4669

Columbia, SC
(803) 765–5904

Nashville, TN
(615) 781–5423

Austin, TX
(512) 916–5783 (5788)

Corpus Christi, TX
(361) 888–3420

Dallas, TX
(214) 320–2400 (2558)

El Paso, TX
(915) 534–6251

Fort Worth, TX
(817) 428–2470 (485–7647)

Houston, TX
(281) 591–2438 (2787)

Houston, TX
(281) 286–0583/0584 (5922)

Lubbock, TX
(806) 472–7681 (7685)

30

Salt Lake City, UT
(801) 530–6901

Norfolk, VA
(757) 441–3820

Bellevue, WA
(206) 553–7520

Appleton, WI
(920) 734–4521

Eau Claire, WI
(715) 832–9019

Madison, WI
(608) 264–5388

Milwaukee, WI
(414) 297–3315

Charleston, WV
(304) 347–5937

OSHA-Approved Safety and Health Plans

Alaska

Alaska Department of Labor and Workforce Development

Commissioner
(907) 465–2700
FAX: (907) 465–2784

Program Director
(907) 269–4904
FAX: (907) 269–4915

Arizona

Industrial Commission of Arizona

Director, ICA
(602) 542–4411
FAX: (602) 542–1614

Program Director
(602) 542–5795
FAX: (602) 542–1614

California

California Department of Industrial Relations

Director
(415) 703–5050
FAX: (415) 703–5114

Chief
(415) 703–5100
FAX: (415) 703–5114

Manager, Cal/OSHA Program Office
(415) 703–5177
FAX: (415) 703–5114

Connecticut

Connecticut Department of Labor

Commissioner
(860) 566–5123
FAX: (860) 566–1520

Conn-OSHA Director
(860) 566–4550
FAX: (860) 566–6916

Hawaii

Hawaii Department of Labor and Industrial Relations

Director
(808) 586–8844
FAX: (808) 586–9099

Administrator
(808) 586–9116
FAX: (808) 586–9104

Indiana

Indiana Department of Labor

Commissioner
(317) 232–2378
FAX: (317) 233–3790

Deputy Commissioner
(317) 232–3325
FAX: (317) 233–3790

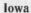

Iowa

Iowa Division of Labor
Commissioner
(515) 281–6432
FAX: (515) 281–4698
Administrator
(515) 281–3469
FAX: (515) 281–7995

Kentucky

Kentucky Labor Cabinet
Secretary (502) 564–3070
FAX: (502) 564–5387

Federal\State Coordinator
(502) 564–3070 ext.240
FAX: (502) 564–1682

Maryland

Maryland Division of Labor
and Industry

Commissioner
(410) 767–2999
FAX: (410) 767–2300

Deputy Commissioner
(410) 767–2992
FAX: (410) 767–2003

Assistant Commissioner, MOSH
(410) 767–2215
FAX: (410) 767–2003

Michigan

Michigan Department of
Consumer and Industry Services

Director
(517) 322–1814
FAX: (517) 322–1775

Minnesota

Minnesota Department of
Labor and Industry

Commissioner
(651) 296–2342
FAX: (651) 282–5405

Assistant Commissioner
(651) 296–6529
FAX: (651) 282–5293

Administrative Director,
OSHA Management Team
(651) 282–5772
FAX: (651) 297–2527

Nevada

Nevada Division of
Industrial Relations

Administrator
(775) 687–3032
FAX: (775) 687–6305

Chief Administrative Officer
(702) 486–9044
FAX: (702) 990–0358
[Las Vegas (702) 687–5240]

New Jersey

New Jersey Department of Labor

Commissioner
(609) 292–2975
FAX: (609) 633–9271

Assistant Commissioner
(609) 292–2313
FAX: (609) 292–1314

Program Director, PEOSH
(609) 292–3923
FAX: (609) 292–4409

New Mexico

New Mexico Environment
Department

Secretary
(505) 827–2850
FAX: (505) 827–2836

Chief
(505) 827–4230
FAX: (505) 827–4422

New York

New York Department of Labor

Acting Commissioner
(518) 457–2741
FAX: (518) 457–6908

Division Director
(518) 457–3518
FAX: (518) 457–6908

North Carolina

North Carolina Department
of Labor

Commissioner
(919) 807–2900
FAX: (919) 807–2855

Deputy Commissioner,
OSH Director
(919) 807–2861
FAX: (919) 807–2855

OSH Assistant Director
(919) 807–2863
FAX: (919) 807–2856

Oregon

Oregon Occupational Safety
and Health Division

Administrator
(503) 378–3272
FAX: (503) 947–7461

Deputy Administrator for Policy
(503) 378–3272
FAX: (503) 947–7461

Deputy Administrator
for Operations
(503) 378–3272
FAX: (503) 947–7461

Puerto Rico

Puerto Rico Department of
Labor and Human Resources

Secretary
(787) 754–2119
FAX: (787) 753–9550

Assistant Secretary for
Occupational Safety and Health
(787) 756–1100,
1106 / 754–2171
FAX: (787) 767–6051

Deputy Director for
Occupational Safety and Health
(787) 756–1100/1106,
754–2188
FAX: (787) 767–6051

South Carolina

South Carolina Department of
Labor, Licensing, and
Regulation

Director
(803) 896–4300
FAX: (803) 896–4393

Program Director
(803) 734–9644
FAX: (803) 734–9772

Tennessee

Tennessee Department of Labor

Commissioner
(615) 741–2582
FAX: (615) 741–5078

Acting Program Director
(615) 741–2793
FAX: (615) 741–3325

Utah

Utah Labor Commission

Commissioner
(801) 530–6901
FAX: (801) 530–7906

Administrator
(801) 530–6898
FAX: (801) 530–6390

Vermont

Vermont Department of
Labor and Industry

Commissioner
(802) 828–2288
FAX: (802) 828–2748

Project Manager
(802) 828–2765
FAX: (802) 828–2195

Virgin Islands

Virgin Islands Department
of Labor

Acting Commissioner
(340) 773–1990
FAX: (340) 773–1858

Program Director
(340) 772–1315
FAX: (340) 772–4323

Virginia

Virginia Department of Labor
and Industry

Commissioner
(804) 786–2377
FAX: (804) 371–6524

Director, Office of Legal Support
(804) 786–9873
FAX: (804) 786–8418

Washington

Washington Department of
Labor and Industries

Director
(360) 902–4200
FAX: (360) 902–4202

Assistant Director
(360) 902–5495
FAX: (360) 902–5529

Program Manager,
Federal–State Operations
(360) 902–5430
FAX: (360) 902–5529

Wyoming

Wyoming Department of
Employment

Safety Administrator
(307) 777–7786
FAX: (307) 777–3646

OSHA Consultation Projects

Anchorage, AK (907) 269–4957	Boise, ID (208) 426–3283
Tuscaloosa, AL (205) 348–3033	Chicago, IL (312) 814–2337
Little Rock, AR (501) 682–4522	Indianapolis, IN (317) 232–2688
Phoenix, AZ (602) 542–1695	Topeka, KS (785) 296–2251
Sacramento, CA (916) 263–2856	Frankfort, KY (502) 564–6895
Fort Collins, CO (970) 491–6151	Baton Rouge, LA (225) 342–9601
Wethersfield, CT (860) 566–4550	West Newton, MA (617) 727–3982
Washington, DC (202) 541–3727	Laurel, MD (410) 880–4970
Wilmington, DE (302) 761–8219	Augusta, ME (207) 624–6400
Tampa, FL (813) 974–9962	Lansing, MI (517) 322–1809
Atlanta, GA (404) 894–2643	Saint Paul, MN (651) 284–5060
Tiyam, GU 9–1–(671) 475–1101	Jefferson City, MO (573) 751–3403
Honolulu, HI (808) 586–9100	Pearl, MS (601) 939–2047
Des Moines, IA (515) 281–7629	Helena, MT (406) 444–6418

36

Raleigh, NC
(919) 807–2905

Columbia, SC
(803) 734–9614

Bismarck, ND
(701) 328–5188

Brookings, SD
(605) 688–4101

Lincoln, NE
(402) 471–4717

Nashville, TN
(615) 741–7036

Concord, NH
(603) 271–2024

Austin, TX
(512) 804–4640

Trenton, NJ
(609) 292–3923

Salt Lake City, UT
(801) 530–6901

Santa Fe, NM
(505) 827–4230

Montpelier, VT
(802) 828–2765

Albany, NY
(518) 457–2238

Richmond, VA
(804) 786–6359

Henderson, NV
(702) 486–9140

Christiansted St. Croix, VI
(809) 772–1315

Columbus, OH
(614) 644–2631

Olympia, WA
(360) 902–5638

Oklahoma City, OK
(405) 528–1500

Madison, WI
(608) 266–9383

Salem, OR
(503) 378–3272

Waukesha, WI
(262) 523–3044

Indiana, PA
(724) 357–2396

Charleston, WV
(304) 558–7890

Hato Rey, PR
(787) 754–2171

Cheyenne, WY
(307) 777–7786

Providence, RI
(401) 222–2438

37

Appendices

Appendix 1
Hazard Control Measures

Information obtained from a job hazard analysis is useless unless hazard control measures recommended in the analysis are incorporated into the tasks. Managers should recognize that not all hazard controls are equal. Some are more effective than others at reducing the risk.

The order of precedence and effectiveness of hazard control is the following:

1. Engineering controls.

2. Administrative controls.

3. Personal protective equipment.

Engineering controls include the following:

- Elimination/minimization of the hazard—Designing the facility, equipment, or process to remove the hazard, or substituting processes, equipment, materials, or other factors to lessen the hazard;

- Enclosure of the hazard using enclosed cabs, enclosures for noisy equipment, or other means;

- Isolation of the hazard with interlocks, machine guards, blast shields, welding curtains, or other means; and

- Removal or redirection of the hazard such as with local and exhaust ventilation.

Administrative controls include the following:

- Written operating procedures, work permits, and safe work practices;

- Exposure time limitations (used most commonly to control temperature extremes and ergonomic hazards);

- Monitoring the use of highly hazardous materials;

- Alarms, signs, and warnings;

- Buddy system; and

- Training.

Personal Protective Equipment—such as respirators, hearing protection, protective clothing, safety glasses, and hardhats—is acceptable as a control method in the following circumstances:

- When engineering controls are not feasible or do not totally eliminate the hazard;

- While engineering controls are being developed;

- When safe work practices do not provide sufficient additional protection; and

- During emergencies when engineering controls may not be feasible.

Use of one hazard control method over another higher in the control precedence may be appropriate for providing interim protection until the hazard is abated permanently. In reality, if the hazard cannot be eliminated entirely, the adopted control measures will likely be a combination of all three items instituted simultaneously.

Appendix 2
Common Hazards and Descriptions

Hazards	Hazard Descriptions
Chemical (Toxic)	A chemical that exposes a person by absorption through the skin, inhalation, or through the blood stream that causes illness, disease, or death. The amount of chemical exposure is critical in determining hazardous effects. Check Material Safety Data Sheets (MSDS), and/or OSHA 1910.1000 for chemical hazard information.
Chemical (Flammable)	A chemical that, when exposed to a heat ignition source, results in combustion. Typically, the lower a chemical's flash point and boiling point, the more flammable the chemical. Check MSDS for flammability information.
Chemical (Corrosive)	A chemical that, when it comes into contact with skin, metal, or other materials, damages the materials. Acids and bases are examples of corrosives.
Explosion (Chemical Reaction)	Self explanatory.
Explosion (Over Pressurization)	Sudden and violent release of a large amount of gas/energy due to a significant pressure difference such as rupture in a boiler or compressed gas cylinder.
Electrical (Shock/ Short Circuit)	Contact with exposed conductors or a device that is incorrectly or inadvertently grounded, such as when a metal ladder comes into contact with power lines. 60Hz alternating current (common house current) is very dangerous because it can stop the heart.

Hazards	Hazard Descriptions
Electrical (Fire)	Use of electrical power that results in electrical overheating or arcing to the point of combustion or ignition of flammables, or electrical component damage.
Electrical (Static/ESD)	The moving or rubbing of wool, nylon, other synthetic fibers, and even flowing liquids can generate static electricity. This creates an excess or deficiency of electrons on the surface of material that discharges (spark) to the ground resulting in the ignition of flammables or damage to electronics or the body's nervous system.
Electrical (Loss of Power)	Safety-critical equipment failure as a result of loss of power.
Ergonomics (Strain)	Damage of tissue due to overexertion (strains and sprains) or repetitive motion.
Ergonomics (Human Error)	A system design, procedure, or equipment that is error-provocative. (A switch goes up to turn something off).
Excavation (Collapse)	Soil collapse in a trench or excavation as a result of improper or inadequate shoring. Soil type is critical in determining the hazard likelihood.
Fall (Slip, Trip)	Conditions that result in falls (impacts) from height or traditional walking surfaces (such as slippery floors, poor housekeeping, uneven walking surfaces, exposed ledges, etc.)
Fire/Heat	Temperatures that can cause burns to the skin or damage to other organs. Fires require a heat source, fuel, and oxygen.
Mechanical/ Vibration (Chaffing/ Fatigue)	Vibration that can cause damage to nerve endings, or material fatigue that results in a safety-critical failure. (Examples are abraded slings and ropes, weakened hoses and belts.)

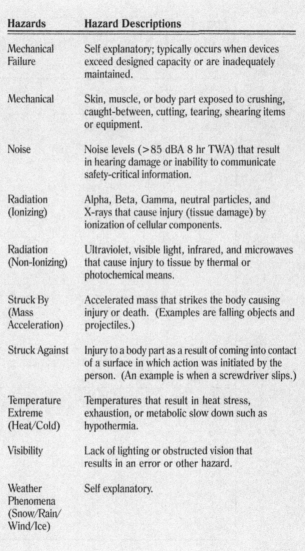

Hazards	Hazard Descriptions
Mechanical Failure	Self explanatory; typically occurs when devices exceed designed capacity or are inadequately maintained.
Mechanical	Skin, muscle, or body part exposed to crushing, caught-between, cutting, tearing, shearing items or equipment.
Noise	Noise levels (>85 dBA 8 hr TWA) that result in hearing damage or inability to communicate safety-critical information.
Radiation (Ionizing)	Alpha, Beta, Gamma, neutral particles, and X-rays that cause injury (tissue damage) by ionization of cellular components.
Radiation (Non-Ionizing)	Ultraviolet, visible light, infrared, and microwaves that cause injury to tissue by thermal or photochemical means.
Struck By (Mass Acceleration)	Accelerated mass that strikes the body causing injury or death. (Examples are falling objects and projectiles.)
Struck Against	Injury to a body part as a result of coming into contact of a surface in which action was initiated by the person. (An example is when a screwdriver slips.)
Temperature Extreme (Heat/Cold)	Temperatures that result in heat stress, exhaustion, or metabolic slow down such as hypothermia.
Visibility	Lack of lighting or obstructed vision that results in an error or other hazard.
Weather Phenomena (Snow/Rain/ Wind/Ice)	Self explanatory.

45

Appendix 3
Sample Job Hazard Analysis Form

Job Title:	Job Location:	Analyst	Date
Task #	Task Description:		
Hazard Type:	Hazard Description:		
Consequence:	Hazard Controls:		
Rational or Comment:			

46

FURTHER READING

Job Hazard Analysis, 3071(2002). *Occupational Safety and Health Administration (OSHA),* Public Domain, Modified and/or Adapt as necessary. Retrieved from http://bit.ly/1ZI1Q7y.

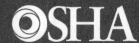

INDEX

A

Ability, 20, 53, 311, 344
ABSS. *See* Activity-based safety system (ABSS)
Action planning, 83
  sample basic action planning forms, 95
Activity-based safety system (ABSS), 42, 266
  activity-based management system, 267
  advantages, 268
  communication links, 266
  elements, 268
    area walkthrough tours, 268
    employee meetings, 268
    employees, one-on-one discussions
      with, 268
    follow-up team, 268
    machine/equipment-specific checklist,
      268
    performance metrics, 268
  roles and responsibilities, 274
    middle management, 274
    safety professional, 275
    senior management, 274
    supervisor/lead person, 274
  safety system, 266
  specifics activities, 266
  success measurement, 276
    safety performance metrics, 276
    safety system elements, 276
  working, 268
Activity hazard analysis, 8, 167, 168, 191, 192
Activity task analysis (ATA), 19, 46
Adapting, to change, 164
Ad hoc sub-committees, 70
Administrative control(s), 159
Administrative process, 109
Administrative structure, 16
Administrator, selecting of, 220
Advanced safety management systems, 350
  ISO 31000 – risk management, 353
  occupational health and safety
    management
    ANSI Z10-2012, 351
    CSA Z1000-06, 351
    ILO-OSH 2001 guidelines, 354
    OHSAS 18001, 352

American Society of Safety Engineers (ASSE)
    Risk Assessment Institute, 199
  establishing task priorities, overview of,
    201
ANSI/AIHA/ASSE/Z10 safety
    management system
  feedback to planning process, 154
  hierarchy of controls, 154
    overview, 157
  interactions with job hazard analysis, 155
  OHSMS policy, 154
  responsibilities and authority, 154
  visualization of various component
    interaction with, 156
Area walkthrough tours, 268
ATA. *See* Activity task analysis (ATA)
At-risk events, 74, 263
  approaches, 53
  contributions, 38–39
  developement, 52
  integrated into JHA process, 41
Audit, 101, 102, 331, 354
  scores, 38
Avoidance, 17, 157, 395

B

Basic stages in conducting job, 287
BBS. *See* Behavior-based safety (BBS)
Behavior, 317
  affective, 319
  approach, 39
  cognitive. *See* Cognitive behaviors
  psychomotor, 318
Behavior-based safety (BBS), 35, 42, 45
  benefits, 35
  guiding principles by DOB, 42
benefits, of doing job, 286
Body language, 111
Body of JHA, 258
Budgets
  adequate, 393
  away from a focus on, 166
  developed based on knowledge, 11
  for implementation of recommended
    hazards and, 16

Printed in the United States
By Bookmasters